Medicinal Chemistry: From Concepts to Applications

Medicinal Chemistry: From Concepts to Applications

Edited by **Erica Helmer**

SYRAWOOD
PUBLISHING HOUSE

New York

Published by Syrawood Publishing House,
750 Third Avenue, 9th Floor,
New York, NY 10017, USA
www.syrawoodpublishinghouse.com

Medicinal Chemistry: From Concepts to Applications
Edited by Erica Helmer

International Standard Book Number: 978-1-68286-096-0 (Hardback)

Printed in the United States of America.

Contents

Preface

This book aims to highlight the current researches and provides a platform to further the scope of innovations in this area. This book is a product of the combined efforts of many researchers and scientists from different parts of the world. The objective of this book is to provide the readers with the latest information in the field.

Medicinal chemistry is an evolving field of science that deals with the development and design of pharmaceutical drugs. It has aided the discovery and development of new drugs for curing severe diseases. The main objective of this book is to give a general overview of different areas of synthetic organic chemistry, structural biology, chemical biology, etc. This book will prove to be beneficial for students and professionals alike.

I would like to express my sincere thanks to the authors for their dedicated efforts in the completion of this book. I acknowledge the efforts of the publisher for providing constant support. Lastly, I would like to thank my family for their support in all academic endeavors.

Editor

Chemical composition and antibacterial activity of the essential oils from *Launaea resedifolia* L

Amar Zellagui[1], Noureddine Gherraf[1*], Segni Ladjel[2] and Samir Hameurlaine[2]

Abstract

Background: Several species of the genus *Launaea* are used in folk medicine such as in bitter stomachic, skin diseases, and reported to have antitumor, insecticide, and cytotoxic activities. The antimicrobial activities of coumarin constituents and the neuropharmacological properties have been investigated as well. In this study, the chemical composition of essential oils from *Launaea resedifolia* L. has been identified using the ordinary GC-MS technique to reveal the presence of 19 compounds dominated by dioctyl phthalate. Moreover, the antibacterial activity of the crude oil has been carried out using disk diffusion method against seven bacteria strains.

Results: Nineteen compounds of essential oil of *L. resedifolia* L. were identified, representing 86.68% of the total oil. The compounds were identified by spectral comparison to be mainly esters, alcohols, ketones, and terpenes. The principal constituents are dioctyl phthalate (39.84%), Decanoic acid, decyl ester (12.09%), 11-Octadecenal (11.24%), and Eucalyptol (07.31%), while others were present in relatively small amounts. As far as antibacterial essays are concerned, it was found that the oils are active against most of the tested bacterial strains.

Conclusion: A major constituent in visible parts was Dioctyl phthalate (39.84%) and the yield of essential oils was 0.9%. These extracts reveal *in vitro* antibacterial activity on the studied bacterial, confirmed by the inhibition zone diameter ranging from 11 to 37 mm and a MIC value between 0.09 and 0.69 depending on the microorganism being tested.

Keywords: chemical composition, antibacterial activity, essential oils, *Launaea resedifolia*

1. Background

The genus *Launaea* (Asteraceae) is represented in the flora of Algeria by nine species, namely, *Launaea acanthoclada, Launaea angustifolia, Launaea anomala, Launaea arborescens, Launaea cassiniana, Launaea glomerata, Launaea nudicaulis, Launaea quercifolia,* and *Launaea resedifolia* [1,2]. *L. resedifolia* (local name "laadid, Azim") is a perennial herb widely distributed in the arid regions of Mediterranean area, where it is abundant in south east of Algeria.

Several species of this genus are used in folk medicine in bitter stomachic, skin diseases, and reported to have antitumor, insecticide and cytotoxic activities [3]. The antimicrobial activities of coumarin constituents [4] and the neuropharmacological properties [5] have been investigated as well.

To the best of the authors' knowledge, there are no reports about the chemical content and biological effect of the essential oils of *L. resedifolia*. There no reports on the essential oils of the species of the genus launaea except that reported by Cheriti et al. [6]. In continuation of our phytochemical and antibacterial studies of the Algerian Sahara medicinal plants [7-11], we report here the findings of our studies on the composition and antimicrobial activity of *L. resedifolia* essential oils. The species was collected during the flowering stage in southeastern Algeria (Ouargla) and identified by Dr. Abdelmadjid Chahma, Biology Department, Ouargla University, Algeria. A voucher specimen was deposited at the herbarium under the code NG 27.

2. Results and discussions

The aerial parts of *L. resedifolia* were collected in March 2010 in the outskirts of Ouargla (600 km south of Algiers). The plant was identified by Dr. Abdelmadjid

* Correspondence: ngherraf@yahoo.com
[1]Laboratory of Biomolecules and Plant Breeding, Life Science and Nature Department, University of Larbi Ben Mhidi Oum El Bouaghi, Algeria
Full list of author information is available at the end of the article

Chahma. A voucher specimen was deposited at the herbarium under the number NG 27.

2.1 Isolation of essential oils

An aliquot of 200 g of the visible parts of *L. resedifolia* was cut into pieces, air-dried under shade, and subjected to hydrodistillation on a Clavenger-type apparatus for 4 h. The distillate was then extracted using diethyl ether. The resulting extract was dried on anhydrous sodium sulphate. Diethyl ether was removed carefully and the essential oil was collected and stored at 4°C until analysis. The oil yield was calculated relative to the dry matter.

2.2 GC-MS analysis

The oil was analyzed by GC/MS using a Agilent 5973EI mass selective detector coupled with an Agilent GC6890A gas chromatograph, equipped with a cross linked 5% PH ME siloxane HP-5MS capillary column (30 m × 0.25 mm, film thickness 0.25 μm). Operating conditions were as follows: carrier gas, helium with a flow rate of 1 mL/min; column temperature 50°C for 1 min, 50-150°C (3°C/mn), 150-250°C (5°C/mn) then isothermal for 5 min.

Injector and detector temperatures: 280°C; split ratio, 1:50.

The MS operating parameters were as follows: ionization potential, 70 eV; ionization current, 2 A; ion source temperature, 200°C; resolution, 1000.

2.3 Identification of components

Identification of oil components was achieved on the basis of their retention indices (RI) (determined with reference to a homologous series of normal alkanes), and by comparison of their mass spectral fragmentation patterns with those reported in the literature [12] and stored on the MS library (NIST database). The concentration of the identified compounds was computed from the GC peak total area without any correction factor.

2.4 Antibacterial activity

In recent years due to an upsurge in antibiotic-resistant infections, the search for novel archetype prescriptions to fight infections is an absolute necessity and in this regard, plant essential oils may offer a great potential and hope. Several studies have reported the efficacy of antibacterials obtained from the essential oils of various plant species [13-15]. In this study, antibacterial activity of essential oil extracted from aerial parts of *L. resedifolia* was tested using different bacterial strains: *Escherichia coli, Staphylococcus aureus, Staphylococcus intermedius, Proteus mirabilis, Streptococcus pyogenes, Pseudomonas aeruginosa,* and *Klebsielle pneumoniae*. In addition, the composition of volatile compounds was also determined.

All bacterial samples were obtained from the bacteriology laboratory SAIDAL, Algeria. The antimicrobial activity tests were carried out using disk diffusion method [15] against seven human pathogenic bacteria, including Gram positive and Gram-negative bacteria. The bacteria strains were first grown on Muller Hinton medium at 37°C for 24 h prior to seeding on to the nutrient agar.

A sterile 6-mm diameter filter disk (Whatman paper n° 3) was placed on the infusion agar seeded with bacteria, and each extract suspended in water was dropped on to each paper disk (40 μL per disk). The treated Petri disks were kept at 4°C for 1 h, and incubated at 37°C for 24 h. The antibacterial activity was assessed by measuring the zone of growth inhibition surrounding the disks. Each experiment was carried out in triplicate [16].

The minimal inhibitory concentration (MIC) was determined by dilution of the essential oil in dimethyl sulphoxide (DMSO) pipetting 0.01 mL of each dilution onto a filter paper disc [17,18]. Dilutions of the oil within a concentration range of 10-420 g/mL were also carried out. MIC was defined as the lowest concentration that inhibited the visible bacterial growth.

A negative control was also included in the test using a filter paper disk saturated with DMSO to check possible activity of this solvent against the bacteria assayed. The experiments were repeated three times.

2.5 Chemical composition

The compounds of aerial parts essential oil of *L. resedifolia* from Algeria are listed in order of their elution on the HP-5MS non-polar column (Table 1). A total of 19 compounds were identified, representing 86.68% of the total oil. The esters made up the largest component of the oil including Dioctyl phthalate (39.84%), Decanoic acid, decyl ester (12.09%) and (E)-2-Heptenoic acid, ethyl ester (5.21%). Aldehydes represent the second largest group (11.45) involving 11-Octadecenal (11.24%) and Heptanal (0.21%).

The monoterpenes represent a relatively low content (8.95%) with eucalyptol as the major constituent (7.31%). A better agreement was found between the oil content of *L. resedifolia* and that of *L. arboresens* as was reported by Cheriti et al. [6]. The slight difference may be due to the geographical location and the harvesting period. It is noteworthy that the results of this study may be considered as the first report on the composition of the essential oils of this endemic species.

2.6 Antimicrobial activity

The quantification of antibacterial activity for *L. resedifolia* essential oils was measured by the agar disk diffusion method. The effectiveness of the essential oil is

Table 1 Chemical content of essential oils of *L. resedifolia* L

	Compound	RT (min)	Percentage
1	Pentanedioic acid, dimetyl ester	14.56	0.13
2	linalool	26.32	1.45
3	Eucalyptol	29.88	7.31
4	Hexadecanol	31.17	2.82
5	Octanol	32.05	0.87
6	α-Limonene diepoxide	32.13	0.19
7	(Z)-6-Octen-2-one	33.23	0.64
8	Heptanal	36.15	0.21
9	3,4-Dimethylcyclohexanol	36.61	0.13
10	bornyl acetate	36.83	0.19
11	caryophyllene oxide	37.68	1.04
12	1,2-Benzenedicarboxylic acid, butyl octyl ester	38.37	0.22
13	Dibutylphthalate	45.51	2.93
14	(Z)-3-Dodecene,	50.38	0.17
15	Hexanedioic acid, dioctyl ester	56.52	Tr.
16	(E)-2-Heptenoic acid, ethyl ester,	60.98	5.21
17	Dioctyl phthalate	61.93	39.84
18	11-Octadecenal	66.81	11.24
19	Decanoic acid, decyl ester	72.39	12.09
	Total		**86.68**
	Esters		60.61
	Aldehydes		11.45
	Oxygene monoterpenes		8.95
	Alcohols		03.82
	Oxygene sesquiterpenes		1.04
	Ketones		0.64
	Alkenes		0.17

demonstrated by the size of the microorganism growth inhibition zone around the filter paper disk, which is typically expressed as the diameter of the inhibition zone in millimeter. Results obtained in the antibacterial study are shown in Table 2. The results indicated that *S. aureus* was the most sensitive strain to the oil of *L. resedifolia* with the strongest inhibition zone (37 mm) and a MIC value of 0.09 mg/mL. The strains *S. intermedius*, *K. pneumoniae*, *S. pyogenes* and *P. mirabilis* were found

Table 2 Inhibition zone diameter (mm)

Microorganisms	Disc diffusion assay (inhibition zone mm)	MIC (mg/mL)
S. aureus	37	0.09
S. intermedius	29	0.13
K. pneumoniae	27	0.21
S. pyogenes	23	0.35
P. mirabilis	20	0.47
E. coli	15	0.54
P. aerugenosa	12	0.69

to be fairly sensitive with inhibition zones of 29, 27, 23, and 20 mm, respectively. Modest activities were observed against *E. coli* and *Pseudomonas aerugenosa* with inhibition zones of 15 and 12 mm. Against *S. intermedius*, *K. pneumoniae*, *S. pyogenes*, *P. mirabilis*, *E. coli* and, *P. aerugenosa*, the oils showed MIC values of 0.13, 0.21, 0.35, 0.47, 0.54, and 0.69 mg/mL, respectively.

3. Conclusions

The chemical analyses by GC/MS allowed the identification of 86.68% of the total volatile products for *L. resedifolia* and 19 volatile compounds. A major constituent in visible parts was Dioctyl phthalate (39.84%) and the yield of essential oils was 0.9%. These extracts reveal *in vitro* antibacterial activity on the studied bacterial, confirmed by the inhibition zone diameter ranging from 11 to 37 mm and a MIC value between 0.09 and 0.69 depending on the microorganism being tested. Antibacterial activities of these essential oils were due to abundance of overall chemical constituents. The antibacterial activity besides several biological activities can be used in place of costly antibiotics for effective control of the food pathogens.

Author details
[1]Laboratory of Biomolecules and Plant Breeding, Life Science and Nature Department, University of Larbi Ben Mhidi Oum El Bouaghi, Algeria [2]Kasdi Merbah University, Ouargla, Algeria

Competing interests
The authors declare that they have no competing interests.

References
1. Ozenda P (1983) Flore du Sahara. CNRS, Paris
2. Quezel P, Santa S (1963) Nouvelle flore d'Algérie et des régions désertique méridionales. CNRS, Paris 2:162
3. Rashid S, Ashraf M, Bibi S, Anjum R (2000) Insecticidal and cytotoxic activities of *Launaea Nudicaulis* (Roxb.) and *Launaea Resedifolia* (Linn.). Pak J Biol Sci 3(5):808–809
4. Ashraf AE, Nabil AA (2006) Antibacterial coumarins isolated from *Launaea resedifolia*. Chem Plant Raw Mater 1:65–68
5. Abdu Raazag A, Auzi , Najat T, Hawisa M, Sherif F, Atyajit D, Sarker (2007) Neuropharmacological properties of *Launaea resedifolia*. Braz J Phamacognosy 17(2):160–165
6. Cheriti A, Saad A, Belboukhari N, Ghezali S (2006) Chemical composition of the essential oil of *Launaea arborescens* from Algerian Sahara. Chem Nat Compounds 42(3):360–361. doi:10.1007/s10600-006-0123-5.
7. Kalla A, Gherraf N, Belkacemi D, Ladjel S, Zellagui A, Hameurelain S, Chihi S, Labed B (2009) Composition of the essential oil of *Rhanterium adpressum* Coss. and *Durieu* from Algeria. Arch Appl Sci Res 1(2):115–118
8. Gherraf N, Zellagui A, Mohamed NS, Hussien TA, Mohamed TA, Hegazy ME, Rhouati S, Moustafa MF, El-Sayed MA, Mohamed Ael-H (2010) Triterpenes from *Euphorbia rigida* . Pharmacognosy Res 2(3):159–162
9. Kalla A, Belkacemi D, Gherraf N, Zellagui A, Messai L, Ladjel S, Hameurelaine S, Labed B, Chihi S (2010) Seasonal variability of essential oil content of *Pituranthos scoparius*. Asian J Chem 22(4):3065–3068
10. Labed B, Gherraf N, Hameurlaine S, Ladjel S, Zellagui A (2010) The antibacterial activity of water extracts of *Traganum nudatum* Del (Chenopodiaceae) growing in Algeria. Der Pharmacia Lettre 2(6):142–145

11. Kendour Z, Ladjel S, Gherraf N, Ouahrani MR (2010) Antimicrobial activity of nine medicinal plants growing in the south of Algeria. Ann Biol Res 1(4):145–147

12. Adams RP (2007) Identification of essential oil components by Gas chromatography/mass spectrometry. Allured Publishing Corporation, Carol Stream, 4

13. Mouhssen L (2001) Methods to study the photochemistry and bioactivity of essential oils. Phytother Res 18:435–448

14. Saet Byoul Lee., *et al* (2007) The antimicrobial activity of essential oil from *Dracocephalum foetidum* against pathogenic microorganisms. J Microbiol 45(1):53–57

15. Derwich E, Benziane Z, Abdellatif B (2010) GC:MS analysis and antibacterial activity of the essential oil of *Mentha. Pulegium* grown in Morocco. Res J Agric Biol Sci 6(3):191–198

16. Bauer AW, Kirby WMM, Sherris JC, Turck M (1966) Antibiotic susceptibility testing by a standardized single disk method. Am J Clin Pathol 45:493–496

17. Iscan G, Demirci F, Kirimer N (2002) Antimicrobial screening: Mentha *piperita* essential oil. J Agric Food Chem 50:3943–3946. doi:10.1021/jf011476k.

18. Demirci F, Guven K, Demirci B, Dadandi MY, Baser KHC (2008) Antibacterial activity of two Phlomis essential oils against food pathogens. Food Control 19:1159–1164. doi:10.1016/j.foodcont.2008.01.001.

Seven naphtho-γ-pyrones from the marine-derived fungus *Alternaria alternata*: structure elucidation and biological properties

Mohamed Shaaban[1,2*†], Khaled A Shaaban[2†] and Mohamed S Abdel-Aziz[3]

Abstract

Eight bioactive pyrone derivatives were identified from the culture of *Alternaria alternata* strain D2006, isolated from the marine soft coral *Denderonephthya hemprichi*, which was selected as its profound antimicrobial activities. The compounds were assigned as pyrophen (**1**), rubrofusarin B (**2**), fonsecin (**3**), and fonsecin B (**5**) beside to the four dimeric naphtho-γ-pyrones; aurasperone A (**6**), aurasperone B (**7**), aurasperone C (**8**), and aurasperone F (**9**). Structures of the isolated compounds were identified on the basis of 1D and 2D NMR spectroscopy and mass (EI, ESI, HRESI) data, and by comparison with the literature. Configuration of the four dimeric naphtho-γ-pyrones **6-9** was analyzed by CD spectra, exhibiting an identical stereochemistry.

Keywords: pyrone derivatives, *Alternaria alternata*, marine fungi, biological activity

1. Background

Infectional diseases and drug resistance phenomena are the most effective reasons for the death of ca. 20 millions yearly. For example, tuberculosis (TB) was the leading cause of ca. two million deaths due to a bacterial pathogen, *Mycobacterium tuberculosis*, among them more than 80% of TB patients living in sub-Africa and Asia [1-4]. Thus, new and more-powerful drugs are necessary to solve these problems. Marine microorganisms, especially fungi, are still a less investigated resource of bioactive substances [5,6]; recent investigations indicated their tremendous potential as source of new drugs [7-13].

In this article, a report on the antimicrobial activity of naphtho-γ-pyrones (naphthopyran-4-ones) attracted our interest [14]. During the investigation of fungal strains for the production of structurally novel active compounds from marine microorganisms, we found that the EtOAc extract of the marine-derived fungal strain *Alternaria alternata* D2006 (isolated from a red soft coral, *Denderonephthya hemprichi*, collected from the Red Sea at Safaga coasts, Egypt) was selected due to its distinctive features in the chemical and biological assays. We therefore performed a bioassay-guided fractionation.

The crude extract possessed in the agar diffusion test potent activity against *Pseudomonas aeruginosa*, *Staphylococcus aureus* and *Candida albicans*. For isolation of the bioactive constituents, *A. alternata* D2006 was upscaled as a shaker-culture using GYMP medium [15] (100% seawater) for 10 days. Thereafter, the obtained black broth was worked up [16] and separated by a series of chromatographic steps, yielding colourless semisolid of pyrophen (**1**) and seven naphtho-γ-pyrones (**2**, **3**, **5-9**) as yellow solids, among them four dimeric analogues (**6-9**). Herein, we describe their separation, structure elucidation (using 1D and 2D NMR and MS (EI, ESI, HRESI) data and antimicrobial properties.

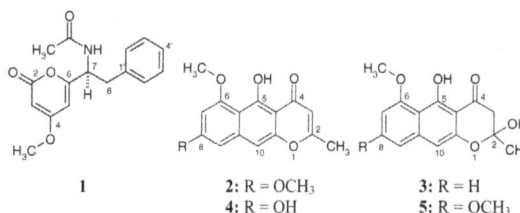

1

2: R = OCH₃
4: R = OH

3: R = H
5: R = OCH₃

* Correspondence: mshaaba_99@yahoo.com
† Contributed equally
[1]Chemistry of Natural Compounds Department, Pharmaceutical Industries Division, National Research Centre, El-Behoos St., Dokki-Cairo 12622, Egypt
Full list of author information is available at the end of the article

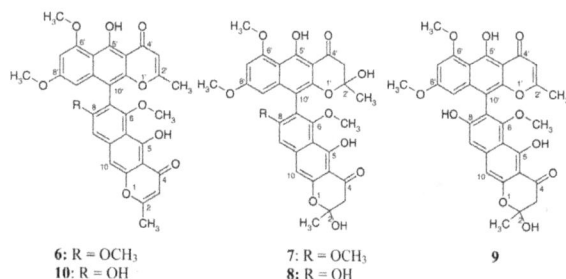

6: R = OCH₃
10: R = OH

7: R = OCH₃
8: R = OH

9

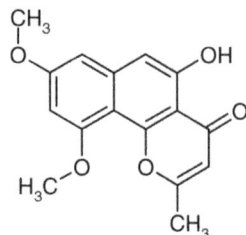

11

2. Taxonomy and characterization

The fungal isolate was identified as *A. alternata* (Dematiaceae) according to Barnett [17]. Microscopically, the conidiophores were dark, simple, rather short or elongate and contained simple or branched chains of conidia. Conidia were dark, typically with both cross and longitudinal septa, with various shapes, obclavate to elliptical or ovoid. The fungal spores were multicellular, dark and having thick cell walls.

3. Results and discussion

The fungal extract showed several UV absorbing (254 nm) yellow bands, exhibiting yellowish-green UV fluorescence at 366 nm. On spraying with anisaldehyde/sulphuric acid and heating they turned orange to dark red, but showed no colour change with sodium hydroxide, thus excluding *peri*-hydroxyquinones.

The molecular formula of compound **1** was determined by HRMS as $C_{16}H_{17}NO_4$; the ^1H NMR spectrum revealed signals for a phenyl residue, an amino NH doublet, and two *m*-coupled methines (δ 5.90, 5.43). Further signals were a methine quartet, a methylene 2H multiplet and two methyl singlets. The ^{13}C NMR/ HMQC spectra indicated the existence of 16 carbons corresponding to a phenyl residue, 2 up-field sp^2 methines (δ100.6, 88.0), 4 quaternary sp^2 atoms (δ171.0-161.9), representing carbonyls or phenolic carbons, and 4 sp^3 carbon signals (δ55.7-22.3). According to these data, compound **1** was identified as pyrophen (**1**) [5], which was isolated and reported previously from *Aspergillus niger* [18,19] and elucidated by crystal structure analysis. Here, we report the full NMR assignments data

for **1** using the 2D NMR experiments for the first time (Figure 1 and Table 1 [see Additional file 1]).

Compound **2** showed a molecular weight of *m/z* 287.09137 (HRESI MS), corresponding to the molecular formula $C_{16}H_{15}O_5$ [M+H]⁺. The ^1H NMR spectra (Table 2) displayed a chelated hydroxyl group (δ 14.96), two *m*-coupled doublets (δ 6.56, 6.38) and two singlets (δ 6.94 and 5.98), along with two methoxy signals (δ 3.99, 3.91) and an sp^2 linked methyl (δ 2.35). The ^{13}C/ HMQC spectra (Table 2) indicated the presence of 16 carbon signals, including 4 sp^2 methines (δ 107.3-97.2), 3 sp^2-oxy carbons (δ 162.6-160.6), 1 carbonyl of γ -lactone (δ 184.2) [20], 5 non-oxygenated sp^2, 2 aromatic-attached methyl ethers (δ 56.0, 55.4) and 1 sp^2-attached methyl (δ 20.6). Full assignment of the 2D NMR experiments (Figure 2 and Table 2) established the structure of **2** as rubrofusarin B, and excluded the structure of the isomeric asperxanthon (**11**) in the same way [21]. Structure of **2** was not fully assigned using 2D NMR before, which we report her to first time (see Additional file 2).

The closely related compound **3** afforded a molecular weight of 290 Da ($C_{15}H_{12}O_5$ by HRESI MS); EI MS gave easily an ion peak at *m/z* 272 by expulsion of water molecule. The ^1H NMR spectrum exhibited aromatic *m*-coupled doublets (δ 6.47, 6.31, $J \sim$ 1.1 Hz) and a methine singlet (δ 6.41), but in contrast to **2**, two phenolic hydroxy signals (δ 14.19, 10.18), and only one methoxy signal (δ 3.84). In addition, an AB signal of diastereotopic methylene protons (δ 3.14, 2.72, $J \sim$ 16.8) and a methyl singlet (δ 1.60) were visible. Based on ^{13}C/ HMQC spectra (Table 2) and HMBC experiment (as it was not fully assigned before using 2D NMR) (Figure 2),

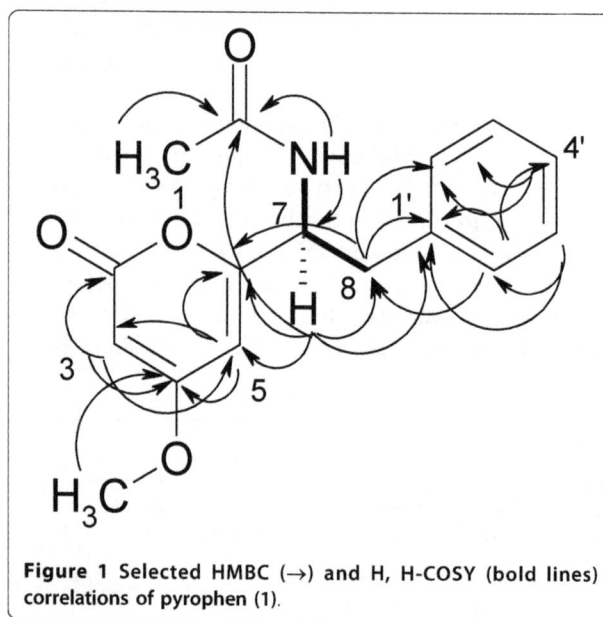

Figure 1 Selected HMBC (→) and H, H-COSY (bold lines) correlations of pyrophen (1).

Table 1 ^{13}C and ^1H NMR data of pyrophen (1) in $CDCl_3$ (J in [Hz])

Number	δ_c	δ_h	Number	δ_c	δ_h
2	164.7	-	7-NHCOCH₃	170.3	-
3	88.0	5.43 (d, 2.2)	7-NHCOCH₃	22.3	1.95 (s)
4	171.0	-	8	38.1	3.09 (m)
4-OCH₃	55.7	3.73 (s)	1'	136.0	-
5	100.6	5.90 (d, 2.2)	2',6'	128.6	7.16 (m)
6	161.9	-	3',5'	128.2	7.25 (m)
7	52.3	4.98 (q, 7.8)	4'	126.5	7.21 (m)
7-NHCOCH₃	-	7.79 (d, 8.4)			

compound **3** was finally established as fonsecin (**3**) (see Additional file 3). The facile loss of water by EI MS corresponded to the formation of TMC-256 A1 (**4**).

Compound **5** displayed similar chromatographic properties and the same ^1H NMR pattern as **3**. The molecular weight of **5** was deduced as 304 Da, which is 14 *amu* higher than that of **3**, attributing to the methylation of the phenolic hydroxyl group at 8-position, hence compound **5** was identified as fonsecin B [22] (see Additional file 4)

3.1. Aurasperones A-C and F
Compound **6** was obtained from fraction II as middle polar yellow solid, displaying a molecular weight at *m/z* 570. The expectation of a dimeric rubrofusarin B (**2**) was confirmed by ^1H NMR spectra, where six sp^2

Table 2 ^{13}C and ^1H NMR data of rubrofusarin B (2) and fonsecin (3) in $CDCl_3$ (J in [Hz])

Number	2		3	
	δ_c	δ_H	δ_c	δ_H
2	167.4	-	100.0	-
2-CH₃	20.6	2.35 (s)	27.6	1.60 (s)
2-OH	-	-	-	6.95 (brs)
3	107.3	5.98 (s)	47.6	3.14 (d, 16.8), 2.72 (d, 16.8)
4	184.2	-	197.5	-
4a	104.3	-	102.5	-
5	162.6	-	164.2	-
5-OH	-	14.96 (s)	-	14.19 (s)
5a	108.4	-	105.2	-
6	160.6	-	161.4	-
6-OCH3	56.0	3.99 (s)	55.6	3.84 (s)
7	97.2	6.38 (d, 2.2)	96.6	6.31 (brd, 1.1)
8	161.5	-	160.7	-
8-OH	-	-	-	10.18 (brs)
8-OCH3	55.4	3.91 (s)	-	-
9	97.8	6.56 (d, 2.2)	101.5	6.47 (s)
9a	141.0	-	142.9	-
10	101.0	6.94 (s)	101.0	6.41 (s)
10a	153.3	-	153.4	-

methine protons were visible, which were classified into two *m*-coupled protons, two α-methines of the consequent γ-pyrones (δ 6.15, 6.08) and two singlet methines (δ 7.35 and 7.24), together with six methyls, among them four methoxy signals. Based on these data and search in literature, compound **6** was identified as aurasperone A [22] (see Additional file 5)

Compound **7** exhibited a close structural similarity with fonsecin B (**5**); the molecular weight was determined as 606 Da, corresponding to the molecular formula $C_{32}H_{30}O_{12}$ (HRESI MS). EI MS of **7** displayed an ion signal at *m/z* 570 as base peak, resulting from the expulsion of two water molecules, affording the molecular weight of aurasperone A (**6**). The ^1H NMR spectrum established a dimeric pattern of fonsecin B (**5**), where four sp^2 methines protons being of two *m*-coupled protons and two singlet methines; two methylene signals (δ 3.02 and 2.89) instead of the two α-methines of the consequent-γ-pyrones shown in **6**, along with six methyls, among them four methoxy signals and two sp^3-bounded methyl signals (δ 1.79, 1.46). In accordance, structure of **7** was assigned as aurasperone B (**7**) [22]. (see Additional file 6)

A third dimer **8** had a molecular weight of 592 Da and a corresponding molecular formula $C_{31}H_{28}O_{12}$. Three consecutive fragment ions (*m/z* 574, 556 and 525) on EI MS corresponded to the expulsion of one H_2O molecule (to afford aurasperone F, **9**), two H_2O (dianhydroaurasperone C, **10**) and $2H_2O + OCH_3$, respectively. The ^1H NMR spectrum displayed the same pattern as in aurasperone B (**7**), except that the methoxy signal (δ 3.78) of 8-OCH₃ in **7** was replaced by a phenolic hydroxyl group, pointing to aurasperone C (**8**) [23]. (see Additional file 7)

Compound **9** was a fourth dimer with a molecular formula $C_{31}H_{26}O_{11}$; on EI MS, it displayed a fragment ion at *m/z* 556 corresponding to an aromatized structural analogue (dianhydroaurasperone C, **10**), and a further fragment at *m/z* 286 corresponded to rubrofusarin B (**2**). The ^1H NMR spectra displayed five sp^2 methines (δ 6.87-6.08), one less than in **6**, replaced by an *AB* signal of a methylene group (δ 3.35-3.25). Accordingly, one of the β-bounded methyls of the lactones was up-field shifted (δ 1.65), while the other one was retained at δ 2.16 as in **6**. In contrast to **6**, only three methoxy signals (δ 3.95-3.43) were visible, while the fourth one was replaced by a phenolic OH. Based on these spectroscopic features, structure **9** was confirmed as aurasperone F [24] (see Additional file 8)

The four dimeric naphtho-γ-pyrones (**6-9**) were presently constructed from two naphtho-γ-pyrone units, which are not symmetrically linked; i.e. the first pyrone (above) unit is linked *via* a middle aromatic moiety (10'-position) to a terminal aromatic residue (7-position) of the second pyrone (down) unit.

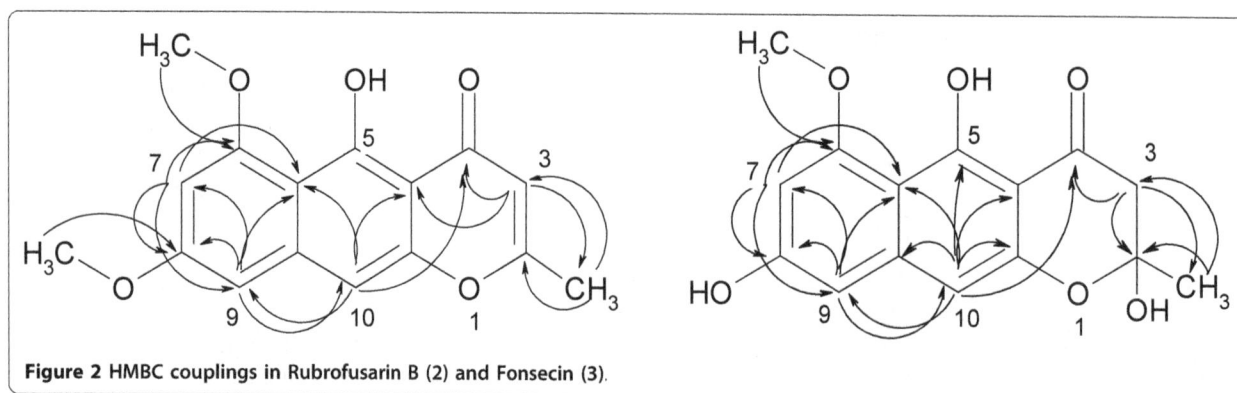

Figure 2 HMBC couplings in Rubrofusarin B (2) and Fonsecin (3).

The optical rotations of the dimers had the same negative sign and similar values indicating that the optical rotation value was dominated by the chiral axes between the two naphthopyranone moieties (atropisomerism). The absolute configurations of dimeric naphtho-γ-pyrones have been determined by circular-dichroism (CD). According to the literature [25], (S)-configured dimeric naphtho-γ-pyrones exhibit a first positive Cotton Effect in the long-wavelength region, a negative Cotton Effect at middle wavelength and then a positive Cotton Effect at shorter one. In our experimental data, the CD spectra for three representative dimeric naphtho-γ-pyrones (6-8) showed closely related values with pronounced Cotton Effects, recognizing them to have the same patterns. In accordance, the ellipticity of aurasperones A-C (6-8) showed three Cotton Effects, one peak was shown firstly in the region of $[\theta]_{284-285}$ +359274-22843.4, then one trough between $[\theta]_{270-267}$ -151670-339938 and the last elliptical peak was shown at $[\theta]_{227-219}$ +107899-5629. As the dimer 6 has no further chiral elements, the chiral axis is dominating the absolute configuration. Based on the revealed features from the CD spectroscopic data, the four dimeric compounds (6-9) have identical (S)-configurations around their corresponding axis between C-10' and C-7 (see Additional file 9)

3.2. Biological activities

The antibiotic activity of compounds 1-8 was examined against 11 microbial test organisms using the agar diffusion method (40 μg/disc) (Table 3). According to the antimicrobial assay, the crude extract of the fungal strain exhibited high activity against bacteria and yeasts (Table 4). Nevertheless, only three of the isolated metabolites were found to exhibited activity: pyrophen (1) and rubrofusarin B (2) displayed high (28 mm) and moderate (12 mm) activity against *C. albicans*, respectively, while aurosperone A (6) was active (13 mm) against the plant pathogenic fungi, *Rhizoctonia solani*. In the brine shrimp assay (10 μg/mL), all

studied compounds here showed weak cytotoxicity (approx. 4-11%).

4. Experimental

The NMR spectra were measured on a Bruker AMX 300 (300.135 MHz), a Varian Unity 300 (300.145 MHz) and Varian Inova 500 (499.876 MHz) spectrometers. EI mass spectra were recorded on a Finnigan MAT 95 spectrometer (70 eV). ESI MS was recorded on a Finnigan LCQ with quaternary pump Rheos 4000 (Flux Instrument). HRMS were recorded by ESI MS on an Apex IV 7 Tesla Fourier-Transform Ion Cyclotron Resonance Mass Spectrometer (Bruker Daltonics, Billerica, MA, USA). Optical rotation was measured on a Perkin-Elmer Polarimeter, model 343. Flash chromatography was carried out on silica gel (230-400 mesh). R_f values were measured on Polygram SIL G/UV$_{254}$ (Macherey-Nagel & Co., Düren, Germany). Size exclusion chromatography was done on Sephadex LH-20 (Lipophilic Sephadex, Amersham Biosciences Ltd.; purchased from Sigma-Aldrich Chemie, Steinheim, Germany).

4.1. Sampling and isolation of the fungal strain

The reddish soft coral *D. hemprichi* was collected from the Red Sea; approx. 30 km offshore from Safaga (east Egypt) at a depth of approx. 30 m. Pieces of the coral were rinsed three times with sterile seawater and then aseptically cut into smaller pieces and shaken for 2 h. The aqueous supernatant was serially diluted, and each 200 μL were inoculated onto 15-cm Petri dishes, each containing 50 mL of yeast extract/starch agar (yeast extract 0.2 g/L, soluble starch 1.0 g/L, agar 20 g/L, chloramphenicol 50 mg/L natural seawater at pH 6.0) [7]. The black single colonies were picked from the plates after inoculation for 25 days at 30°C and subcultured on the same medium without chloramphenicol. The strain is deposited in the culture collection of the Department of Microbial Chemistry, NRC, Cairo, Egypt.

Table 3 Antimicrobial (40 μg/disc (∅ 9 mm; [mm]) and cytotoxic (10 μg/mL) activities of compounds 1-8

Compound number	BS[a]	SA[b]	SV[c]	EC[d]	CA[e]	MM[f]	CV[g]	CS[h]	SS[i]	PS[j]	PU[k]	Brine shrimp
1	ND	ND	ND	ND	28	ND	ND	ND	ND	ND	ND	4.2%
2	ND	ND	ND	ND	12	ND	ND	ND	ND	ND	ND	11%
3	ND	ND	ND	ND	ND	ND	ND	ND	ND	13	ND	Nt
4	ND	ND	ND	ND	ND	ND	ND	ND	ND	ND	ND	8.8%
5	ND	ND	ND	ND	ND	ND	ND	ND	ND	ND	ND	5.0%
6	ND	ND	ND	ND	ND	ND	ND	ND	ND	ND	ND	9.7%
7	ND	ND	ND	ND	ND	ND	ND	ND	ND	ND	ND	6.4%
8	ND	ND	ND	ND	ND	ND	ND	ND	ND	ND	ND	9.7%

[a]*Bacillus subtilis*, [b]*S. aureus*, [c]*Streptomyces viridochromogenes* (Tü 57), [d]*Escherichia coli*, [e]*C. albicans*, [f]*Mucor miehi*, [g]*Chlorella vulgaris*, [h]*Chlorella sorokiniana*, [i]*Scenedesmus subspicatus*, [j]*R. solani*; [k]*Pythium ultimum*
ND, not detected.

4.2. Fermentation and working up

The well-grown single colonies of *A. alternata* were inoculated in subculture agar slants containing malt extract medium: malt extract (30 g/L), peptone 5 g/L), agar (20 g/L), natural sea water (1000 mL); at pH approx. 5.5 for 7 days at 30°C). The obtained grown agar slants were served to inoculate 500-mL Erlenmeyer flasks, each containing 100 mL of GYMP medium (g/L): malt extract (3), yeast extract (3), peptone (5), glucose (10) and 1000 mL natural seawater at pH approx. 6.5 at 30°C. The culture media was in turn applied to cultivation on a rotary shaker (10 days). After harvesting, the afforded black broth was centrifuged (7,000 rpm for 15 min), and the obtained two phases, mycelial cake and supernatant, were individually extracted with ethyl acetate. The obtained unique black organic extracts were applied to biological and chemical screenings.

The well-grown agar slants of the fungal strain D2006 were served to inoculate 60 of 1-L Erlenmeyer flasks, each containing 300-mL of GYMP medium (g/L): malt extract (3), yeast extract (3), peptone (5), glucose (10), agar (20) and 1000 mL of 100% seawater at pH approx. 6.5. The inoculated media was applied to additional cultivation using a rotary shaker (150 rpm) for 10 days. After harvesting, the obtained black culture broth was mixed with celite (approx. 1.5 kg) and then filtered *in vacuo*. The afforded two phases, filtrate and mycelium, were applied to exhaustive extraction by ethyl acetate. TLC of both organic extracts recognized their unique,

Table 4 Antimicrobial activities of the fugal extract (60 μg/disc (5-mm diameter)

Test organism	Extract activity (mm)
P. aeruginosa	17
S. aureus	23
C. albicans	20
A. niger	ND

ND, not detected.

and they were combined therefore, and concentrated *in vacuo*, affording 5.5 g as black crude extract.

4.3. Isolation of the active constituents

The obtained extract was applied to column chromatography on silica gel eluted by CH_2Cl_2-MeOH gradient and monitored by TLC to afford five fractions: I (0.62 g), II (1.21 g), III (0.71 g), IV (1.52 g) and V (0.22 g). Fraction I was re-purified on silica gel column (DCM) followed by Sephadex LH-20 (DCM/40% MeOH) to afford a colourless semisolid of phyrophen (1) (468.0 mg). Application of Fraction II to PTLC (DCM/3% MeOH) followed by purification on Sephadex LH-20 (DCM/40% MeOH) lead to isolation of two yellow solids of rubrofusarin B (2, 11.0 mg) and aurosperone A (6, 13.0 mg), respectively. Fraction III was purified using a silica gel column (DCM-MeOH) followed by Sephadex LH-20 (DCM/40% MeOH) to give a yellow solid of aurasperone F (9, 15.0 mg). Purification of the middle polar fraction IV *via* PTLC (DCM/5% MeOH) followed by Sephadex LH-20 (MeOH) yielded three yellow solids of aurasperone B (7, 8.0 mg), aurasperone C (8, 14.0 mg) and fonsecin (3, 11.5 mg). As the same for IV, the polar fraction V afforded three yellow solids of fonsecin B (5, 12.0 mg), aurasperone B (7, 3.4 mg) and aurasperone C (8, 4.1 mg).

Pyrophen (1)
Colourless semisolid, UV-absorbing, no colour reaction on spraying with anisaldehyde/sulphuric acid; R_f = 0.86 (CH_2Cl_2/5% MeOH); **^{1}H NMR** (300 MHz, CDCl$_3$) and **^{13}C NMR** (125 MHz, CDCl$_3$) see Table 1; **EI MS** *m/z* (%) = 287.2 ([M]$^+$, 28), 228.1 (8), 196.1 (40), 154.2 (100), 125.1 (16), 111.1 (6), 91.1 (12), 43.1 (11); **(+)-ESI MS** *m/z* (%) = 596.9 ([2M+Na]$^+$, 85), 310 [M+Na]$^+$, 36), 288 ([M+H]$^+$, 100); **(-)-ESI MS** *m/z* 286 [M+H]$^-$; **(+)-HRESI MS** *m/z* 288.12301 ([M+H]$^+$, calcd: 288.12303 for $C_{16}H_{18}NO_4$); 310.10490 ([M+Na]$^+$, calcd: 310.10497 for $C_{16}H_{17}NO_4Na$).

Rubrofusarin B (2)
Yellow solid, UV-green fluorescence (365 nm), orange with anisaldehyde/sulphuric acid; R_f = 0.78 (CH_2Cl_2/5%

MeOH); ^1H **NMR** (300 MHz, CDCl$_3$) and ^{13}C **NMR** (125 MHz, CDCl$_3$) see Table 2; **EI MS** m/z (%) = 286.2 ([M]$^{+\cdot}$, 100), 268.1 ([M-H$_2$O]$^+$, 12), 257.2 ([M-CHO]$^+$, 44), 240.2 (8) 213.2 (5), 43.1 (7); **(+)-ESI MS** m/z (%) = 594.9 ([2M+Na]$^+$, 14), 287 ([M+H]$^+$, 100); **(+)-HRESI MS** m/z 287.09137 ([M+H]$^+$, calcd: 287.09139 for C$_{16}$H$_{15}$O$_5$).

Fonsecin (3)

Yellow solid, UV-green fluorescence (365 nm), turned dark red with anisaldehyde/sulphuric acid; R_f = 0.38 (CH$_2$Cl$_2$/5% MeOH); ^1H **NMR** (300 MHz, CDCl$_3$) and ^{13}C **NMR** (125 MHz, CDCl$_3$) see Table 2; **EI MS** m/z (%) = 290.2 ([M]$^+$, 24), 272.2 ([M-H$_2$O]$^+$, 16), 243.2 (8), 232.1 (21), 189.1 (7), 175.1 (16), 101.1 (15), 85.1 (22), 59.1 (36), 43.1 (100); **(+)-ESI MS** m/z (%) = 291 ([M+H]$^+$); **(-)-ESI MS** m/z (%) = 289 ([M-H]$^-$); **(+)-HRESI MS** m/z 291.08631 ([M+H]$^+$, calcd: 291.08631 for C$_{16}$H$_{15}$O$_6$).

Fonsecin B (5)

Yellow solid, UV-green fluorescence (365 nm), turned dark red with anisaldehyde/sulphuric acid; R_f = 0.44 (CH$_2$Cl$_2$/5% MeOH); ^1H **NMR** (300 MHz, DMSO-d_6) δ = 14.09 (brs, 1H, 5-OH), 7.00 (brs, 1H, 2-OH), 6.68 (brd, 1H, J ~ 1.1 Hz, H-9), 6.55 (s, 1H, H-10), 6.38 (brd, 1H, J ~ 1.1 Hz, H-9), 3.84 (s, 6H, 6,8-OCH$_3$), 3.14 (d, 1H, J ~ 16.8 Hz, H-3a), 2.72 (d, 1H, J ~ 16.8 Hz, H-3b), 1.61 (s, 3H, 2-CH$_3$); **EI MS** m/z (%) = 304.3 ([M]$^+$, 56), 286.3 ([M-H$_2$O]$^+$, 8), 262.3 (8), 247.2 (28), 246.2 (60), 220.2 (20), 218.2 (10), 149.2 (20), 145.2 (34), 127.2 (12), 116.2 (64), 101.2 (48), 84.1 (36), 66.1 (24), 59.1 (63), 43.1 (100).

Aurasperone A (6)

Yellow solid, UV-green fluorescence (365 nm), turned orange with anisaldehyde/sulphuric acid; R_f = 0.82 (CH$_2$Cl$_2$/5% MeOH); $[\alpha]_D^{20}$ = -18.9 (c = 0.19, MeOH); CD (c 1.1929 × 10^{-5} mol/L [c 6.8 µg/mL], MeOH) $[\theta]_{400}$ 0 $[\theta]_{284}$ +22843, $[\theta]_{270}$ -36396, $[\theta]_{219}$ +5629; ^1H **NMR** (300 MHz, CD$_3$OD) δ = 7.35 (s, 1H, H-10), 7.25 (s, 1H, H-9), 6.51 (brd, 1H, J ~ 1.1 Hz, H-7'), 6.23 (brd, 1H, J ~ 1.1 Hz, H-7), 6.15 (s, 1H, H-3), 6.08 (s, 1H, H-3'), 3.95 (s, 3H, 6'-OCH$_3$), 3.79 (s, 3H, 8-OCH$_3$), 3.59 (s, 3H, 8'-OCH$_3$), 3.46 (s, 3H, 6-OCH$_3$), 2.42 (s, 3H, 2-CH$_3$), 2.13 (s, 3H, 2'-CH$_3$); **EI MS** m/z (%) = 570.5 ([M]$^+$, 44), 539.5 ([M-OCH$_3$]$^+$, 10), 513.4 (5), 286 (7), 167.2 (7), 145.2 (44), 116.2 (100), 85.1 (39), 55.1 (22), 43.1 (24).

Aurasperone B (7)

Yellow solid, UV-green fluorescence (365 nm), turned orange with anisaldehyde/sulphuric acid; R_f = 0.48 (CH$_2$Cl$_2$/5% MeOH); $[\alpha]_D^{20}$ = -18.3 (c = 0.12, MeOH); CD (c 2.83 × 10^{-5} mol/L [c 17.2 µg/mL], MeOH) $[\theta]_{400}$ 0, $[\theta]_{284}$ +143232, $[\theta]_{267}$ -151670, $[\theta]_{227}$ +46610; ^1H **NMR** (300 MHz, CDCl$_3$) δ = 14.51 (brs, 1H, 5'-OH), 14.08 (brs, 1H, 5-OH), 6.84 (s, 1H, H-9), 6.72 (s, 1H, H-9), 6.37 (d, 1H, J ~ 1.1 Hz, H-7'), 6.14 (d, 1H, J ~ 1.1

Hz, H-9'), 3.99 (s, 3H, 6'-OCH$_3$), 3.78 (s, 3H, 8-OCH$_3$), 3.63 (s, 3H, 8'-OCH$_3$), 3.39 (s, 3H, 6-OCH$_3$), 3.02, (d, 2H, J ~ 16.3 Hz, 3-H$_2$), 2.89 (m, 2H, 3'-H$_2$), 1.79 (s, 3H, 2-CH$_3$), 1.46 (s, 3H, 2'-CH$_3$); **EI MS** m/z (%) = 570.3 ([M-2H$_2$O]$^+$, 100), 539.4 ([M-(2H$_2$O+OCH$_3$)]$^+$, 74), 524.3 (5), 299.2 (12), 272.2 (13), 269.7 (24), 230.2 (18), 193.1 (12), 154.2 (14), 149.1 (19), 130.1 (48), 91.1 (54), 57.1 (30), 43.1 (57); **(+)-HRESI MS** m/z 607.18100 ([M +H]$^+$, calcd: 607.18100 for C$_{32}$H$_{31}$O$_{12}$), m/z 629.16294 ([M+Na]$^+$, calcd: 629.16295 for C$_{32}$H$_{30}$O$_{12}$Na).

Aurasperone C (8)

Yellow solid, UV-green fluorescence (365 nm), turned orange with anisaldehyde/sulphuric acid; R_f = 0.26 (CH$_2$Cl$_2$/5% MeOH); $[\alpha]_D^{20}$ = -33.5 (c = 0.17, MeOH); CD (c 4.29 × 10^{-5} mol/L [c 24 µg/mL], MeOH) $[\theta]_{400}$ 0, $[\theta]_{285}$ +359273, $[\theta]_{268}$ -339938, $[\theta]_{226}$ +107899.87; ^1H **NMR** (300 MHz, CD$_3$OD): δ = 6.84 (s, 1H, H-10), 6.57 (s, 1H, H-9), 6.38 (d, 1H, J ~ 1.2 Hz, H-9'), 6.20 (d, 1H, J ~ 1.2 Hz, H-7'), 3.93 (s, 3H, 6'-OCH$_3$), 3.60 (s, 3H, 8'-OCH$_3$), 3.50 (s, 3H, 6-OCH$_3$), 3.30-3.29 (m, 4H, 3,3'-H$_2$), 1.69 (s, 3H, 2-CH$_3$), 1.49 (s, 3H, 2'-CH$_3$); **EI MS** m/z (%) = 574.3 ([M-H$_2$O]$^+$, 6), 556.3 ([M-2H$_2$O]$^+$, 42), 525.3 ([M-(2H$_2$O+OCH$_3$)]$^+$, 32), 264.2 (7) 58.2 (28), 43.1 (100); **(+)-HRESI MS** m/z 615.14779 ([M+Na]$^+$, calcd: 615.14729 for C$_{31}$H$_{28}$O$_{12}$Na), m/z 593.16570 ([M+H]$^+$, calcd: 593.16534 for C$_{31}$H$_{29}$O$_{12}$).

Aurasperone F (9)

Yellow solid, UV-green fluorescence (365 nm), turned orange with anisaldehyde/sulphuric acid; R_f = 0.55 (CH$_2$Cl$_2$/5% MeOH); ^1H **NMR** (300 MHz, CD$_3$OD) δ = 6.87 (s, 1H, H-10), 6.55 (s, 1H, H-9), 6.51 (d, 1H, J ~ 1.1 Hz, H-9'), 6.36 (brd, 1H, J ~ 1.1 Hz, H-7'), 6.08 (s, 1H, H-3'), 3.95 (s, 3H, 6'-OCH$_3$), 3.63 (s, 3H, 8'-OCH$_3$), 3.43 (s, 3H, 6-OCH$_3$), 3.35-3.25, (m, 2H, 3-H$_2$), 2.16 (s, 3H, 2'-CH$_3$), 1.65 (s, 3H, 2-CH$_3$); **EI MS** m/z (%) = 556.5 ([M-H$_2$O]$^+$, 5), 286.3 ([rubrofusarin B (2)]$^+$, 8), 84.1 (12), 57.2 (10), 44.1 (100); **(+)-ESI MS** m/z (%) = 1172 ([2M+Na+H]$^+$, 19), 575 ([M+H]$^+$, 100); **(-)-ESI MS** m/z (%) = 1721 ([3M-H]$^-$, 31), 1147 ([2M-H]$^-$, 22), 573 ([M-H]$^-$, 100).

4.4. Biological activities

Antimicrobial activity

Compounds **1-8** were dissolved in CH$_2$Cl$_2$/10% MeOH at a concentration of 1 mg/mL. Aliquots of 40 µL were soaked on filter paper discs (9 mm Ø, no. 2668, Schleicher & Schüll GmbH, Germany) and dried for 1 h at room temperature under sterilized conditions. The paper discs were placed on inoculated agar plats and incubated for 24 h at 38°C for bacterial and 48 h (30°C) for the fungal isolates, while the algal test strains were incubated at room temperature in day light.

For the fungal extract examination, representative test microbes; *P.aeruginosa, S. aureus, C. albicans* and *A.*

niger were used. Both bacterial and yeast strains were grown on nutrient agar medium (g/L): Beef extract 3; peptone, 10; and agar, 20. The pH was adjusted to 7.2. The fungal strain was grown on Czapek-Dox medium (g/l): Sucrose, 30; $NaNO_3$, 3; $MgSO_4.7H_2O$, 0.5l; KCl, 0.5; $FeSO_4$, 0.01; K_2HPO_4, 1; and agar, 20. The pH was maintained at 6.0. The disc diffusion test has been done according to Collins and Lyne [26]. Filter paper discs (5 mm diameter) were saturated with 200 μ*g* from the culture extract, and located on the surface of the agar plates (150 mm diameter containing 50 mL of solidified media). The paper discs were placed on inoculated agar plats and incubated for 24 h at 38°C (bacteria and yeast) and 48 h at 30°C (fungi).

Brine shrimp microwell cytotoxicity assay

The cytotoxic assay was performed according to Takahashi et al. [27] and Sajid et al. [28].

5. Conclusions

In this research article, eight bioactive pyrone derivatives were identified from the culture of *A. alternata* strain D2006, isolated from the marine soft coral *D. hemprichi*. Selection of the strain was based on its profound antibiotic and antimicrobial activities. Structures of the isolated compounds were identified on the basis of 1D and 2D NMR spectroscopy and mass (EI, ESI, HRESI) data, and by comparison with the literature. Configuration of the four dimeric naphtha-γ-pyrones **6-9** was analyzed by CD spectra, exhibiting an identical stereochemistry. The biological activity (antimicrobial and cytotoxicity) of the fungal extract and its corresponding isolated compounds were comparatively studied. This is as a trial to find out new leading drugs to overcome some of the recently discovered diseases.

Additional material

Additional file 1: Spectral data of Pyrophen (1). Ten charts (chart 1-10) containing the mass (ESI, HRESI, EI MS) and NMR (^{1}HNMR, ^{13}CNMR, H, H COSY, HMQC, HSQC, HMBC) spectral data of Pyrophen (**1**).

Additional file 2: Spectral data of Rubrofusarin B (2). Thirteen charts (chart 11-23) containing the mass (ESI, EI, HRESI MS) and NMR (^{1}HNMR, ^{13}CNMR, H, H COSY, HMQC, HSQC, HMBC) spectral data of Rubrofusarin B (**2**).

Additional file 3: Spectral data of Fonsecin (3). Nine charts (chart 24-32) containing the mass (ESI, EI MS) and NMR (^{1}HNMR, ^{13}CNMR, H, H COSY, HMQC, HSQC, HMBC) spectral data of Fonsecin (**3**).

Additional file 4: Spectral data of Fonsecin B (5). Two charts (chart 33-34) containing the mass (EI MS) and NMR (^{1}HNMR) spectral data of Fonsecin B (**5**).

Additional file 5: Spectral data of Aurasperone A (6). Two charts (chart 35-36) containing the mass (EI MS) and NMR (^{1}HNMR) spectral data of Aurasperone A (**6**)

Additional file 6: Spectral data of Aurasperone B (7). Three charts (chart 37-39) containing the mass (HRESI, EI MS) and NMR (^{1}HNMR) spectral data of Aurasperone B (**7**)

Additional file 7: Spectral data of Aurasperone C (8). Four charts (chart 40-43) containing the mass (ESI, HRESI MS) and NMR (^{1}HNMR) spectral data of Aurasperone C (**8**)

Additional file 8: Spectral data of Aurasperone F (9). Three charts (chart 44-46) containing the mass (ESI, EI MS) and NMR (^{1}HNMR) spectral data of Aurasperone F (**9**)

Additional file 9: CD Spectra of Aurasperones A-C (6-8). Three charts (chart 47-49) containing the CD spectral data of Aurasperones A-C (**6-8**).

Acknowledgements

The authors are deeply thankful to Prof. H. Laatsch for his Lab facilities and unlimited support. We are appreciated greatly R. Machinek for the NMR spectra, Dr. H. Frauendorf for the mass measurements, F. Lissy for biological activity tests and A. Kohl for technical assistance. Dr. Mohamed Shaaban is deeply thankful to the DAAD offices in Cairo and Bonn for kindly financing of the project during the visiting period in Germany.
Supplementary Information accompanying this paper includes MS, NMR and CD spectra.

Author details

^{1}Chemistry of Natural Compounds Department, Pharmaceutical Industries Division, National Research Centre, El-Behoos St., Dokki-Cairo 12622, Egypt ^{2}Institute of Organic and Biomolecular Chemistry, University of Göttingen, Tammannstrasse 2, D-37077 Göttingen, Germany ^{3}Department of Microbial Chemistry, Genetic Engineering and Biotechnology Division, National Research Centre, El-Behoos St., Dokki-Cairo 12622, Egypt

Competing interests

The authors declare that they have no competing interests.

References

1. DWHO Report (2006) Global tuberculosis control: surveillance, planning, financing E. World Health Organization, Geneva p 1
2. Alland D, Kalkut GE, Moss AR, McAdam RA, Hahn JA, Bosworth W, Drucker E, Bloom BR (1994) Transmission of tuberculosis in New York City. An analysis by DNA fingerprinting and conventional epidemiologic methods. N Engl J Med 330(24):1710–1716. doi:10.1056/NEJM199406163302403.
3. Whalen C, Horsburgh CR, Hom D, Lahart C, Simberkoff M, Ellner J (1995) Accelerated course of human immunodeficiency virus infection after tuberculosis. Am J Respir Crit Care Med 151(1):129–135
4. Zumla A, Grange J (1998) Tuberculosis. BMJ 316(719):1962–1964
5. Laatsch H *AntiBase*, a data base for rapid structural determination of microbial natural products, and annual updates, chemical concepts, Weinheim, Germany.http://wwwuser.gwdg.de/~hlaatsc/antibase.htm
6. Laatsch H (2006) Marine bacterial metabolites. In: Proksch P, Müller WEG (ed) Frontiers in marine biotechnology. Horizon Bioscience, Norfolk, UK pp 225–288. ISBN 1-904933-18-1
7. Shiono Y, Tsuchinari M, Shimanuki K, Miyajima T, Murayama T, Koseki T, Laatsch H, Takanami K, Suzuki K (2007) Fusaristatins A and B, two new cyclic lipopeptides from an endophytic *Fusarium* sp. J Antibiot 60(5):309–316. doi:10.1038/ja.2007.39.
8. Al-Zereini W, Schuhmann I, Laatsch H, Helmke E, Anke H (2007) New aromatic nitro compounds from *Salegentibacter* sp. T436, an Arctic sea ice bacterium. Taxonomy, fermentation, isolation and biological activities. J Antibiot 60(5):301–308. doi:10.1038/ja.2007.38.
9. Namikoshi M, Akano K, Kobayashi H, Koike Y, Kitazawa A, Rondonuwu AB, Pratasik SB (2002) Distribution of marine filamentous fungi associated with marine sponges in coral reefs of Palau and Bunaken Island, Indonesia. J Tokyo Univ Fish 88:15–20
10. Lange L (1996) Microbial metabolites–an infinite source of novel chemistry. Pure Appl Chem 68(2):745–748
11. Hawksworth DL, Rossman AY (1997) Where are all the undescribed fungi? Phytopathology 87(9):888–891. doi:10.1094/PHYTO.1997.87.9.888.

12. Abdelazim A (2004) Secondary metabolites of marine-derived fungi: natural product chemistry and biological activity. PhD Thesis, Rheinischen Friedrich-University, Bonn, Germany

13. Feofilova EP (2001) The kingdom fungi: heterogeneity of physiological and biochemical properties and relationships with plants, animals, and prokaryotes (Review). Appl Biochem Microbiol 37(2):124–137. (Translated from Prikladnaya Biokhimiya i Mikrobiologiya 2001, 37(2):141-155). doi:10.1023/A:1002863311534.

14. James GG, Zhang HJ, Susan LP, Bernard DS, Andrew DM, Fernando C, Norman RF (2004) Antimycobacterial naphthopyrones from *Senna obliqua*. J Nat Prod 67(2):225–227. doi:10.1021/np030348i.

15. Masoud W, Kaltoft CH (2006) The effects of yeasts involved in the fermentation of *Coffea arabica* in East Africa on growth and ochratoxin A (OTA) production by *Aspergillus ochraceus*. Int J Food Microbiol 106(2):229–234. doi:10.1016/j.ijfoodmicro.2005.06.015.

16. Bibani MAF, Baake M, Lovisetto B, Laatsch H, Helmke E, Weyland H (1998) Marine bacteria. X. Anthranilamides: new antimicroalgal active substances from a marine Streptomyces sp. J Antibiot 51(3):333–340. doi:10.7164/antibiotics.51.333.

17. Barnett HL (1972) Illustrated genera of imperfect fungi. Burgess Publishing Company, Minneapolis, 2

18. Barnes CL, Steiner JR, Torres E, Pacheco R, Marquez H (1990) Structure and absolute configuration of pyrophen, a novel pyrone derivative of L-phenylalanine from *Aspergillus niger*. Int J Pept Protein Res 36(3):292–296

19. Varoglu M, Crews P (2000) Biosynthetically diverse compounds from a saltwater culture of sponge-derived *Aspergillus niger*. J Nat Prod 63(1):41–43. doi:10.1021/np9902892.

20. Abd-Alla HI, Shaaban M, Shaaban KA, Abu-Gabal NS, Shalaby NMM, Laatsch H (2009) New bioactive compounds from *Aloe hijazensis*. Nat Prod Res 23(11):1035–1049. doi:10.1080/14786410802242851.

21. Sakurai M, Kohno J, Yamamoto K, Okuda T, Nishio M, Kawano K, Ohnuki T (2002) TMC-256A1 and C1, new inhibitors of IL-4 signal transduction produced by *Aspergillus niger var niger* TC 1629. J Antibiot 55(8):685–692. doi:10.7164/antibiotics.55.685.

22. Priestap HA (1984) New naphthopyrones from *Aspergillus fonsecaeus*. Tetrahedron 40(19):3617–3624. doi:10.1016/S0040-4020(01)88792-5.

23. Tanaka H, Wang P, Namiki M (1972) Structure of Aurasperone C. Agric Biol Chem 36(13):2511–2517. doi:10.1271/bbb1961.36.2511.

24. Bouras N, Mathieu F, Coppel Y, Lebrihi A (2005) Aurasperone F–a new member of the naphtho-gamma-pyrone class isolated from a cultured microfungus, *Aspergillus niger* C-433. Nat Prod Res 19(7):653–659. doi:10.1080/14786410412331286955.

25. Zhang Y, Ling S, Fang Y, Zhu T, Gu Q, Zhu WM (2008) Isolation, structure elucidation, and antimycobacterial properties of dimeric naphtho-γ-pyrones from the marine-derived fungus *Aspergillus carbonarius*. Chem Biodivers 5(1):93–100. doi:10.1002/cbdv.200890017.

26. Collins CH, Lyne PM (1985) Microbiological methods. Butterworth and Co. Publishers Ltd., London, 5 pp 167–181

27. Takahashi A, Kurasawa S, Ikeda D, Okami Y, Takeuchi T (1989) Altemicidin, a new acaricidal and antitumor substance. I. Taxonomy, fermentation, isolation and physico-chemical and biological properties. J Antibiot 42(11):1556–1561. doi:10.7164/antibiotics.42.1556.

28. Sajid I, Fondja Yao CB, Shaaban KA, Hasnain S, Laatsch H (2009) Antifungal and antibacterial activities of indigenous *Streptomyces* isolates from saline farmlands: prescreening, ribotyping and metabolic diversity. World J Microbiol Biotechnol 25(4):601–610. doi:10.1007/s11274-008-9928-7.

3

Size-controlled green synthesis of silver nanoparticles mediated by gum ghatti (*Anogeissus latifolia*) and its biological activity

Aruna Jyothi Kora[1], Sashidhar Rao Beedu[2*] and Arunachalam Jayaraman[1]

Abstract

Background: Gum ghatti is a proteinaceous edible, exudate tree gum of India and is also used in traditional medicine. A facile and ecofriendly green method has been developed for the synthesis of silver nanoparticles from silver nitrate using gum ghatti (*Anogeissus latifolia*) as a reducing and stabilizing agent. The influence of concentration of gum and reaction time on the synthesis of nanoparticles was studied. UV–visible spectroscopy, transmission electron microscopy and X-ray diffraction analytical techniques were used to characterize the synthesized nanoparticles.

Results: By optimizing the reaction conditions, we could achieve nearly monodispersed and size controlled spherical nanoparticles of around 5.7 ± 0.2 nm. A possible mechanism involved in the reduction and stabilization of nanoparticles has been investigated using Fourier transform infrared spectroscopy and Raman spectroscopy.

Conclusions: The synthesized silver nanoparticles had significant antibacterial action on both the Gram classes of bacteria. As the silver nanoparticles are encapsulated with functional group rich gum, they can be easily integrated for various biological applications.

Keywords: Antibacterial, Autoclaving, Gum ghatti, Silver nanoparticles, Surface-Enhanced Raman Scattering (SERS)

Background

A survey of earlier literature suggests that various natural polymers such as starch [1], chitosan [2], and tannic acid [3] have been reported as reducing agents for the synthesis of silver and gold nanoparticles. It has been demonstrated that the plant-based exudate gums such as gum *Acacia* [4] and gum kondagogu [5] can be utilized as reducing and stabilizing agents for the silver nanoparticle biosynthesis. Gum gellan, a microbial heteropolysaccharide, was employed for similar purpose in the case of gold nanoparticles [6]. Gum ghatti is a naturally occurring water soluble, complex polysaccharide derived as an exudate from the bark of *Anogeissus latifolia* (Combretaceae family), a native tree of the Indian sub-continent. The name gum ghatti has originated from its transportation through mountain passes or ghats. This native Indian gum is collected from the forests by the tribals and

marketed through government organizations such as Girijan Co-operative Corporation Ltd., Visakhapatnam, India. The world production of gum ghatti is about 1,000–1,500 MT/year [7,8]. This biopolymer is an arabinogalactan type of natural gum and its morphological, structural, physico-chemical, compositional, solution, thermal, rheological, and emulsifying properties have been well documented and studied [9-17]. This biopolymer is a high-arabinose, protein rich, acidic heteropolysaccharide, occurring in nature as mixed calcium, magnesium, potassium, and sodium salt [12-14,16]. The primary structure of this gum is composed of sugars such as, L-arabinose, D-galactose, D-mannose, D-xylose, and D-glucuronic acid in a molar ratio of 48:29:10:5:10 and < 1% of rhamnose, which is present as non-reducing end-groups. The gum contains alternating 4-*O*-substituted and 2-*O*-substituted α-D-mannopyranose units and chains of $1 \rightarrow 6$ linked β-D-galactopyranose units with side chains of L-arabinofuranose residues. Six percent of rhamnose in the polysaccharide is linked to the galactose backbone as α-Rhap-$(1 \rightarrow 4)$ β-galactopyranose

* Correspondence: sashi_rao@yahoo.com
[2]Department of Biochemistry, University College of Science, Osmania University, Hyderabad 500 007, AP, India
Full list of author information is available at the end of the article

side chain. It has a molecular weight of 8.94×10^7 g/mol [12,13,15,16].

The gum ghatti with a CAS number 9000-28-6 is recognized as "generally recognized as safe" (GRAS) and approved as a food ingredient (Code 184.1333) by the Food and Drug Administration, USA, under the function of emulsifier and emulsifier salt. Its use in food is also approved in Japan, China, South Korea, Singapore, Russia, Australia, South Africa, Iran, Saudi Arabia, Latin America, and other countries. But, it is not approved as a food additive in European Union and not been accorded a European food safety E number. It is considered as a food grade additives of food by the Bureau of Indian Standards, India under Indian Standard IS 7239:1974 [13,15,16]. In India, the application of this hydrocolloid in traditional medicine and food preparations is well known for centuries. The gum is fed to the lactating mothers in the form of *laddu* to enhance the nutrients in milk as well as to prevent the post-delivery backache [18]. The gum *laddu* is also eaten as a heating agent during winter season [18,19]. The gum ghatti is comprised of around 80% soluble dietary fiber and acts a prebiotic by supplying the matrix required to sustain the bacterial flora of the human colon. This hydrocolloid is resistant to gastrointestinal enzymes and known to be degraded enzymatically only by the specific microflora of the colon such as *Bifidobacterium longum*, thereby aiding in bifidus fermentation [20-22]. This gum is also given for the treatment of diarrhea and diabetes [23]. Earlier studies on gum ghatti fed white leghorn cockerels and albino rats have established the hypolipidemic activity of gum ghatti [24,25]. Recent studies have established that gum ghatti has a potential application as a release modifier for controlled drug delivery [26]. Gum ghatti has long been used in non-food applications, such as, calico printing, explosives, varnishes, car polishes, ceramics, cosmetics; and in pharmaceutical, textile, paper, petroleum, and mining industries. Also, this biopolymer aids in various photoelectric determinations [7,8,13,16,23].

The attractive features of gum ghatti prompted us to use this biopolymer for the synthesis and stabilization of silver nanoparticles due to its (i) edible nature and GRAS [13]; (ii) natural availability and low cost [23]; (iii) intermediate viscosity between gum arabic and gum karaya [14,15]; (iv) greater stability to pH acidification, electrolyte addition, and high-pressure treatment [15,17]; (v) higher emulsification ability and superior emulsion storage stability at lower concentrations [15], and (vi) exceptional interfacial characteristics with faster kinetics [17]. The green synthesis of inherently safer silver nanoparticles depends on the adoption of the basic requirements of green chemistry; the solvent medium, the benign reducing agent, and the non-hazardous stabilizing agent [1,27]. In this context, we have explored and developed a facile and green synthetic route for the production of silver nanoparticles using a proteinaceous, edible, renewable natural plant polymer, gum ghatti as both the reducing and stabilizing agents. Being a natural polymer, gum ghatti is amenable for biodegradation. The synthesis was carried out in aqueous medium by autoclaving, without the addition of any external chemical reducing agent. In this study, autoclaving was adopted as a synthetic route to produce sterile silver nanoparticles that are completely free from bacteria, viruses, and spores, which would suit biological applications. The focus of this study was on (i) the synthesis, (ii) characterization, and (iii) capping and stabilization of silver nanoparticles. In addition, we have also demonstrated the antibacterial activity of the prepared nanoparticles on Gram-positive and Gram-negative bacteria for finding out the potential of the generated nanoparticles for various environmental and biomedical applications.

Methods
Characterization of synthesized silver nanoparticles
In order to study the formation of silver nanoparticles, the UV–Visible absorption spectra of the prepared colloidal solutions were recorded using an Elico SL 196 spectrophotometer (Hyderabad, India), from 250 to 800 nm, against autoclaved gum blank. The absorption spectra of gum before and after autoclaving were also recorded against ultra pure water blank. The size and shape of the nanoparticles were obtained with Hitachi H 7500 (Tokyo, Japan) and JEOL 3010 (Tokyo, Japan) transmission electron microscopes (TEM), operating at 80 and 200 kV, respectively. Samples were prepared by depositing a drop of colloidal solution on a carbon-coated copper grid and drying at room temperature. The X-ray diffraction (XRD) analysis was conducted with a Rigaku, Ultima IV diffractometer (Tokyo, Japan) using monochromatic Cu Kα radiation ($\lambda = 1.5406$ Å) running at 40 kV and 30 mA. The intensity data for the nanoparticle solution deposited on a glass slide were collected over a 2θ range of 35–85° with a scan rate of 1°/min. The nanoparticles were recovered from the synthesized solutions by centrifugation and made into powders using a FTS Systems, Dura-Dry^{TM} MP freeze dryer (New York, USA). The IR spectra of the lyophilized samples were recorded using a Bruker Optics, TENSOR 27 FT-IR spectrometer (Ettlingen, Germany); over a spectral range of 400–4000 cm^{-1}. The Raman spectrum of the synthesized nanoparticles was recorded at room temperature using the 532-nm line from a SUWTECH, G-SLM diode laser (Shanghai, China). The scattered light was collected and detected using a CCD-based monochromator, covering a spectral range of 150–1700 cm^{-1}. The sample solution was taken in a standard 1 cm × 1 cm cuvette and placed in the path of the laser beam.

Results and discussion
Synthesis of silver nanoparticles
The present experimental investigation reports the green synthesis of silver nanoparticles using gum ghatti by autoclaving. This method utilizes a proteinaceous, edible, renewable, and water soluble biopolymer; gum ghatti which functions as both reducing and stabilizing agents during synthesis. By virtue of being a natural polymer, this gum is also amenable for biodegradation. The process of autoclaving makes the silver nanoparticles intrinsically safe and sterile, in environmentally benign solvent water. Moreover, generation of gum–silver nanoparticles by autoclaving is a prerequisite for biological applications. Thus, the adopted method is meeting the requirements of green chemistry principles.

Proposed mechanism of reduction
During autoclaving at 121°C under the influence of temperature and pressure (103 kPa), this biopolymer expands and becomes more accessible for the silver ions to interact with the available functional groups on the gum as observed earlier for starch [1]. The gum has been categorized under arabinogalactan due to the abundance of arabinose and galactose. This acidic heteropolysaccharide is known to be rich in uronic acid content and shows a pH of 4.5–5.5 [8,14-17]. The presence of hydroxyl and carboxylic groups on this biopolymer [28] facilitates the complexation of silver ions. Subsequently, these silver ions oxidize the hydroxyl groups to carbonyl groups, during which the silver ions are reduced to elemental silver. In addition to this inherent oxidation, the dissolved air may also causes oxidation of the existing hydroxyl groups to carbonyl groups such as aldehydes and carboxylates. In turn, these powerful reducing aldehyde groups along with the other existing carbonyl groups reduce more and more of silver ions to elemental silver. Further, these nanoparticles are probably capped and stabilized by the polysaccharides along with the proteins present in the gum. As these carbohydrate polymers are very complex, it is most likely that more than one mechanism is involved in the complexation and subsequent reduction of silver ions by gum ghatti during autoclaving. Silver ion complexation by hydroxyl groups and its subsequent reduction by aldehyde groups are reported for starch, in which silver nanoparticles were produced by autoclaving [1]. Silver nanoparticles produced using gum *Acacia*, carboxylate groups involving complexation of silver ions and its subsequent reduction by hydroxyl groups were reported [4].

The reduction of silver ions by this gum even at room temperature was observed. But, the formed nanoparticles were not stable and aggregated due to lack of stabilization of the synthesized nanoparticles. It was noticed that the autoclaving at 121°C and 103 kPa of

pressure, increased the extent of synthesis and stabilization of the nanoparticles. It is known that elevated temperature and pressure accelerate the synthesis of nanoparticles [1]. Besides, this process complexly eliminates the microbial contamination possibly acquired during gum secretion, collection, handling, and transportation.

Characterization of synthesized silver nanoparticles
UV–Visible spectroscopy
The UV–Vis absorption spectroscopy is one of the most widely used simple and sensitive techniques for the observation of nanoparticle synthesis. In order to monitor the formation of silver nanoparticles, the absorption spectra of synthesized silver nanoparticles were recorded against respective autoclaved gum blanks. Figure 1 is indicating (a) gum tears of grade 1 quality, (b) gum powder sieved to 38 μm particle size, and (c) centrifuged gum solution of 0.5%. To optimize the nanoparticle synthesis, the influence of parameters such as concentration of gum and reaction time was studied. The role of gum concentration on the synthesis was studied by autoclaving these gum solutions (0.1–0.5%) containing 1 mM of silver nitrate for 30 min. Figure 2a shows the UV–Vis spectra of the produced silver nanoparticles with different concentrations of gum (0.1–0.5%) at 1 mM $AgNO_3$ and 30 min of autoclaving. After autoclaving the silver nitrate containing gum solutions, the appearance of yellow color in the reaction mixtures was observed. This is a clear indication for the formation of silver nanoparticles by the gum. It reveals that the efficiency of nanoparticle synthesis increases with increasing concentration of gum. The synthesis was also evaluated by varying the reaction time (10–60 min) and reduction was studied with 0.5% gum at 1 mM $AgNO_3$ (Figure 2b). It was noticed that the reduction capacity of the gum increased with reaction time. As the autoclaving time increases, possibly more and more of hydroxyl groups are being converted to carbonyl groups by air oxidation, which in turn reduce the silver ions. In the UV-Vis spectra a single strong peak with a maximum around 412 nm was observed, which corresponds to the typical surface plasmon resonance (SPR) of conducting electrons from the surface of silver nanoparticles. The SPR absorption of metal nanoparticles like gold and silver is very sensitive to the changes of the size and shape of the nanoparticles formed [29].

Transmission electron microscopy
Figure 3 shows the TEM images of the silver nanoparticles synthesized with 0.5% gum and 1 mM $AgNO_3$ autoclaved for 30 min. These nanoparticles are spherical, polydisperse, aggregated, and the average particle size obtained from these micrographs was about 31.6±21.7 nm (Figure 3c). The

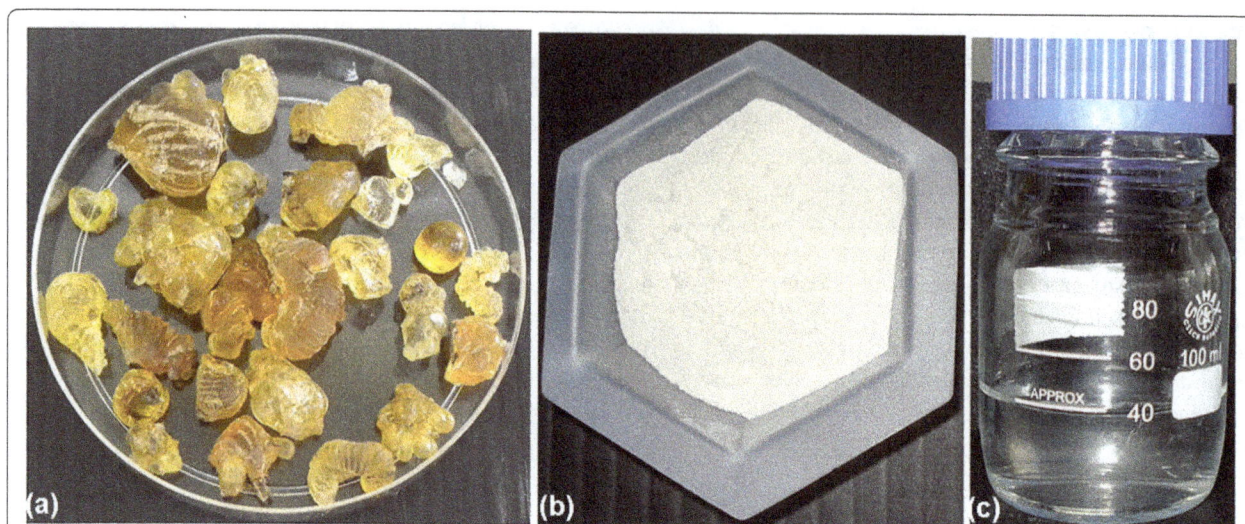

Figure 1 A digital photograph showing (a) Gum tears of grade 1 quality, (b) gum powder sieved to 38 μm particle size, and (c) centrifuged gum solution of 0.5% (w/v).

influence of gum concentration on the morphology of the nanoparticles was investigated with 0.1% gum and 1 mM $AgNO_3$, autoclaved for 30 min (Figure 4). These nanoparticles were spherical in shape and nearly isotropic in nature. The average particle size obtained from the corresponding diameter distribution was about 5.7 ± 0.2 nm (Figure 4e). The effect of autoclaving time on the shape and size of the nanoparticles was confirmed with 0.1% gum solution, autoclaved for 60 min at 1 mM $AgNO_3$ (Figure 5). The TEM observations of this sample indicate the shape anisotropy and the nanoparticles display a rich variety of shapes in

varying sizes. In addition to nanospheres, hexagonal, and polygonal nanoprisms, ellipsoidal and uneven shaped nanoparticles were observed. These nanoparticles are polydisperse, aggregated, and the average particle size obtained from these micrographs was about 27.2 ± 11.5 nm, for 60 min of reaction time (Figure 5e). The selected-area electron diffraction (SAED) patterns depicted in Figures 4d and 5d exhibit concentric rings with intermittent bright dots, indicating that these nanoparticles are highly crystalline in nature. These rings can be attributed to the diffraction from the (111), (200), (220), and (311) planes of face-centered

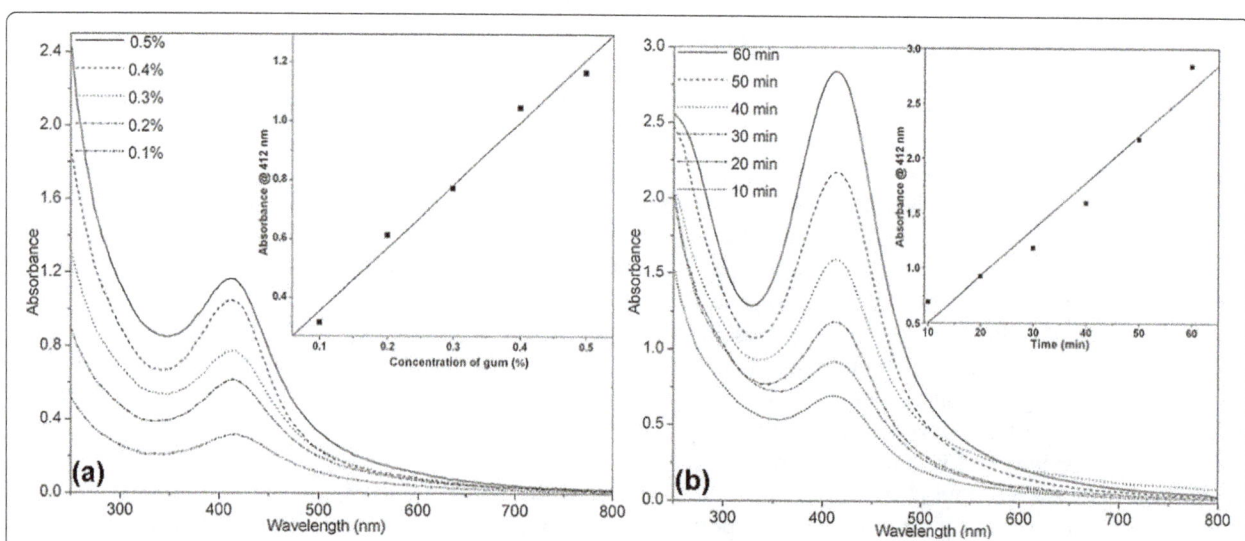

Figure 2 The UV–Vis absorption spectra of silver nanoparticles synthesized: (a) by autoclaving different concentrations of gum ghatti solutions at 1 mM $AgNO_3$ concentration for 30 min; inset plot of A_{max} versus gum concentration and (b) with 0.5% (w/v) gum ghatti solutions at 1 mM $AgNO_3$ concentration for different durations of autoclaving; inset plot of A_{max} versus autoclaving time.

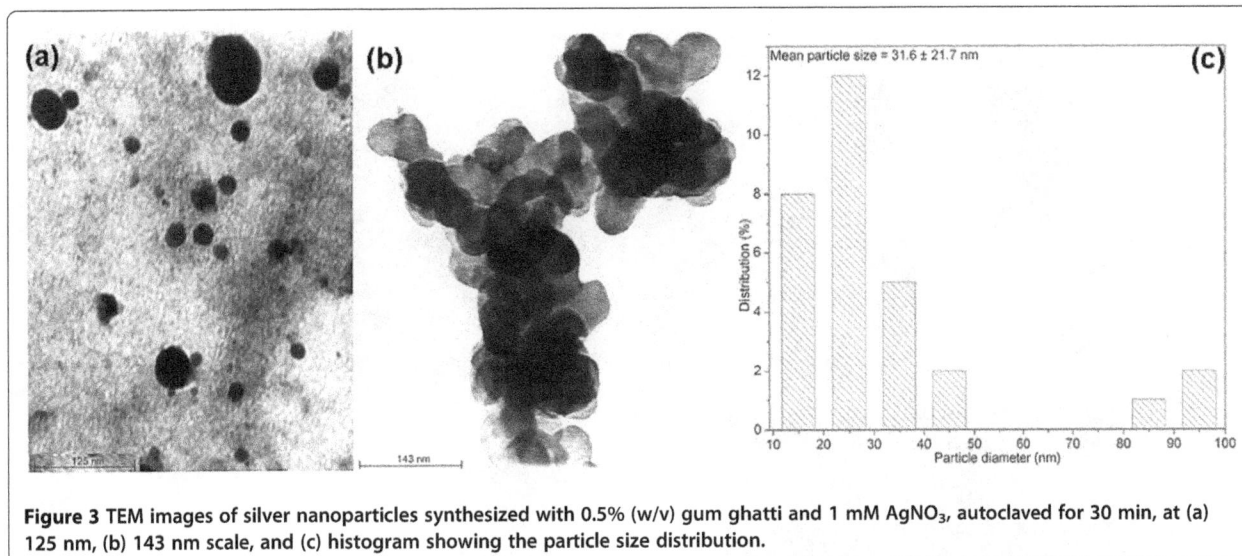

Figure 3 TEM images of silver nanoparticles synthesized with 0.5% (w/v) gum ghatti and 1 mM AgNO₃, autoclaved for 30 min, at (a) 125 nm, (b) 143 nm scale, and (c) histogram showing the particle size distribution.

cubic (fcc) silver. The crystallinity of the synthesized nanoparticles was also supported from the observed clear lattice fringes in high-resolution images (Figures 4c and 5c). Interestingly at 0.1% gum and 1 mM of AgNO₃ concentration with 30 min of autoclaving, nearly 70% of the nanoparticles formed were in the size of 5.7 nm (Figure 4e). When the concentration of gum was decreased from 0.5 to 0.1%, the average particle size of the silver nanoparticles formed

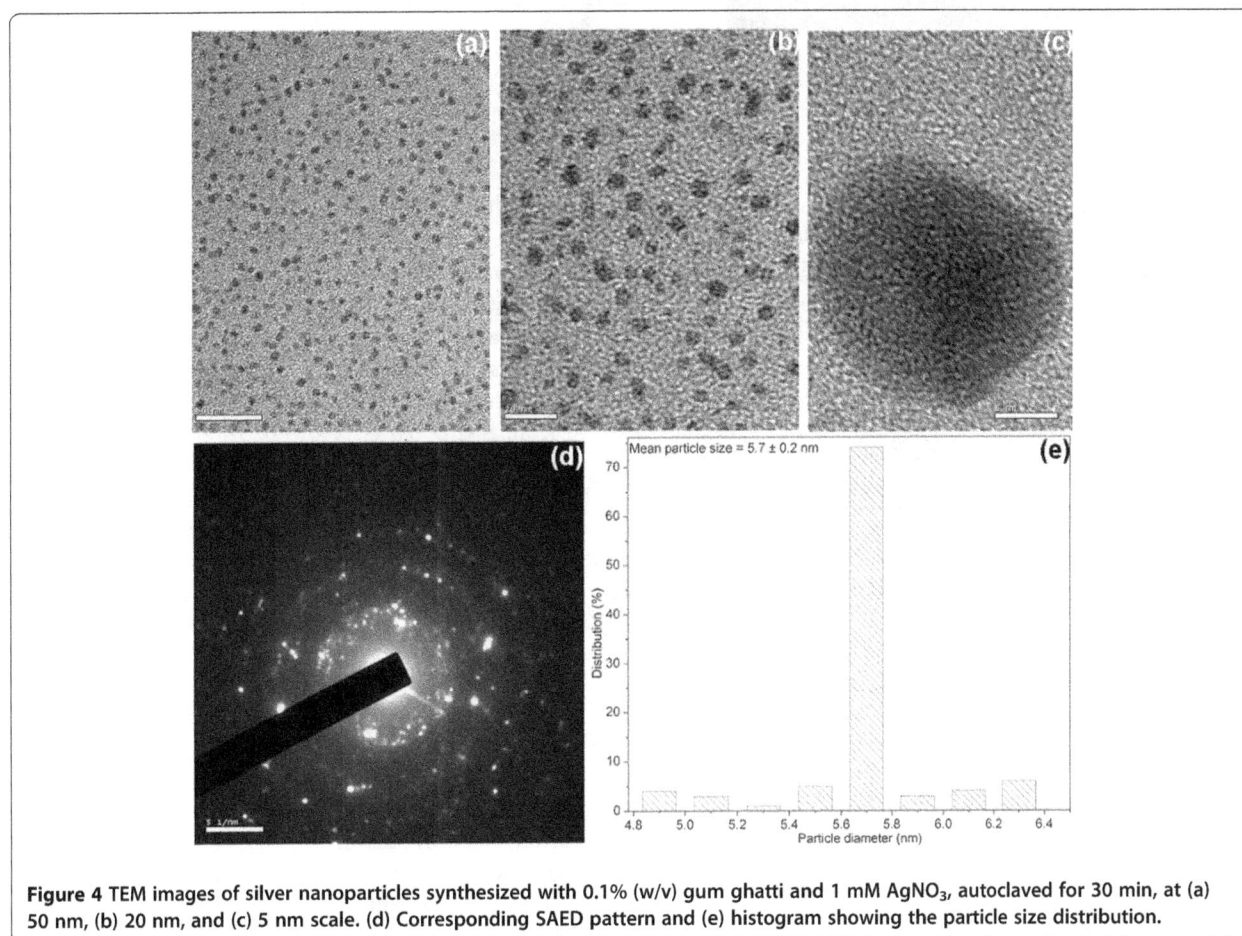

Figure 4 TEM images of silver nanoparticles synthesized with 0.1% (w/v) gum ghatti and 1 mM AgNO₃, autoclaved for 30 min, at (a) 50 nm, (b) 20 nm, and (c) 5 nm scale. (d) Corresponding SAED pattern and (e) histogram showing the particle size distribution.

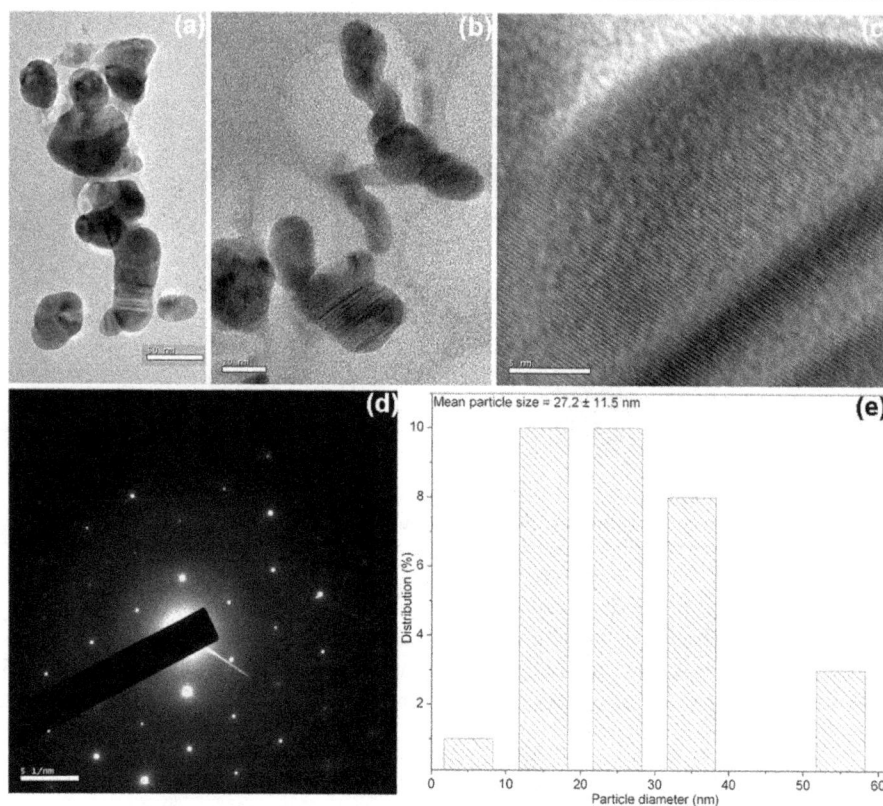

Figure 5 TEM images of silver nanoparticles synthesized with 0.1% (w/v) gum ghatti and 1 mM AgNO₃, autoclaved for 60 min, at (a) 50 nm, (b) 20 nm, and (c) 5 nm scale. (d) Corresponding SAED pattern and (e) histogram showing the particle size distribution.

decreased. This was also confirmed in a previous study on size controllable synthesis of silver nanoparticles with tannic acid, in which the concentration of the polyphenol decreased from 23.5 to 1.8 μM [3]. The decrease in polydispersity with decrease in the concentration of gum was also evident from the TEM images (Figures 3 and 4). It is worth noting that the shape of the particles changed from spheres to anisotropic nanostructures, when the reaction time was increased to 60 min at 0.1% of gum concentration (Figures 4 and 5). This is most likely due to the continual growth of nanoparticles during longer period of autoclaving. This study indicates that the particle size of the silver nanoparticles can be controlled by varying the concentration of gum and reaction time. As a result, nanoparticles with near monodispersity were obtained with 0.1% gum and 30 min of reaction time at 1 mM of silver nitrate concentration.

X-ray diffraction

The XRD technique was used to determine and confirm the crystal structure of silver nanoparticles. The XRD pattern of the silver nanoparticles is shown in Figure 6. There were five well-defined characteristic diffraction peaks at 38.3°, 44.6°, 64.8°, 77.6°, and 81.9°, respectively,

corresponding to (111), (200), (220), (311), and (222) planes of fcc crystal structure of metallic silver. The interplanar spacing (d_{hkl}) values (2.348, 2.030, 1.437, 1.229, and 1.175 Å) calculated from the XRD spectrum of silver nanoparticles was in agreement with the standard silver values. Thus, the XRD pattern further corroborates the highly crystalline nature of nanoparticles observed from SAED patterns and high-resolution TEM images (Figures 4 and 5). The lattice constant calculated from this pattern was 4.061 Å, a value which is in agreement with the value reported in literature for silver (JCPDS PDF card 04–0783). Also, the broadening of the diffraction peaks was observed owing to the effect of nano-sized particles. As the nanoparticles are capped by the moieties of gum, the background observed was high.

Fourier transform infrared spectroscopy (FTIR)

The FTIR spectra of the gum and nanoparticles were recorded in order to identify the functional groups of gum involved in the reduction and capping/stabilization of the synthesized nanoparticles. Figure 7 shows the FTIR spectra of the lyophilized gum and silver nanoparticles. The major absorbance bands present in the

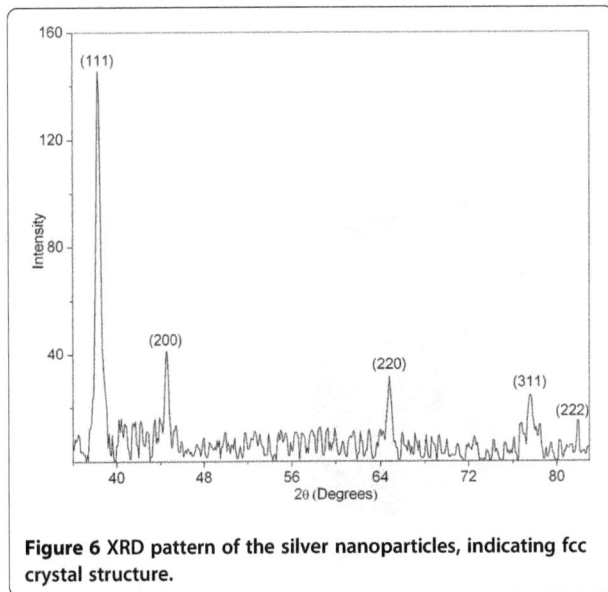

Figure 6 XRD pattern of the silver nanoparticles, indicating fcc crystal structure.

spectrum of gum ghatti were at 3425, 2928, 2368, 2341, 2122, 1635, 1406, 1311, 1234, 1068, and 1028 cm^{-1}. The broad band observed at 3425 cm^{-1} could be assigned to stretching vibrations of O–H groups in gum ghatti. The bands at 2928, 1406, and 1234 cm^{-1} correspond to asymmetric stretching, scissoring; and twisting and rocking vibrations of methylene groups, respectively. The broad band at 2122 cm^{-1} only appeared in the spectrum of gum could be assigned to various carbonyl species. The stronger band found at 1635 cm^{-1} could be assigned to characteristic asymmetrical stretch of carboxylate group. The symmetrical stretch of carboxylate group can be attributed to the band present at 1311 cm^{-1}. The peaks at 1068 and 1028 cm^{-1} were due to the C–O stretching

vibration of ether and alcoholic groups, respectively [28]. While, the spectrum of lyophilized nanoparticles showed characteristic absorbance bands at 3431, 2964, 2345, 2304, 1728, 1632, 1385, 1260, and 1024 cm^{-1}. In the IR spectrum of nanoparticles, a shift in the absorbance peaks was observed from 3425 to 3431 cm^{-1} and 1635 to 1632 cm^{-1}, and 1311 to 1385 cm^{-1}, suggesting the binding of silver ions with hydroxyl and carboxylate groups, respectively. It is pertinent to note that nanoparticles shows a new band at 1728 cm^{-1} corresponding to carbonyl stretching vibrations in aldehydes, ketones, and carboxylic acids [2]. Further, the occurrence of the peak at 1728 cm^{-1} and disappearance of the peak at 2122 cm^{-1} confirm that the reduction of the silver ions is coupled to the oxidation of the hydroxyl and carbonyl groups, indicative of more extensively oxidized nature of the gum. Based on the band shift in the hydroxyl and carbonyl groups and the loss of existing carbonyls and appearance of a new carbonyl peak, it can be inferred that both hydroxyl and carbonyl groups of gum are involved in the synthesis of silver nanoparticles. The variations in the shape and peak position of the hydroxyl and carboxylate groups have been reported, where silver nanoparticles were synthesized using another polysaccharide, gum *Acacia* [4].

Raman spectroscopy

In order to find out the possible functional groups of capping agents associated in the stabilization of silver nanoparticles, Raman spectrum of the nanoparticles was recorded. Figure 8 gives the selective enhancement of Raman bands of the organic capping agents bound to the nanoparticles. The spectrum shows a strong and sharp band at 240 cm^{-1}, which can be attributed to the stretching vibrations of Ag–N [30,31] and Ag–O bonds [32]. This

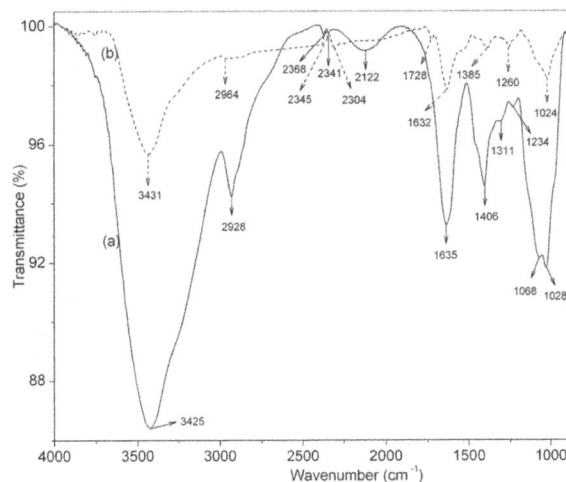

Figure 7 FTIR spectra of freeze dried (a) gum ghatti and (b) silver nanoparticles.

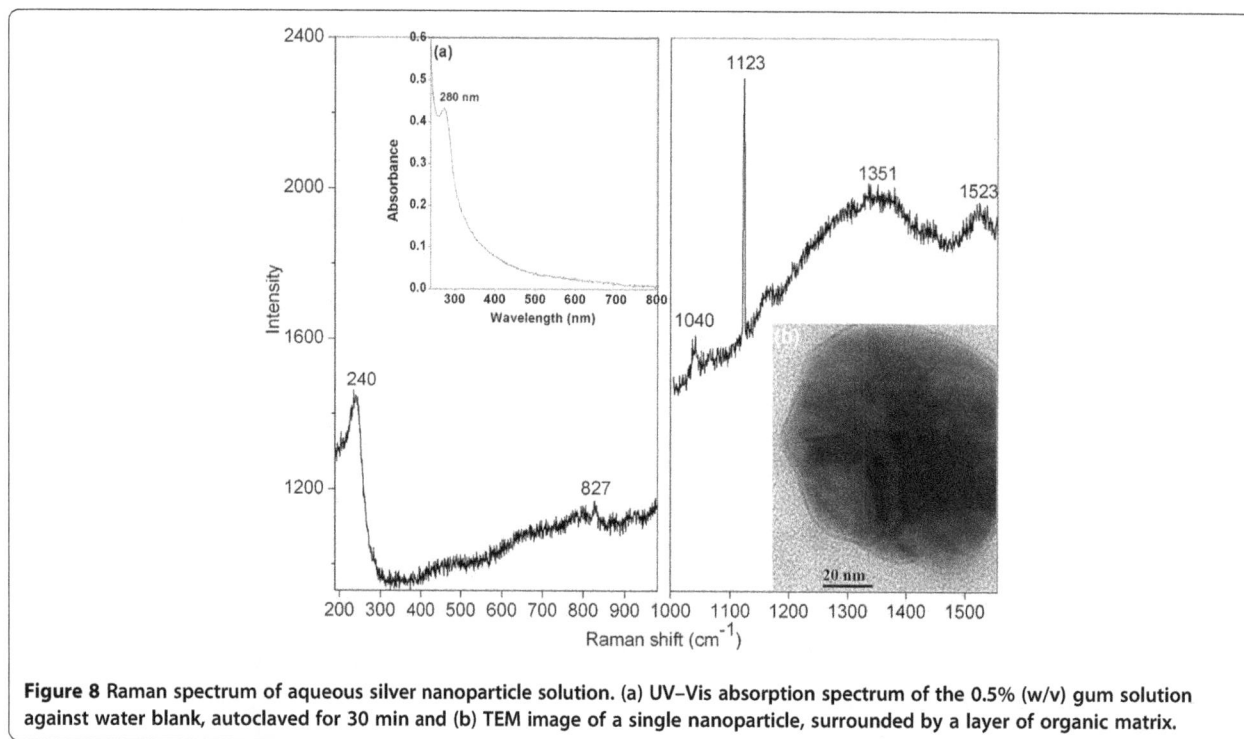

Figure 8 Raman spectrum of aqueous silver nanoparticle solution. (a) UV–Vis absorption spectrum of the 0.5% (w/v) gum solution against water blank, autoclaved for 30 min and (b) TEM image of a single nanoparticle, surrounded by a layer of organic matrix.

peak indicates the formation of a chemical bond between silver and amino nitrogen [31]; and silver and carboxylate groups [32] of gum molecules. It confirms that the gum is bound to the silver nanoparticle surface either through amino or carboxylate group or both. It is known to have close frequencies for the Ag–N and Ag–O stretching vibrations and the involvement of both N and O atoms in binding result in surface-enhanced Raman scattering (SERS) band broadening [30]. The broad ones at 1351 and 1523 cm^{-1} correspond to symmetric and asymmetric $C = O$ stretching vibrations of carboxylate group, respectively [31]. The enhancement in the intensity of the CO_2 stretching vibration suggests the direct binding of the COO^- group with the silver surface [32]. The broad band at 1040 and a sharp peak at 1123 cm^{-1}; the one at 827 cm^{-1} comes from the C–H in plane bending and out of plane wag, respectively [30], from the saccharide structure of gum. Thus, from the preferential enhancement of these bands; it can be concluded that both amino and carboxylate groups of the gum are involved in the capping of the silver nanoparticles. These results are in concurrence with earlier biosynthesis of silver nanoparticles carried out with non-pathogenic fungus *Trichoderma asperellum* [31]. It was reported earlier that the carboxylate groups of glycoprotein of gum *Acacia* were involved in binding of silver nanoparticles [4]. It is known that proteins can bind to nanoparticles either through free amino groups or by electrostatic interaction of negatively charged carboxylate groups [33]. The gum ghatti is known to contain protein and the protein content was reported to be in

the range of 2.8–3.7% [13-17]. This observation is further substantiated by the measured protein concentration of 2.7% for the gum and the UV–Vis absorption spectrum of the 0.5% gum solution against water blank, autoclaved for 30 min, given in Figure 8a. An absorption peak at 280 nm is clearly visible and is attributed to electronic excitations in tryptophan and tyrosine residues in the proteins [1,33], which are present in the gum. The stabilization of nanoparticles by capping agents is also validated from the TEM image showing a single nanoparticle that is surrounded by a layer of organic matrix (Figure 8b). Thus, one can conclude that once the silver ions are reduced to silver nanoparticles by the polyhydroxylated gum, proteins present in the gum subsequently encapsulate and stabilize these particles along with saccharide molecules. Based on these observations, these silver nanoparticles can be used as a possible substrate for SERS. As observed in IR spectra (Figure 7), gum ghatti is rich in various functional groups; and their capping on silver nanoparticles provides surface reactivity. It is reported that the functional unit used as a capping agent plays an important role and determines the tissue distribution profile of gold nanoparticles [34]. Thus, these functionalized nanoparticles are useful for various applications such as drug delivery [6], targeted biological interactions [34], and biological labels [35].

Antibacterial assay

For checking the antibacterial activity, silver nanoparticles with an average size of 5.7 ± 0.2 nm were used. These nanoparticles were prepared with 0.1% gum solution containing

1 mM AgNO₃, autoclaved for 30 min. After 24 h of incubation at 37°C, growth suppression was observed in plates loaded with 5 μg of silver nanoparticles. Whereas, the negative control plates loaded with autoclaved gum did not produce any ZOI. Gum–silver nanoparticles showed growth inhibition around the wells against the tested bacteria. ZOI of around 12.25 mm diameter was observed for the Gram-positive bacterial strain *S. aureus* ATCC 25923. In the case of Gram-negative bacterial strains *E. coli* ATCC 25922, *E. coli* ATCC 35218, and *P. aeruginosa* ATCC 27853, the detected ZOI were 9.0, 8.0, and 11.0 mm, respectively. As expected, the positive control plates loaded with silver nitrate exhibited inhibition zones (Table 1). The ZOI values noted for different bacterial strains with silver nanoparticles are comparable with the positive controls. Based on these results, it can be concluded that the synthesized silver nanoparticles had significant antibacterial action on both the Gram classes of bacteria.

Experimental

Synthesis of silver nanoparticles

Silver nitrate (AgNO₃) (E. Merck, Mumbai, India) of analytical reagent grade was used for the synthesis. "Gum ghatti" grade-1 was purchased from Girijan Cooperative Corporation Ltd., Hyderabad, India. All the solutions were prepared in ultra pure water. Gum ghatti was powdered in a Prestige high-speed mechanical blender (Bengaluru, India) and sieved to obtain a mean particle size of 38 μm. Then, 0.5% (w/v) of homogenous gum stock solution was prepared by adding this powder to reagent bottle containing ultra pure water and stirring overnight at room temperature. Then this solution was centrifuged to remove the insoluble materials and the supernatant was used for all the experiments. The protein concentration in the gum solution was quantified by Lowry's method using a Bangalore Genei™ protein estimation kit, Cat No 105560 (Bengaluru, India). The silver nanoparticles were synthesized by autoclaving the silver nitrate solutions containing various concentrations of gum ghatti at 121°C and 103 kPa of pressure for different durations of time, under dark conditions. The effect of concentration of gum and reaction time on nanoparticle synthesis was studied.

Antibacterial assay

The well-diffusion method was used to study the antibacterial activity of the synthesized silver nanoparticles.

All the glassware, media, and reagents used were sterilized in an autoclave at 121°C, 103 kPa of pressure for 20 min. *Staphylococcus aureus* (ATCC 25923); and *Escherichia coli* (ATCC 25922), *E. coli* (ATCC 35218), and *Pseudomonas aeruginosa* (ATCC 27853) were used as model test strains for Gram-positive and Gram-negative bacteria, respectively. Bacterial suspension was prepared by growing a single colony overnight in nutrient broth and by adjusting the turbidity to 0.5 McFarland standard [36]. Mueller Hinton agar plates were inoculated with this bacterial suspension and 5 μg of silver nanoparticles was added to the center well with a diameter of 6 mm. The nanoparticles used were prepared with 0.1% gum solution containing 1 mM AgNO₃, autoclaved for 30 min. Negative control plates were maintained with autoclaved gum-loaded wells. The culture plates loaded with silver nitrate at a silver concentration of 5 μg were included as positive controls. These plates were incubated at 37°C for 24 h in a bacteriological incubator and the zone of inhibition (ZOI) was measured by subtracting the well diameter from the total inhibition zone diameter. Three independent experiments were carried out with each bacterial strain.

Conclusions

This study reports the facile synthesis of silver nanoparticles from silver nitrate using gum ghatti. The adopted method is compatible with green chemistry principles as the gum serves as a dual functional reductant and stabilizer for the synthesis of nanoparticles. At a given gum concentration, the efficiency of nanoparticle synthesis increases with reaction time, a property attributable to the large reduction capacity of the gum. As the particle size of the nanoparticles can be controlled, this method can be implemented for the large-scale production of monodispersed and spherical nanoparticles of around 5.7 nm due to the availability of low-cost plant-derived biopolymer. The hydroxyl and carboxylate groups of the gum facilitate the complexation of silver ions during autoclaving. Subsequently, these silver ions are reduced to elemental silver possibly by *in situ* oxidation of hydroxyl groups; and by the intrinsic carbonyl groups in addition to those produced by the air oxidation. This proposed mechanism is also substantiated by the FTIR data. Further, the formed silver nanoparticles had significant antibacterial action on both the Gram classes of bacteria. The surface reactivity provided by

Table 1 Inhibition zones (mm) observed with different bacterial culture plates loaded with silver nanoparticles and silver nitrate at a silver concentration of 5 μg

Test compound	*S. aureus* 25923	*E. coli* 25922	*E. coli* 35218	*P. aeruginosa* 27853
Silver nanoparticles	12.25	9.0	8.0	11.0
Silver nitrate	13.5	11.0	7.6	12.0

capping enables these functionalized nanoparticles as promising candidates for various pharmaceutical, biomedical, and environmental applications. Notably, the selective enhancement of Raman bands of the organic capping agents bound to the silver colloids allows these nanoparticles as suitable substrates for SERS. In view of this, further studies are envisaged to explore the other potential applications of this gum-based nanoparticles.

Competing interests

The authors declare that they have no competing interests.

Acknowledgments

We thank Dr. S. V. Narasimhan, Associate Director and Dr. Tulsi Mukherjee, Director, Chemistry Group, BARC, for their constant support and encouragement for this study. The support rendered for high-resolution TEM measurements by the DST unit on Nanoscience, Sophisticated Analytical Instrument Facility (SAIF) at IIT-Madras, Chennai, is gratefully acknowledged.

Author details

[1]National Centre for Compositional Characterisation of Materials (NCCCM), Bhabha Atomic Research Centre, ECIL PO, Hyderabad 500 062AP, India. [2]Department of Biochemistry, University College of Science, Osmania University, Hyderabad 500 007, AP, India.

References

1. Vigneshwaran N, Nachane RP, Balasubramanya RH, Varadarajan PV (2006) A novel one-pot 'green' synthesis of stable silver nanoparticles using soluble starch. Carbohydr Res 341:2012–2018
2. Wei D, Qian W (2008) Facile synthesis of Ag and Au nanoparticles utilizing chitosan as a mediator agent. Colloids Surf B 62:136–142
3. Dadosh T (2009) Synthesis of uniform silver nanoparticles with a controllable size. Mater Lett 63:2236–2238
4. Mohan YM, Raju KM, Sambasivudu K, Singh S, Sreedhar B (2007) Preparation of acacia-stabilized silver nanoparticles: a green approach. J Appl Polym Sci 106:3375–3381
5. Kora AJ, Sashidhar RB, Arunachalam J (2010) Gum kondagogu (Cochlospermum gossypium): a template for the green synthesis and stabilization of silver nanoparticles with antibacterial application. Carbohydr Polym 82:670–679
6. Dhar S, Reddy EM, Shiras A, Pokharkar V, Prasad BLV (2008) Natural gum reduced/stabilized gold nanoparticles for drug delivery formulations. Chem Eur J 14:10244–10250
7. Panda H (2003) Gum ghatti. In: The complete technology book on natural products (Forest based). National Institute of Industrial Research, Delhi, pp 1–9
8. Nussinovitch A (2010) Miscellaneous uses of plant exudates. In: Plant gum exudates of the world: sources, distribution, properties and applications. CRC Press, Taylor and Francis, Boca Raton, USA, pp 347–368
9. Srivastava VK, Rai RS (1963) Physico-chemical studies on gum Dhawa (Anogeissus latifolia wall.). Colloid Polym Sci 190:140–143
10. Aspinall GO, Bhavanadan VP, Christensen TB (1965) Gum ghatti (Indian gum). Part V. Degradation of the periodate-oxidised gum. J Chem Soc 2677–2684
11. Jefferies M, Pass G, Phillips GO (1977) Viscosity of aqueous solutions of gum ghatti. J Sci Food Agric 28:173–179
12. Tischer CA, Iacomini M, Wagner R, Gorin PAJ (2002) New structural features of the polysaccharide from gum ghatti (Anogeissus latifola). Carbohydr Res 337:2205–2210
13. Amar V, Al-Assaf S, Phillips GO (2006) An introduction to gum ghatti: another proteinaceous gum. Foods Food Ingredients J Jpn 211:275–280
14. Katayama T, Ido T, Sasaki Y, Ogasawara T, Al-Assaf S, Phillips GO (2008) Characteristics of the adsorbed component of gum ghatti responsible for its oil–water interface advantages. Foods Food Ingredients J Jpn 213:372–376

15. Ido T, Ogasawara T, Katayama T, Sasaki Y, Al-Assaf S, Phillips GO (2008) Emulsification properties of GATIFOLIA (Gum ghatti) used for emulsions in food products. Foods Food Ingredients J Jpn 213:365–371
16. Kaur L, Singh J, Singh H (2009) Characterization of gum ghatti (Anogeissus latifolia): a structural and rheological approach. J Food Sci 74:E328–E332
17. Castellani O, Gaillard C, Vié V, Al-Assaf S, Axelos M, Phillips GO, Anton M (2010) Hydrocolloids with emulsifying capacity. Part 3: adsorption and structural properties at the air–water surface. Food Hydrocolloids 24:131–141
18. Shahane J (2006) Dinkache ladu-remembrance of things past. http://thecookscottagetypepad.com/curry/2006/03/dinkache_ladure.html. Accessed 17 March 2010
19. Meena KL, Yadav BL (2010) Some ethnomedicinal plants of southern Rajasthan. Indian J Tradit Knowl 9:169–172
20. Crociani F, Alessandrini A, Mucci MM, Biavati B (1994) Degradation of complex carbohydrates by Bifidobacterium spp. Int J Food Microbiol 24:199–210
21. Hill MJ (1995) Bacterial fermentation of complex carbohydrate in the human colon. Eur J Cancer Prevent 4:353–358
22. Ramberg J, Gardiner T (2002) Ghatti gum—Anogeissus latifolis stem gum (ghatti gum). GlycoEssential 7 Ingredients. http://www.glyconutrients-center.org/ghatti-gum.php. Accessed 17 March 2010
23. Mishra A, Raikwar A (2005) Anogeissus latifolia (ghatti gum): the edible gum. Vaniki Sandesh 29:27–28
24. Fahrenbach MJ, Riccardi BA, Grant WC (1966) Hypocholesterolemic activity of mucilaginous polysaccharides in white leghorn cockerels. Proc Soc Exp Biol Med 123:321–326
25. Parvathi KMM, Ramesh CK, Krishna V, Paramesha M, Kuppast IJ (2009) Hypolipidemic activity of gum ghatti of Anogeissus latifolia. Phcog Mag 5:11–14
26. Joshi MG, Setty CM, Deshmukh AS, Bhatt YA (2010) Gum ghatti: a new release modifier for zero-order release in 3-layered tablets of diltiazem hydrochloride. Indian J Pharm Educ Res 44:78–85
27. Raveendran P, Fu J, Wallen SL (2003) Completely "green" synthesis and stabilization of metal nanoparticles. J Am Chem Soc 125:13940–13941
28. Edwards HGM, Falk MJ, Sibley MG, Alvarez-Benedi J, Rull F (1998) FT-Raman spectroscopy of gums of technological significance. Spectrochim Acta A 54:903–920
29. Huanga NM, Lim HN, Radiman S, Khiew PS, Chiu WS, Hashim R, Chia CH (2010) Sucrose ester micellar-mediated synthesis of Ag nanoparticles and the antibacterial properties. Colloids Surf A 353:69–76
30. Chowdhury J, Ghosh M (2004) Concentration-dependent surface-enhanced Raman scattering of 2-benzoylpyridine adsorbed on colloidal silver particles. J Colloid Interface Sci 277:121–127
31. Mukherjee P, Roy M, Mandal BP, Dey GK, Mukherjee PK, Ghatak J, Tyagi AK, Kale SP (2008) Green synthesis of highly stabilized nanocrystalline silver particles by a non-pathogenic and agriculturally important fungus T. asperellum. Nanotechnology 19:075103–075109
32. Biswas N, Kapoor S, Mahal HS, Mukherjee T (2007) Adsorption of CGA on colloidal silver particles: DFT and SERS study. Chem Phys Lett 444:338–345
33. Vigneshwaran N, Ashtaputre NM, Varadarajan PV, Nachane RP, Paralikar KM, Balasubramanya RH (2007) Biological synthesis of silver nanoparticles using the fungus Aspergillus flavus. Mater Lett 61:1413–1418
34. Genevieve MF, Stan WC, Dae Young K, Raghuraman K, Kavita K, Nripen C, Kattesh K (2009) Biodistribution of maltose and gum arabic hybrid gold nanoparticles after intravenous injection in juvenile swine. Nanomed: Nanotech Biol Med 5:128–135
35. Schrand AM, Braydich-Stolle LK, Schlager JJ, Dai L, Hussain SM (2008) Can silver nanoparticles be useful as potential biological labels? Nanotechnology 19:235104–235116
36. Kora AJ, Manjusha R, Arunachalam J (2009) Superior bactericidal activity of SDS capped silver nanoparticles: Synthesis and characterization. Mater Sci Eng C 29:2104–2109

4

Development of 4H-pyridopyrimidines: a class of selective bacterial protein synthesis inhibitors

Joseph W Guiles[1,3], Andras Toro[1,4], Urs A Ochsner[1,5] and James M Bullard[1,2*]

Abstract

Background: We have identified a series of compounds that inhibit protein synthesis in bacteria. Initial IC_{50}'s in aminoacylation/translation (A/T) assays ranged from 3 to14 μM. This series of compounds are variations on a 5,6,7,8-tetrahydropyrido[4,3-d]pyrimidin-4-ol scaffold (e.g., 4H-pyridopyrimidine).

Methods: Greater than 80 analogs were prepared to investigate the structure-activity relationship (SAR). Structural modifications included changes in the central ring and substituent modifications in its periphery focusing on the 2- and 6-positions. An A/T system was used to determine IC_{50} values for activity of the analogs in biochemical assays. Minimum inhibitory concentrations (MIC) were determined for each analog against cultures of *Enterococcus faecalis*, *Moraxella catarrhalis*, *Haemophilus influenzae*, *Streptococcus pneumoniae*, *Staphylococcus aureus*, *Escherichia coli tolC* mutants and *E. coli* modified with PMBN.

Results: Modifications to the 2-(pyridin-2-yl) ring resulted in complete inactivation of the compounds. However, certain modifications at the 6-position resulted in increased antimicrobial potency. The optimized compounds inhibited the growth of *E. faecalis*, *M. catarrhalis*, *H. influenzae*, *S. pneumoniae*, *S. aureus*, *E. coli tolC*, mutants and *E. coli* modified with PMBN with MIC values of 4, ≤ 0.12, 1, 2, 4, 1, 1 μg/ml, respectively. IC_{50} values in biochemical assay were reduced to mid-nanomolar range.

Conclusion: 4H-pyridopyrimidine analogs demonstrate broad-spectrum inhibition of bacterial growth and modification of the compounds establishes SAR.

Keywords: antibiotic, drug discovery, structure-activity relationship (SAR), protein synthesis, inhibitor, *Staphylococcus aureus*, *Streptococcus pneumoniae*

1. Background

Bacterial infections continue to represent a major worldwide health hazard. Our health care systems are increasingly confronted with drug-resistant hospital and community-acquired infections [1]. With the recent emergence of numerous, clinically important, drug-resistant bacteria including *Staphylococcus aureus*, *Streptococcus pneumoniae*, *Enterococcus faecalis*, *Mycobacterium tuberculosis*, enhanced-spectrum β-lactamase producing *Escherichia coli* and *Klebsiella sp.* and *Pseudomonas aeruginosa*, an emergency is becoming apparent. Antibacterials kill bacteria by interfering with processes of cellular function that are essential for their survival. The majority of clinically important antibiotics target the ribosome and protein synthesis in general [2,3] and most of these are naturally occurring antibiotics or derivatives of naturally occurring antibiotics [4,5].

We have developed an aminoacylation/translation (A/T) system for screening for inhibitors of protein synthesis and in high throughput screens (HTS) of focused chemical compounds we identified a class of selective bacterial protein synthesis inhibitors, 5,6,7,8-tetrahydropyrido[4,3-d]pyrimidin-4-ol (e.g., 4H-pyridopyrimidine) [6]. Two compounds, 321525 and 321528 (Figure 1), were found to exhibit the greatest inhibitory activity in the initial HTS using the A/T assays and subsequently antibacterial activity was confirmed against *S. pneumoniae*, *S. aureus*, and *E. coli tolC* mutants. The compounds 321525 and 321528 were retested in the A/T assay and inhibited protein synthesis with IC_{50}'s of 2.8 and 1.2 μM, respectively. Minimum inhibitory concentrations (MIC) were determined

* Correspondence: bullardj@utpa.edu
[1]Replidyne, Inc., Louisville, CO, USA
Full list of author information is available at the end of the article

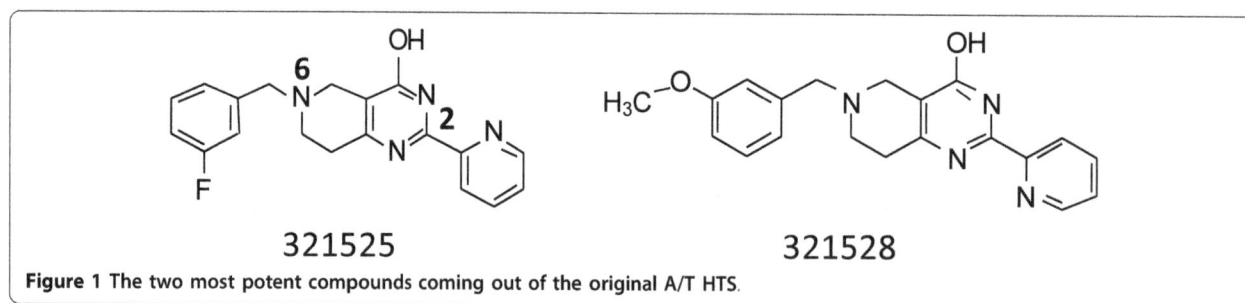

Figure 1 The two most potent compounds coming out of the original A/T HTS.

321525   321528

for a panel of bacteria including *E. faecalis, Moraxella. catarrhalis, Haemophilus influenzae, S. pneumoniae, S. aureus, E. coli tolC* mutants, and *E. coli* modified with PMBN. The MIC of 321525 and 321528 against these pathogens was 32, 0.25, 4, 8, 32, 8, 32, and 128, 2, 8, 32, > 128, 128, 32 μg/ml, respectively [6]. The inhibitory activity of these two compounds encouraged us to initiate structure-activity relationship (SAR) studies. Previously, minimum bactericidal concentration testing of the 4H-pyridopyrimidines initially indicated that the compounds were bactericidal against *H. influenzae*, but only bacteriostatic against *S. pneumoniae* [6,7]. Also, we previously conducted macromolecular synthesis (MMS) assays to test compounds to determine if RNA, DNA, or protein synthesis was inhibited in bacterial cultures. Assays were carried out in cultures containing the *E. coli tolC* mutant and also in cultures of *S. aureus*. The MMS data for two representative compounds, REP323219 and REP323370, indicate that the 4H-pyridopyrimidines are specific inhibitors of protein synthesis in the cell [6]. We report here the results of an in-depth SAR study of the inhibitory compound series.

2. Methods and materials
The original hit compounds were from a chemical compound library containing 2100 compounds from Asinex (Moscow, Russia). All analogs of the original hit compounds were prepared by Asinex. Biochemical analysis and determination of IC_{50} values of the original compounds and testing of the analogs were carried out using the A/T assay as described [6]. Broth microdilution MIC testing was performed in 96-well microtiter plates according to Clinical Laboratory Standards Institute (CLSI; formerly NCCLS) document M7-A6 [8]. MIC values were determined for *E. faecalis, M. catarrhalis, H. influenzae, S. pneumoniae, S. aureus, E. coli tolC* mutants, and *E. coli* modified with PMBN. MMS assays were performed in cultures of *E. coli tolC* mutants as described [6,9].

3. Results and discussion
We re-evaluated 321376, 321386, 321388, 321378, 321521, 321522, 321524, 321526, 321527, and 321529 from the initial library obtained from Asinex (Figure 2).

These compounds are similar to 321525 and 321528. The first four were identical to the original compounds with the exception that the nitrogen in the 2-pyridin-2-yl was walked around the pyridine ring to the 3-yl and 4-yl positions (Figure 2). Movement of the nitrogen resulted in complete loss of inhibitory activity, both biochemical and biological (Table 1). Similarly, in the final six compounds, the effect of the 3-fluoro- and 3-methoxy-benzyl substitution at the 6-position were tested by removing or walking around these functional groups on their parent 6-benzyl group. These initial compounds also contained 2- and 3-hydroxy substitutions at the 6-position. In the initial HTS, these compounds exhibited activity, but fell below the cutoff that defined a hit compound. When these compounds were re-assayed in triplicate they exhibited similar IC_{50} values as the original two compounds (Table 1). When tested against the panel of bacteria, these compounds also showed similar bacterial growth inhibition as 321525 and 321528, with the exception of 321526 which exhibited little or no anti-bacterial activity.

To determine how critical the structure of the 2-pyridin-2-yl ring was to the activity of the compound series, we introduced two moderate changes to 321521 (Figure 3). First, a methyl group was added next to the nitrogen in the pyridine ring (332052) and second, the pyridine ring was replaced with a pyrazine ring (323354) (Figure 3). The compound 323354 reduced potency tenfold and 332052 completely abolished activity in the A/T assay. Both compounds lost anti-bacterial activity against all bacteria in the panel, except against *M. catarrhalis* where the MIC values increased 120- and 60-fold, respectively. Next, the pyridine ring at the 2-position was replaced with a furan (332053), or a thiophene (332057), or a methyl thiazole (323356) (Figure 3). The furan and methyl thiazole replacements abolished all biochemical activity in the A/T assay, while biochemical activity of the thiophene replacement was reduced over 40-fold. Only the methyl thiazole replacement exhibited slight antibacterial activity. More analogs will be required to complete a comprehensive study of this part of the compound series, but from these preliminary results all changes were

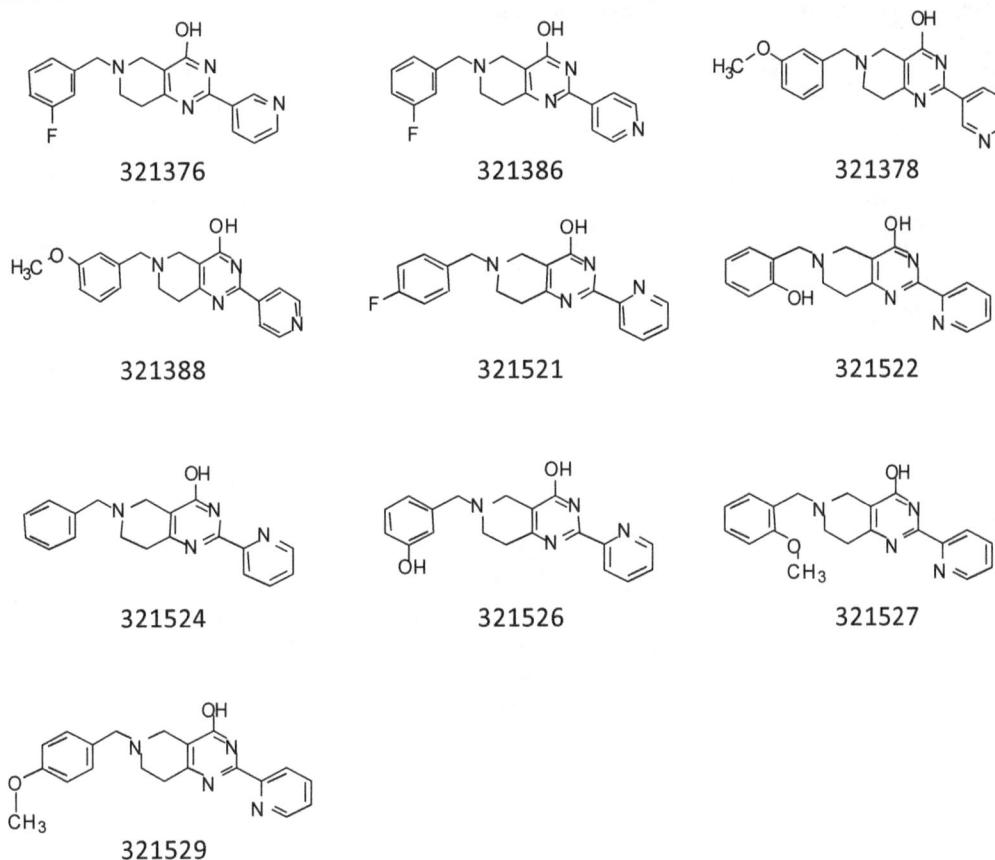

Figure 2 Additional compounds identified in the original compound library.

observed to be deleterious to the activity of the compound series.

Fifty-eight new compounds were prepared in which the phenyl ring at the 6-position of the core structure was modified (Figure 4). In the instances that the modification contained a hydroxyl or a carbonyl group (323196, 323197, 323200, 323204, 323206, 323210, 323211, 323213, 323214, 323215, 323217, 323222, 323224, 323225, 323231, 323232, 323236, 323238), the biochemical potency was maintained or increased; however, in each case the microbiological inhibition was lost (Table 1). For example, compound 323200 in which the benzene ring was modified to a 2-(2-methoxyphenoxy) acetamide, the IC_{50} was improved three to sevenfold yet the MIC was above maximum testing concentrations for the entire panel of bacteria. When the phenyl ring contained multiple methyl or methoxy substitutions (323191, 323202, 323209, 323221, 323223, 323226) an overall increase in the IC_{50} and MIC values (decrease in potency) was observed. In the case of 323221, the 3,4,5-trimethoxy substitution abolished both biochemical and microbiological activities.

Further five-member ring (323195, 323234, 323239) or six-member ring (323192, 323235) substitutions at the 6-position decreased the potency with the exception of compound 323195 in which the benzene ring was replaced with 1-phenylpyrrolidine. In this case, the activity was observed to be comparable to the original two compounds. Next, five member-ring structures were fused to the benzene ring to form five benzodioxoles (323199, 323205, 323207, 323227, 323233) and one benzimidazol (323213) (Figure 4). These compounds all tended to decrease potency of the compound series with the exception of 323227. When the benzene ring was replaced with 5-chloro-1,3-benzodioxole in 323227 a three to sevenfold improvement in the IC_{50} was observed.

A 4-dimethylamino substitution (323218) to the phenyl ring resulted in a five and tenfold improvement in the IC_{50} but an increase was observed in the MIC for all bacteria tested. When the 4-dimethylamino of 323218 was modified to a 4-dimethylaminomethyl group (323201) or to a 3-diethylaminomethyl group (323193), biochemical activity was maintained however all antibacterial activity was lost.

The most moderate modification to the benzene ring at the 6-position was the attachment of one or two halogens to the ring structure. These changes resulted in increased potency of the compound series in inhibition of bacterial growth. However, not all of this set of

Table 1 IC$_{50}$ and MIC values of compounds against pathogenic bacteria

Compound	IC$_{50}$ (µM)	E. fae* (µg/ml)	M. cat (µg/ml)	H. flu (µg/ml)	S. pneumo (µg/ml)	S. aureus (µg/ml)	E. coli tolC (µg/ml)	E. coli +PMBP (µg/ml)
321376	> 300	N/D	N/D	N/D	N/D	> 128	> 128	N/D
321578	> 300	> 128	> 128	> 128	> 128	> 128	> 128	> 128
321386	> 300	> 128	> 128	> 128	> 128	> 128	> 128	> 128
321388	> 300	> 128	> 128	> 128	> 128	> 128	> 128	> 128
321521	2.4	16	0.5	4	16	128	16	64
321522	2.6	16	1	2	16	128	32	64
321524	2.0	16	1	4	16	128	16	64
321526	3.5	> 128	64	> 128	> 128	> 128	> 128	> 128
321527	1.8	64	2	16	32	> 128	64	> 128
321529	2.6	128	2	8	32	> 128	32	128
323191	> 300	128	4	32	32	> 128	128	64
323192	> 300	128	4	64	32	> 128	128	64
323193	4.1	> 128	> 128	> 128	> 128	> 128	> 128	> 128
323194	3.4	64	1	8	8	64	16	16
323195	1.5	64	2	16	32	64	32	16
323196	1.6	32	128	> 128	> 128	> 128	> 128	> 128
323197	4.4	> 128	16	32	128	> 128	> 128	> 128
323198	2.7	> 128	1	8	16	> 128	32	64
323199	1.1	128	1	16	16	128	32	32
323200	0.4	> 128	> 128	> 128	> 128	> 128	> 128	> 128
323201	2.1	> 128	> 128	> 128	> 128	> 128	> 128	> 128
323202	4.3	32	0.25	4	4	16	8	32
323203	2.0	64	1	8	4	16	8	16
323204	2.1	> 128	64	32	128	> 128	> 128	> 128
323205	> 300	128	4	16	32	> 128	64	64
323206	> 300	> 128	> 128	> 128	> 128	> 128	> 128	> 128
323207	> 300	> 128	> 128	> 128	> 128	> 128	> 128	> 128
323208	2.7	> 128	4	64	32	> 128	64	64
323209	1.5	> 128	4	64	32	> 128	64	64
323210	3.2	> 128	> 128	> 128	> 128	> 128	> 128	> 128
323211	1.6	> 128	64	> 128	> 128	> 128	> 128	> 128
323212	3.4	128	1	> 128	4	64	8	16
323213	2.4	> 128	> 128	> 128	> 128	> 128	> 128	> 128
323214	> 300	> 128	> 128	> 128	> 128	> 128	> 128	> 128
323215	2.1	> 128	128	64	> 128	> 128	> 128	> 128
323216	1.1	32	≤0.12	2	4	16	8	8
323217	4.8	> 128	32	32	> 128	> 128	> 128	> 128
323218	0.24	> 128	4	16	32	> 128	128	64
323219	3.0	32	≤0.12	4	4	16	8	16
323220	2.1	32	≤0.12	2	4	16	8	8
323221	> 300	> 128	> 128	> 128	> 128	> 128	> 128	> 128
323222	> 300	> 128	> 128	> 128	> 128	> 128	> 128	> 128
323223	14.7	> 128	4	32	32	> 128	128	64
323224	4.9	> 128	16	8	> 128	> 128	> 128	128
323225	17.1	> 128	2	8	128	> 128	> 128	> 128
323226	8.0	> 128	64	> 128	> 128	> 128	> 128	> 128
323227	0.37	> 128	8	32	64	> 128	64	> 128
323228	0.30	64	0.5	4	8	31	16	16
323229	0.53	64	0.5	8	8	64	16	16
323230	2.0	32	0.5	8	8	32	16	16
323231	5.9	128	128	128	128	> 128	> 128	> 128

Table 1 IC$_{50}$ and MIC values of compounds against pathogenic bacteria *(Continued)*

323232	3.2	> 128	8	> 128	> 128	> 128	128	> 128
323233	> 300	128	4	16	32	> 128	64	64
323234	5.8	128	16	128	128	> 128	> 128	64
323235	37.9	> 128	8	64	64	> 128	128	128
323236	7.8	> 128	> 128	> 128	> 128	> 128	> 128	> 128
323237	2.8	64	0.5	4	8	32	8	16
323238	2.1	> 128	16	32	> 128	> 128	> 128	> 128
323239	3.0	64	8	64	> 128	> 128	64	128
323338	64.4	16	≤0.12	2	4	16	4	8
323339	19.0	64	≤0.12	8	4	32	2	2
323340	> 300	16	≤0.12	1	2	4	1	2
323341	41.4	32	≤0.12	2	4	16	8	16
323342	28.9	32	≤0.12	2	2	32	4	16
323343	8.24	32	≤0.12	1	2	8	4	2
323344	11.6	32	≤0.12	4	2	8	1	4
323345	> 300	> 128	32	64	128	> 128	128	128
323353	1.7	> 128	8	32	128	> 128	128	128
323354	21.6	> 128	16	> 128	> 128	> 128	> 128	> 128
323355	32.1	> 128	4	64	64	128	64	64
323356	> 300	128	8	64	128	> 128	128	> 128
323365	2.27	16	≤0.12	4	4	8	4	4
323366	2.47	8	≤0.12	4	2	8	4	2
323367	1.89	4	≤0.12	1	2	8	2	8
323368	0.47	> 128	> 128	> 128	> 128	> 128	> 128	> 128
323369	2.01	64	4	16	64	128	64	32
323370	0.28	16	≤0.12	2	4	16	8	8
332052	> 300	> 128	32	> 64	> 128	> 128	> 128	> 128
332053	> 300	> 128	> 128	> 64	> 128	> 128	> 128	> 128
332054	7.4	8	≤0.12	1	2	4	2	1
332055	16.4	64	32	16	128	> 128	128	64
332057	101	> 128	> 128	> 128	> 128	> 128	> 128	> 128
332058	0.56	16	≤0.12	0.5	2	16	4	4

E. faecalis, M. catarrhalis, H. influenzae, S. pneumoniae, S. aureus, E. coli tolC mutants, and *E. coli* modified with PMBN

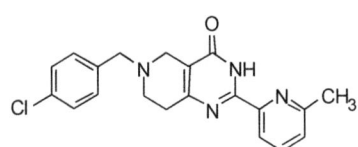

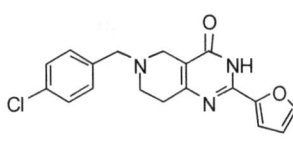

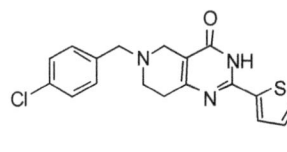

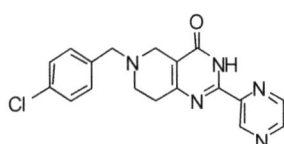

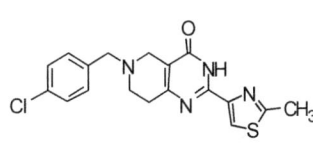

Figure 3 Compounds in which the pyridine ring attached to the central scaffold/core in the 2-position was modified.

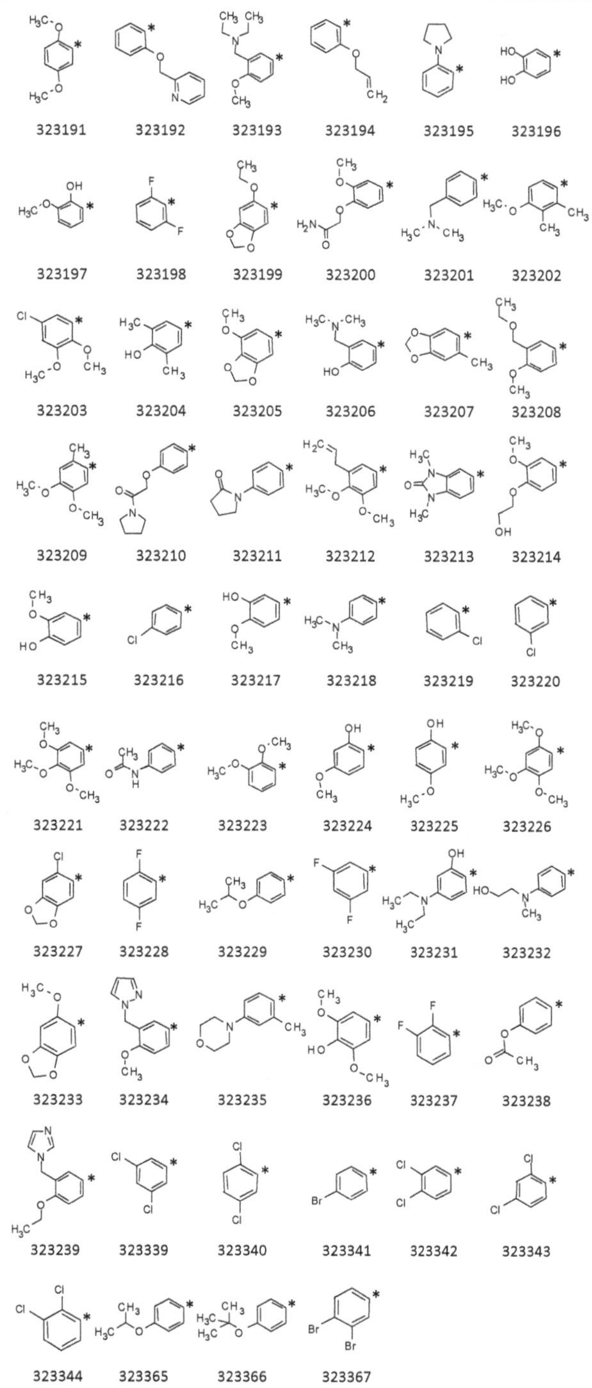

Figure 4 Compounds in which the benzene ring attached at the 6-position of the core structure was modified. Asterisk represents the point of attachment to the core structure.

decreased with compounds in which two chlorine atoms (323339, 323340, 323342, 323343, and 323344) were walked around the phenyl ring. Compounds containing a 3-bromobenzene or a 2,3-dibromobenzene at the 6-position (323341, 323367) also decreased biochemical potency. Even though a moderate decrease in biochemical potency was observed for a subset of these compounds as a whole they exhibited some of the greatest increases in potency for inhibiting bacterial growth. The 2,3-dimethoxy-5-chloro substitution in 323203 maintained biochemical and enhanced antibacterial potency.

The remaining four compounds (323194, 323208, 323212, and 323229) contained 2-(ethenyloxy)benzene, 2-(ethoxymethyl)-3-(methoxybenzene, 2,3-dimethoxy-4 (prop-2-en-1-yl)benzene and 3-(propan-2-yl ether)benzene at the 6-position, respectively. Variations of alkyl, alkenyl, alkoxyl, and alkenoxy groups exhibited no extreme shifts in either the IC_{50} or MIC values, although all four were potent compounds.

Next, based on compound 323216 (Figure 4), changes to the 5,6,7,8-tetrahydropyrido[4,3-*d*]pyrimidin-4-ol core were implemented (Figure 5). Removal of the carbonyl group from the pyrimidine ring of the core (323355) resulted in moderate increase of both IC_{50} and the MIC values. Attachment of a 3-methyl group onto the tetrahydropyrido[4,3-*d*]pyrimidin (323345) abolished most biochemical and antibacterial activities, whereas addition of an 8-methyl group (332054) enhanced antibacterial activity. Oxidation of the tetrahydropyrido[4,3-d]pyrimidin core (332055) resulted in a negative effect on the activity of the compounds series. Ring enlargement to tetrahydro-3H-pyrimido[5,4-c]azepin (332058) had profound effects on both IC_{50} and MIC values. The IC_{50} was improved to 0.56 μM and the MIC values determined for different bacteria in the panel were improved to the lowest levels observed for any compound tested.

Finally, changes were made in the linker tethering the phenyl ring to the 6-position of the core scaffold (Figure 6). First, the point of attachment of the linker was changed from the 6-position to the 5-position (323338). This resulted in a significant increase in the IC_{50} but a slight improvement in the MIC values. Next, the methylene linker was replaced with a carbonyl carbon (323353) or a carboxamido linker (323368). The insertion of the carbonyl carbon resulted in decreased potency in bacterial cultures. The amide group resulted in an improved IC_{50}, but a complete loss of antibacterial activity was observed. Next, the length of the carbon linker was increased by the addition of a carbonyl carbon (323369) or with an additional carbon (323370). The addition of the carbonyl carbon significantly increased the MIC. Insertion of an additional carbon however improved the IC_{50} to one of the lowest values recorded and maintained low MIC values.

compounds improved the IC_{50} values. When two fluorine atoms (323198, 323228, 323230, and 323237) or one chlorine atom (323216, 323219, and 323220) were walked around the phenyl ring at the 6-position on the core structure, the biochemical potency was maintained or increased. However, the biochemical potency was

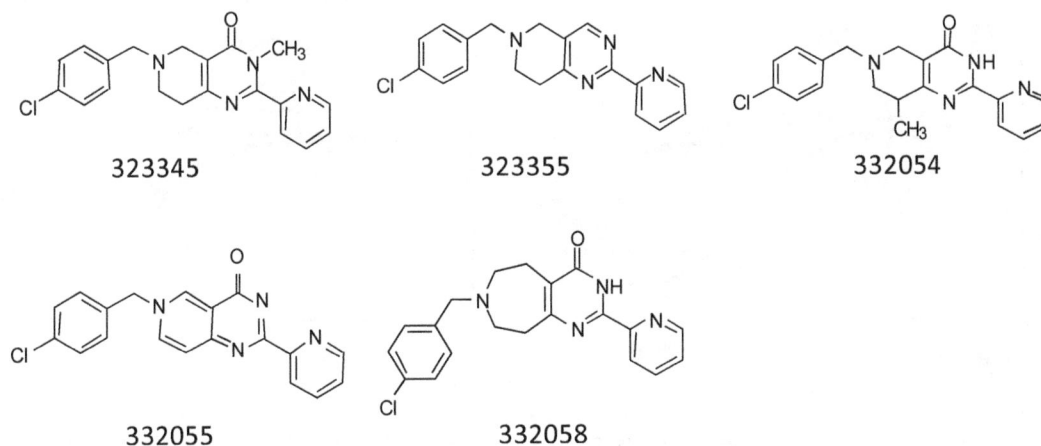

Figure 5 Compounds in which the central scaffolds/cores were modified.

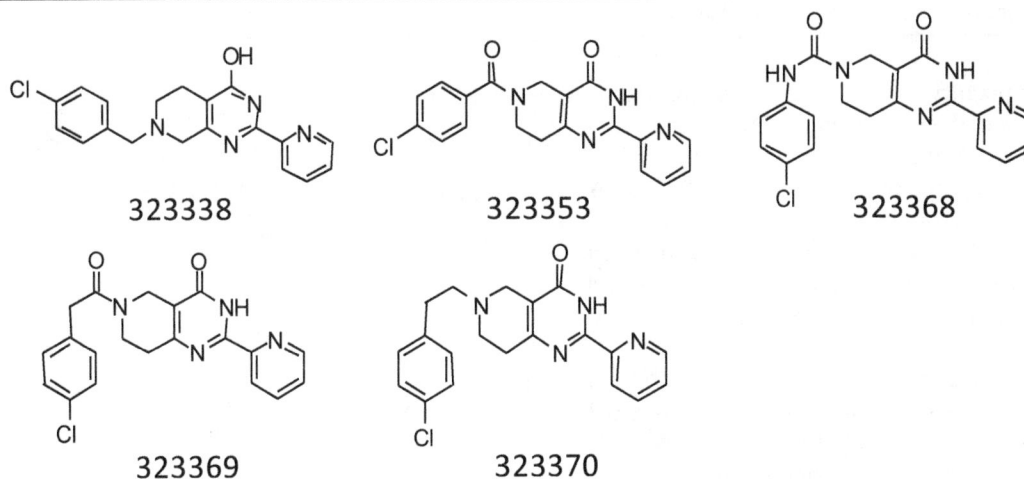

Figure 6 Compounds in which the linker connecting the benzene ring attached at the 6-position of the core structures were modified.

4. Conclusion

In summary, this library of compounds allows a determination of what kind and where changes in the compound series will be allowed. It is obvious that almost any change in the pyridine ring at the 2-position of the core will not be tolerated. Changes to the benzene ring tethered to the 6-position of the core are permitted but

Table 2 Comparison of good IC$_{50}$ to MIC values

Compound	IC$_{50}$ μM	MIC
323218	0.24	+
323227	0.37	+
323228	0.30	++
323229	0.53	++
323368	0.47	-
323370	0.28	+++
332058	0.56	+++

+, poor; ++, moderate; +++, good antibacterial activity.

Table 3 Comparison of good MIC to IC$_{50}$ values

Compound	MIC	IC$_{50}$ μM
323338	+++	64.4
323339	+++	19.0
323340	+++	> 300
323341	+++	41.4
323342	+++	28.9
323343	+++	8.24
323344	+++	11.6
323365	+++	2.27
323366	+++	2.47
323367	+++	1.89
323370	+++	0.28
332054	+++	7.40
332058	+++	0.56

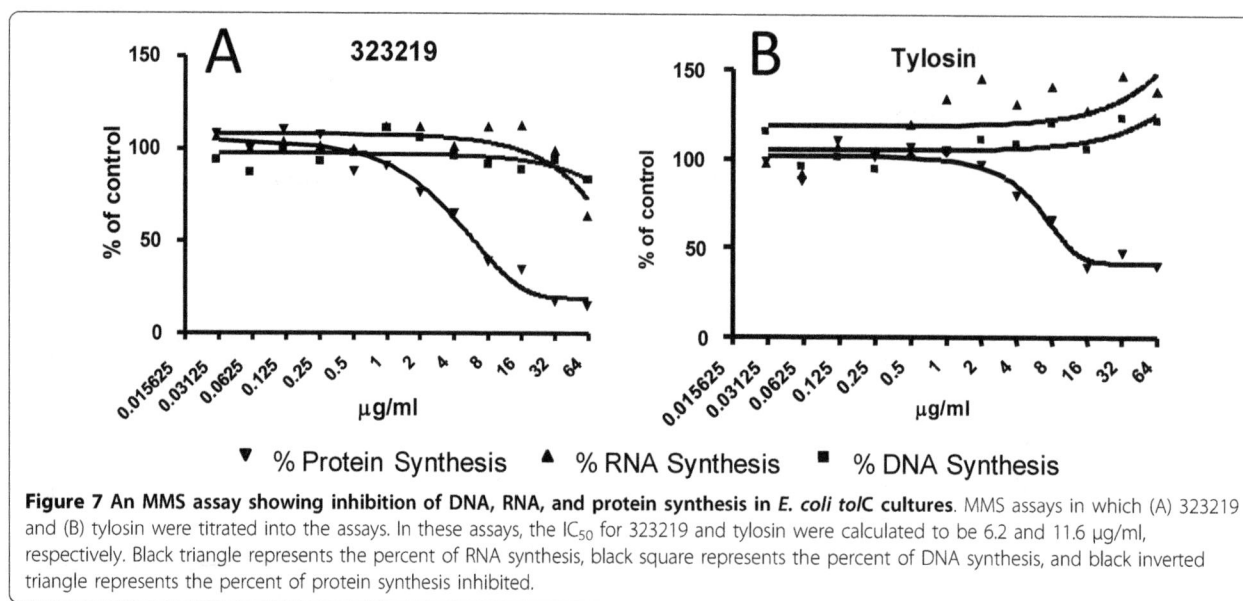

Figure 7 An MMS assay showing inhibition of DNA, RNA, and protein synthesis in _E. coli tolC_ cultures. MMS assays in which (A) 323219 and (B) tylosin were titrated into the assays. In these assays, the IC_{50} for 323219 and tylosin were calculated to be 6.2 and 11.6 µg/ml, respectively. Black triangle represents the percent of RNA synthesis, black square represents the percent of DNA synthesis, and black inverted triangle represents the percent of protein synthesis inhibited.

tend to increase potency when they are simple in nature. It is possible to lengthen the 6-linker, but adding functional groups to the linker may impede antibacterial activity. Of the compounds tested, the IC_{50} was improved to sub-micromolar values with seven compounds (Table 2). Most of these compounds maintained or increased MIC's when compared to 321525 and 321528; however, one compound completely abolished antibacterial activity (Table 2). In some instances, there was a complete disconnect between IC_{50} and MIC values. Compound 323340 displayed a good antibacterial activity; however, it had no inhibitory effect in the A/T assay suggesting a different mechanism of inhibition (Table 3). When comparing biochemical inhibitory activity and antibacterial activity of the compounds, only two compounds (323370 and 332058) appear in both tables. It is possible that compounds with good biochemical activity that lack antibacterial potency may not be able to enter the bacterial cells, or are effluxed or modified to an inactive state by the bacteria. Also, compounds with good MIC but poor IC_{50} values may exhibit a secondary mode of action that leads to the observed antibacterial activity.

We have demonstrated specific inhibition of protein synthesis in _E. coli tolC_ cells for a number of the compounds described above, including 323202, 323203, 323216, 323219, and 323220. These results indicate that the types of modifications in these compounds are tolerated with regard to maintaining the specific mode of action. When compared with a known inhibitor (tylosin) of bacterial protein synthesis, 323219 exhibited similar inhibition profiles in MMS assays (Figure 7). The other compounds tested yielded similar results.

Author details
[1]Replidyne, Inc., Louisville, CO, USA [2]Chemistry Department, SCIE. 3.320, The University of Texas-Pan American, 1201 W. University Drive, Edinburg, TX 78541, USA [3]CedarburgHauser Pharmaceuticals, Denver, CO, USA [4]Mannkind Corporation, Valencia, CA, USA [5]Crestone, Inc., Boulder, CO, USA

Competing interests
The authors declare that they have no competing interests.

References
1. Overcoming Antimicrobial Resistance (2000) World Health Organization Report on Infectious Diseases (WHO/CDS/2000.2)
2. Hermann T (2005) Drugs targeting the ribosome. Curr Opin Struct Biol 15:355–366. doi:10.1016/j.sbi.2005.05.001.
3. Knowles DJ, Foloppe N, Matassova NB, Murchie AI (2002) The bacterial ribosome, a promising focus for structure-based drug design. Curr Opin Pharmacol 2:501–506. doi:10.1016/S1471-4892(02)00205-9.
4. Bryskier A (2005) Antimicrobial agents: antibacterials and antifungals. ASM Press, Washington, DC
5. Cundiffe E (1990) The ribosome. In: Hill WE, Dahlberg A, Garrett RA, Moore PB, Schlessinger D, Warner JR (eds) Structure, function, and evolution. Am Soc Microbiol, Washington, DC pp. 479–490
6. Ribble W, Hill WE, Jarvis TC, Ochsner UA, Guiles JW, Janjic N, Bullard JM (2010) Discovery and analysis of 4H-Pyridopyrimidines, a class of selective bacterial protein synthesis inhibitors. Antimicrob Agents Chemother 54:4648–4657. doi:10.1128/AAC.00638-10.
7. National Committee for Clinical Laboratory Standards (2002) Methods for determining bactericidal activity of antimicrobial agents: approved guide line M26-A. NCCLS, Wayne, PA
8. National Committee for Clinical Laboratory Standards (2003) Methods for dilution antimicrobial susceptibility test for bacteria that grow aerobically: approved standard M7-A6. NCCLS, Wayne, PA
9. Ochsner UA, Young CL, Stone KC, Dean FB, Janjic N, Critchley IA (2005) Mode of action and biochemical characterization of REP8839, a novel inhibitor of methionyl-tRNA synthetase. Antimicrob Agents Chemother 49:4253–4262. doi:10.1128/AAC.49.10.4253-4262.2005.

5

Bioactive flavanoids from *Glycosmis arborea*

Mohammad Faheem Khan, Nisha Negi, Rajnikant Sharma and Devendra Singh Negi*

Abstract

Background: *Glycosmis* is a genus of evergreen glabrous shrub and distributed all over India. It possesses various medicinal properties and is used in indigenous medicine for cough, rheumatism, anemia, and jaundice. *Glycosmis arborea* is a rich source of alkaloids, terpenoids, coumarins, as well as flavonoids.

Results: The chemical investigation of methanol fraction of the leaves of *G. arborea* led to the isolation of one new flavone C-glycoside along with three known flavanoids, named as 5,7-dihydroxy-2-[4-hydroxy-3-(methoxy methyl) phenyl]-6-C-β-D-glucopyranosyl flavone (4), 5,7,4′-trihydroxy-3′-methoxy flavone (1), 5,4′-dihydroxy-3′-methoxy-7-O-β-D-glucupyranosyl flavanone (2), and 5,4′-dihydroxy-3′-methoxy-7-O-(α-L-rhamnosyl-(1‴→6‴)-β-D-glucopyranosyl) flavanone (3), respectively. The structures of all compounds were elucidated with the help of nuclear magnetic resonance spectrometry. Pure compounds and fractions were evaluated for pest antifeedant and antimicrobial activity.

Conclusion: Four compounds were isolated from the leaves of *G. arborea*. Among them, compound 4 showed significant antimicrobial activity.

Keywords: *Glycosmis arborea*, Rutaceae, Flavone C-glycoside, Antifeedant activity, Antimicrobial activity

Background

Glycosmis is a genus of evergreen glabrous shrub, distributed in warm and temperate regions of the world, and is a rich source of alkaloids and amide; however, terpenoids, coumarins, and flavonoids were also reported [1,2]. Previously, a new carbazole alkaloid, designated as glycoborinine, was isolated from the roots of *Glycosmis arborea*, along with two known alkaloids, carbazole glycozoline and glycozolidine, and two known quinoline alkaloids, *viz.* skimianine and 3-(3′,3′-dimethylallyl)-4,8-dimethoxy-*N*-methylquinolin-2-one [3]. There are about 60 species in the Indo-Malaysia region, and 7 are found in India. In Uttarakhand, *G. arborea* (Hindi-*Ban Nimbu*, Sanskrit-*Ashvashokta*) grows commonly in Sal and miscellaneous forests of Tarai Bhabher at 600-m heights [4].

As a part of our ongoing studies aimed at the phytochemical and pharmacological characterization of this plant, we found that hexane and methanol fractions of the ethanol extract of *G. arborea* leaves showed significant antifeedant and antimicrobial activity. Herein, therefore, we decided to carry out a detailed study to investigate the chemical composition of *G. arborea*. In particular, we

report the isolation and characterization of one new flavone C-glycoside (4) along with three known compounds (1 to 3) (Figure 1) with their antifeedant and antimicrobial activities. The known compounds were identified by using spectroscopic methods including infrared (IR), UV, mass, and 1D and 2D nuclear magnetic resonance (NMR) analysis and also by comparing data already reported in the literature. Methanol fraction yielded one new flavone C-glycoside (4) and three known compounds *viz.* 5,7,4′-trihydroxy-3′-methoxy flavone (1) [5], 5,5′-dihydroxy-4′-methoxy-7-O-β-D-glucupyranosyl flavanone (2) [6], and 5,5′-dihydroxy-4′-methoxy-7-O-(L-rhamnosyl-(1‴→6‴)-β-D-glucopyranosyl) flavanone (3) [7]. Among these, compounds 1 and 2 have been reported for the first time from *G. arborea*.

Methods

Plant material

The *G. arborea* leaves were collected from Rajaji National Park, Rishikesh, Uttarakhand, India during the flowering season and identified by a taxonomist of the Botany Department of HNB Garhwal University Uttarakhand. A voucher specimen is deposited in the Department of Botany, HNB Garhwal University, Uttarakhand.

* Correspondence: devendra_negi@yahoo.com
Department of Chemistry, HNB Garhwal University, Srinagar (Garhwal), Uttarakhand 246174, India

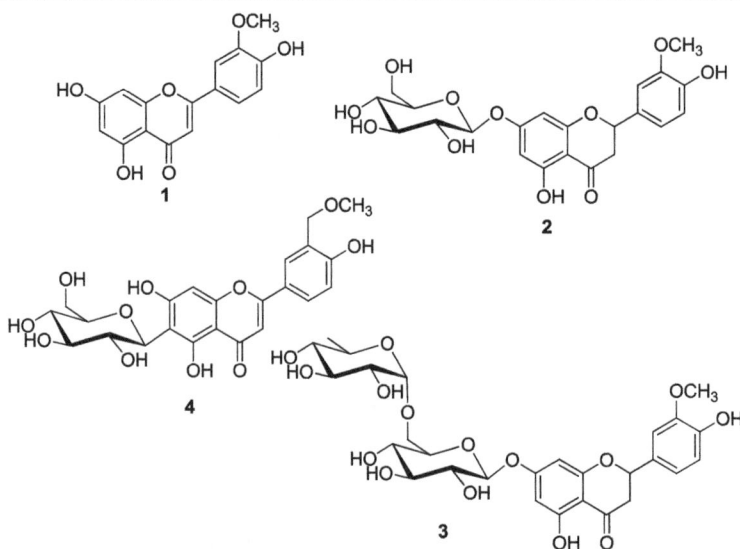

Figure 1 Chemical structure of isolated compounds from *G. arborea* leaves.

Extraction and isolation

Parts of the dried leaves of *G. arborea* (1.8 kg) were air dried, grinded, and refluxed with 90% ethanol. The total ethanol extract was concentrated under reduced pressure at a temperature below 50°C to a dark green viscous mass coded as F001 (120 g) that was partitioned with hexane (F003) (21 g) and *n*-butanol F004 (88 g). The *n*-butanol soluble layer was then successfully fractionated into chloroform (4 g) (F005), ethyl acetate (19 g) (F006), and methanol soluble fraction (63 g) (F007). The methanol soluble fraction (F007) after removal of the solvent was chromatographed over silica gel (800 g) and eluted with mixtures of $CHCl_3$/MeOH as eluents to give four fractions A1 to A4 (9:1, 88:12, 85:15, 82:18). Fraction A2 (2.4 g) was rechromatographed on silica gel with $CHCl_3$/MeOH mixtures (9:1, 85:15) and yielded compounds **1** (70 mg), **2** (90 mg), **3** (46 mg), and **4** (36 mg).

5,7,4′-trihydroxy-3′-methoxy flavone (1, $C_{16}H_{12}O_6$)

M.p. 287°C to 288°C; UV (MeOH) λ_{max} nm: 214, 241, 268, 348; IR (KBr) v_{max} cm^{-1}: 3431, 1634, 1594, 1382, 1351, 1078, 770. ESIMS ($C_{16}H_{12}O_6$) *m/z*: 300 [M]$^+$, 285 [M-CH$_3$]$^+$, 272 [M-CO]$^+$, 257 [M-43]$^+$, 241, 242, 215, 204, 193, 176, 152 [A$_1$]$^+$, 148 [B$_1$]$^+$, 136, 124 [A$_1$-28]$^+$ 107, 105. ^{1}H NMR (400 MHz, DMSO-d_6): δ ppm 6.62 (1H, s, H-3) 6.05 (1H, d, *J* = 2.0 Hz, H-6), 6.38 (1H, d, *J* = 2.0 Hz, H-8), 7.63 (1H, d, *J* = 2.4 Hz, H-2′) 6.87 (1H, d, *J* = 9.0 Hz, H-5), 7.78 (1H, dd, *J* = 2.4, 9.0 Hz, H-6) 3.86 (3H, brd s, OCH$_3$). ^{13}C NMR (100 MHz, DMSO-$d6$): δ ppm 161.02 (C-2) 106.32 (C-3), 182.2 (C-4) 160.9 (C-5), 98.7 (C-6), 164.2 (C-7), 93.9 (C-8), 103.6 (C-4a), 157.1 (C-8a), 124.1 (C-1′), 115.6 (C-2′), 148.4 (C-3′), 145.2 (C-4′), 117.0 (C-5′), 122.3 (C-6′), 56.2 (OCH$_3$).

5,4′-dihydroxy-3′-methoxy-7-O-β-D-glucupyranosyl flavanone (2, $C_{22}H_{24}O_{11}$)

M.p. 264°C; UV (MeOH) λ_{max} nm: 295, 328. IR (KBr) v_{max} cm^{-1}: 3423, 1620, 1594, 1351, 1071, 1012, 974, 921. ESIMS (% int.) ($C_{22}H_{24}O_{11}$) *m/z*: 464 [M]$^+$ (70), 449 [M-CH$_3$]$^+$ (3), 416 [M-OCH$_3$-OH]$^+$ (17), 381 (88), 353 (93), 302 [M-Glu]$^+$ (4), 301 (4), 203 (6). ^{1}H NMR (400 MHz, DMSO-d_6): δ ppm 12.01 (1H, s, OH-5), 9.09 (1H, s, OH-5′), 5.47 (1H, dd, *J* = 6.2, 9.2 Hz, H-2) 2.8 (1H, dd, *J* = 12.4 Hz, H-3a), 3.29 (1H, dd, *J* = 13.0, 17.2 Hz, H-3b), 6.13 (1H, d, *J* = 2.4 Hz, H-6), 6.10 (1H, d, *J* = 2.4 Hz, H-8), 6.92 (1H, dd, *J* = 3.2, 8.0 Hz, H-2′), 6.89 (1H, d, *J* = 8.4 Hz, H-3′), 6.92 (1H, d, *J* = 3.2 Hz, H-6), 4.67 (1H, d, *J* = 7.6 Hz, H-1″), 3.42-3.82 (5H, m, sugar), 3.76 (3H, brd s, OCH$_3$). ^{13}C NMR (100 MHz, DMSO-d_6): δ ppm 78.77 (C-2), 42.4 (C-3), 197.44 (C-4), 165.52 (C-5), 96.3 (C-6), 163.43 (C-7), 95.51 (C-8), 103.69 (C-4a), 162.88 (C-8a), 131.27 (C-1′), 112.2 (C-2′), 118.33 (C-3′), 148.36 (C-4′), 146.83 (C-5′), 114 (C-6′), 100.99 (C-1″), 71 to 76 (C-2″-C-5″), 66.41 (C-6″), 56.05 (OCH$_3$).

5,4′-dihydroxy-3′-methoxy-7-O-(α-L-rhamnosyl-(1‴→6″)-β-D-glucopyranosyl) flavanone (3, $C_{28}H_{34}O_{15}$)

UV (MeOH) λ_{max} nm: 293, 326. IR (KBr) v_{max} cm^{-1}: 3472 (OH), 1630, 1602 (aromatic), 1521, 1352, 1092, 815. ESIMS ($C_{28}H_{34}O_{15}$) (% int.) *m/z*: 610 [M]$^+$, 633 [M + Na]$^+$ (54), 595 (2), 551 (5), 507 (7), 463 (7), 388 (77), 364 (93), 338 (70), 306 (50), 233 (35), 179 (43), 151 (16). ^{1}H NMR (400 MHz, C$_5$H$_5$N-d_5): δ ppm 12.24 (1H, s, OH-5), 8.84 (1H, s, OH-5′), 5.45 (1H, dd, *J* = 6.2, 9.6 Hz, H-2), 2.85 (1H, dd, *J* = 12.4 Hz, H-3a), 3.22 (1H, dd, *J* = 13.0, 17.2 Hz, H-3b), 6.49 (1H, d, *J* = 2.1 Hz, H-6), 6.60 (1H, d, *J* = 2.1 Hz, H-8), 7.11 (1H, dd, *J* = 2.1,

6.3 Hz, H-2′), 6.96 (1H, d, J = 6.3 Hz, H-3′), 7.51 (1H, d, J = 2.1 Hz, H-6), 5.69 (1H, d, J = 7.6 Hz, H-1″), 4.26 to 4.66 (5H, m, H-2″-H-6″), 5.43 (1H, d, J = 3.0 Hz, H-1‴), 4.14 to 4.60 (4H, m, H-2‴-H-5‴), 1.57 (3H, d, J = 5.7 Hz, H-6‴), 3.71 (3H, brd s, OCH$_3$). ^{13}C NMR (100 MHz, C$_5$H$_5$N-d_5): δ ppm 79.50 (C-2), 43.16 (C-3), 197.1 (C-4), 166.48 (C-5), 96.44 (C-6), 164.08 (C-7), 97.32 (C-8), 104.34 (C-4a), 163.49 (C-8a), 132.15 (C-1′), 118.49 (C-2′), 112.31 (C-3′), 148.43 (C-4′), 149.12(C-5′), 115.32 (C-6′), 102.51 (C-1″), 72.79 to 78.45 (C-2″, C-5″), 67.37 (C-6″), 101.55 (C-1‴), 69.83 to 77.24 (C-2″, C-5‴), 18.61 (C-6‴, methyl), 55.89 (OCH$_3$).

5,7-dihydroxy-2-[4-hydroxy-3-(methoxymethyl)phenyl]-6-C-β-D-glucopyranosyl flavone (4, C$_{23}$H$_{24}$O$_{11}$)

UV (MeOH) λ_{max} nm: 208, 306. IR (KBr) ν_{max} cm^{-1}: 3437, 1660, 1590, 1350, 1074, 901, 836. EIMS (C$_{23}$H$_{24}$O$_{11}$) (% int.) m/z: 493 [M + OH]$^+$ (18), 478 [M + 2H]$^+$ (11), 448 [M-CO]$^+$ (14), 455 (94), 444 (11), 433 (9), 413 (22), 301 (4), 260 (3), 203 (2), 136 (2). ^{1}H NMR (400 MHz, DMSO-d_6) and ^{13}C NMR (100 MHz, DMSO-d_6) δ (see Table 1).

Antifeedant assay

The antifeedant activity of the extracts against the polyphagous pest *Spodoptera litura* was tested using the leaf dip method [7]. Five percent concentrations of each extract were prepared by dissolving extracts in a small quantity of ethanol and diluting in water containing 0.05% Triton X-100. The leaf discs of about 5 cm^2 were prepared out of castor leaf (*Ricinus communis* L.) and were dipped for 30 s in an extract or compound separately. The leaf discs dipped only in water containing 0.05% Triton X-100 were used as controls. The leaf discs were air dried, and on each treated leaf disc, 10 larvae of *S. litura* (1 day old) were released. Three replications were maintained for each extract. Larval weight was taken after 4 days of treatment. Antifeedant activity of fractions and the purified compounds were tested against the polyphagous crop pest *S. litura* (Table 2).

Antibacterial assay

The *in vitro* antibacterial activity was tested by the disc diffusion method [8] using pathogenic strains of *Agrobacterium tumifaciens*, *Pseudomonas syringae*, and *Pectobacterium. carotovorum*. Concentrations of 200 and 500 μg/disc of compounds were impregnated on the discs. These discs were placed on the surface of the agar plates already inoculated with pathogenic bacteria. The plates were incubated at 37°C and examined at 48 h for zone of inhibition, if any, around the discs. Gentamicin was used in the assay as a standard control drug. An additional control disc without any sample but impregnated with an equivalent amount of solvent (DMSO)

Table 1 NMR spectroscopic (400 MHz) data of compound 4 in DMSO-d_6

Positions	^{1}H (J in Hz)	^{13}C	HSQC	HMBC	
				^2J	^3J
2	-	161.51	qC		
3	6.77 (s)	103.46	CH	C-4	C-4a,1′,5′
4	-	182.47	qC		
5	-	162.97	qC		
6	-	104.97	qC		
7	-	156.36	qC		
8	6.26 (s)	98.50	CH	C-8a	C-6, 2
4a	-	104.38	qC		
8a	-	160.75	qC		
1′	-	121.98	qC		
2′	8.02 (d, J = 2.4, 8.4)	129.34	CH		C-5′, 8a
3′	6.88 (d, J = 8.4)	116.17	CH		C-1′
4′	-	151.42	qC		
5′	-	164.30	qC		
6′	6.91 (d, J = 2.4)	116.17	CH	C-1′	C-3′
1″	4.65 (d, J = 9.9)	73.74	CH	C-6, 2″	C-3″, 5″, 5, 7
2″	3.82 (dd, J = 9.2,9.6)	70.86	CH	C-1″	
3″	3.24 (t, J = 9.2)	79.01	CH		
4″	3.34 (t, J = 9.2)	71.18	CH		
5″	3.22 (ddd, J = 5.0, 9.2)	82.22	CH		C-1″
6″	3.75 (d, J = 11.6)	61.65	CH$_2$	C-5″	
	3.52 (dd, J = 6.0,12.0)				
1‴	3.17 s	48.97	CH$_2$		
OCH$_3$	3.89	56.8	CH$_3$		C-4′
OH-5	13.15				

was also used in the assay. The result of antibacterial activity indicated that methanol fraction and compound 4 exhibited a mild to moderate activity (Table 3).

Results and discussion
Chemistry

The repeated chromatography of methanol fraction of the leaves of *G. arborea* led to the isolation of four flavonoids by gradient elution with the CHCl$_3$/MeOH mixture of increasing polarity. Compound 4 was isolated as a yellow solid which was further crystallized in acetone.

Table 2 Pest antifeedant activity of *G. arborea* fractions against *S. litura* L

Fractions	Percent feeding index (PFI) 2.5 (μg/cm^2)
Hexane	46.71 ± 4.07
Methanol	50.21 ± 5.21

A concentration of 0.05% Triton X-100 was used as control.

Table 3 Antibacterial activity of *G. arborea* fraction and isolated compound against plant bacterial pathogens

Particular	Concentration (µg/disc)	Zone of inhibition (in mm)		
		Agrobacterium tumifaciens	*Pseudomonas syringae*	*Pectobacterium carotovorum*
Methanol fraction	200	12	-	14
	500	16	6	18
Compound **4**	200	9	-	-
	500	11	-	-

Gentamicin was used as a standard control drug.

It had the composition $C_{23}H_{24}O_{11}$ ($m/z = 476$) as derived from the positive mode of electrospray ionization mass spectrometry (ESIMS) analysis. A positive Shinoda test and color reaction with ferric chloride suggested the presence of free phenolic hydroxyl groups. The UV spectrum exhibited absorption maxima at 208 and 306 nm which are characteristic of a flavone skeleton [9]. Its IR spectrum showed the presence of a hydroxyl group at 3,437 cm^{-1} and a chelated carbon at 1,660 cm^{-1} (γ pyrone nucleus) along with other absorption bands at 1,590 and 838 cm^{-1}, a characteristic of an aromatic nucleus.

The ^{1}H NMR spectrum showed the signals typical for flavone moiety. A double doublet at δ 8.02 ($J = 2.4, 8.4$ Hz) and doublet at 6.88 ($J = 2.4$ Hz) and in the aromatic region with meta-coupling were assigned to H-2' and H-6'. Another doublet at δ 7.92 ($J = 8.4$ Hz) was attributed to H-3' proton. Two sharp singlets at δ 6.77 and 6.26 were ascribed as H-3 and H-8, respectively. The downfield chemical shift at δ 13.15 was assigned to the hydroxyl proton of OH-5. A sharp peak resonated at δ 3.8 due to the methoxy proton. ^{1}H spectra showed upfield signal at δ 3.15 for two protons attributed to aliphatic methylene H-1'''. The ^{13}C NMR spectra showed the signals for 23 carbons which were differentiated into 10 methines, 2 methylenes, 1 methyl, and 10 quaternary carbons on the basis of distortionless enhancement by polarization transfer (DEPT; 90 and 135) experiments. DEPT 135 revealed the presence of two methylene carbons in a molecule resonating at δ 61.65 and 48.97 assigned to C-6' and C-1'''. From ^{1}H spectra, two doublets of one proton resonated at δ 4.65 and 3.75 assigned to H-1'' ($J = 9.9$ Hz, anomeric) and H-6''a. Two doublet of doublets of one proton at δ 3.82 ($J = 9.2, 9.9$ Hz) and 3.52 ($J = 12$ Hz) were attributed to H-2'' and H-6''b. A multiplet at δ 3.22 to 3.34 showed for the remaining three sugar protons.

The exact proton and carbon assignments were made by a combination of 2D NMR experiments such as COSY, heteronuclear single-quantum correlation (HSQC), and heteronuclear multiple bond correlation (HMBC). The position of sugar was confirmed by HMBC long-range correlation in which anomeric H-1'' showed long-range coupling with 162.97 (C-5), 104.97 (C-6), and 156.3 (C-7), suggesting the position of sugar at C-6 of aromatic ring B (Figure 2). The double bond position was confirmed by

coupling of a proton singlet (δ 6.77) with 182.47 (C-4) and 121.98 (C-1'), suggesting that it must be placed at C-3 and assigned as H-3. The 5-hydroxy flavone skeleton was assigned on the basis of ^{13}C NMR data which showed C-4 resonance at δ 182.47, characteristic of 5-hydroxy flavone [10,11]. The signal resonating at δ 56.8 was due to methoxy carbon. The upfield appearance of anomeric carbon (73.74) and proton (4.65) as compared to those of aromatic O-glycoside data and anomeric proton correlation with C-5, C-6, and C-7 in the long-range HMBC experiment exhibited its C-glycosidic nature which was confirmed by its resistance to acidic hydrolysis [12,13]. The remaining HMBC correlations are given in Table 1.

The structure was supported by the mass spectroscopic studies, which showed molecular ion peak at 478 m/z [M$^+$+2H]. Fragment at 445 m/z was due to loss of carbonyl [M$^+$-CO] and further at 433 m/z was due to loss of the methyl group [M$^+$-CO-CH$_3$]. A higher percentage of fragmentation also appeared at 455 m/z [M$^+$-H$_2$O-3H]. Thus, compound **4** was unambiguously identified as 5,7-dihydroxy-2-[4-hydroxy-3-(methoxymethyl) phenyl]-6-C-β-D-glucopyranosyl flavone, a new flavone C-glycoside named as Arboreaside.

Biological studies

Antifeedant activity

All the fractions and compounds were tested for antifeedant activity. Among them, the hexane and methanol fractions showed significant antifeedant action against *S. litura* L. In a dual-choice leaf disc method, hexane and methanol fractions were tested for pesticidal potential.

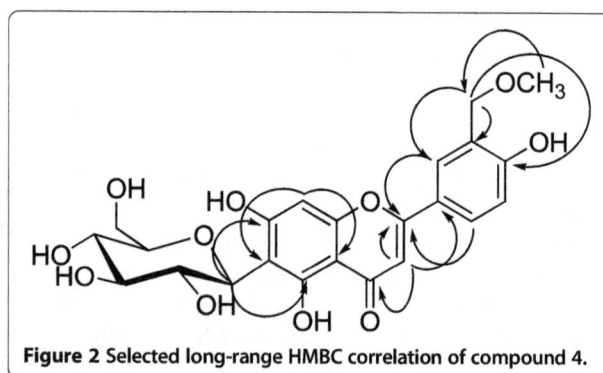

Figure 2 Selected long-range HMBC correlation of compound 4.

The hexane fraction showed a percent feeding index (PFI) of 46.71 ± 4.07, while the methanol fraction showed a PFI of 50.21 ± 5.01 as given in Table 2.

Antibacterial activity

All the fractions and compounds were also tested for antibacterial activity. The methanol fraction and compound 4 showed antimicrobial activity against the plant bacterial pathogens *A. tumifaciens*, *P. syringae*, and *P. carotovorum*. It was found that moderate inhibitory activities were observed against *A. tumifaciens* and *P. carotovorum* at a concentration of 200 µg, whereas *P. syringae* was found to be fatal at 500 µg. Compound 4 showed moderate inhibition against *A. tumifaciens* as shown in the Table 3.

Experimental

All melting points are uncorrected and were taken in open capillaries. The UV spectra were recorded on a PerkinElmer Lambda 15 UV/VIS spectrophotometer (PerkinElmer, Waltham, MA, USA) in methanol as blank. IR spectra were recorded on a PerkinElmer Infrared 15 in KBr pellets and are expressed per centimeter. The ^{1}H and ^{13}C NMR were scanned on a Bruker AVANCE 400 MHz (Bruker Corporation, Billerica, MA, USA) at C_5D_5N-d_5, DMSO-d_6, CD_3OD, and $CDCl_3$ at 400, 300, and 100 MHz with TMS as internal reference. Proton-detected heteronuclear correlations were measured using HMQC (optimized for J_{HC} =14.5 Hz) and HMBC (optimized for J_{HC} =7 Hz). Mass spectra were recorded on a Micromass Quattro II (Micromass UK Ltd., Manchester, UK) at 70 eV for ESIMS. Column chromatography was carried out using silica gel (60 to 120 mesh, Qualigen (Carlsbad, CA, USA)/ Merck (Whitehouse Station, NJ, USA)). Thin layer chromatography was carried out over plates made of silica gel G of Qualigen/Merck.

Conclusion

In conclusion, the present paper has shown the isolation and structure elucidation of one new flavone C-glycoside (4) along with three known compounds (1 to 3) from methanol fraction of *G. arborea* leaves. With regard to bioactivity, all fractions and isolated compounds were evaluated for antifeedant and antibacterial activity. Among them, hexane and methanol fractions showed antifeedant activity, whereas methanol fraction and compound 4 showed significant antibacterial activity.

Competing interests

The authors declare that they have no competing interests.

Acknowledgment

The authors are extremely grateful to Prof. A.D. Kinghorn, USA for the NMR and ESIMS experiments and Dr. S. Narasimhan, AHRF, Chennai for the antifeedant and antibacterial activity. This investigation received financial assistance from CSIR, New Delhi in the form of a network project [02(3286)/12].

References

1. Ito C, Itoigawa M, Sato A, Hasan CM, Rashid NA, Tokuda H, Mukainoka T, Nishino H, Furukawa H (2004) Chemical constituents of *Glycosmis arborea*: three new carbazole alkaloids and their biological activity. J Nat Prod 67:1488–1491
2. Pacher T, Bacher M, Hofer O, Greger H (2001) Stress induced carbazole phytoalexins in *Glycosmis species*. Phytochemistry 58:129–135
3. Chakravarty AK, Sarkar T, Masuda K, Shiojima K (1999) Carbazole alkaloids from roots of *Glycosmis arborea*. Phytochemistry 50:1263–1266
4. Gaur RD (1999) Flora of District Garhwal North West Himalaya. Transmedia Publication, Srinagar, p 380
5. Yahagi T, Daikonva A, Kitanaka S (2012) Flavonol acyl glycosides from flower of *Albizia julibrissin* and their inhibitory effects on lipid accumulation in 3T3-L1 cells. Chem Pharm Bull 60:129–136
6. Yu-Jen K, Yu-Ching Y, Li-Jie Z, Ming-Der W, Li-Ming YK, Yuh-Chi K, Syh-Yuan H, Cheng-Jen C, Kuo-Hsiung L, Hsiu-O H, Yao-Haur K (2010) Flavanone and diphenylpropane glycosides and glycosidic acyl esters from *Viscum articulatum*. J Nat Prod 73:109–114
7. Negi DS, Kumar A, Sharma RK, Shukla N, Negi N, Tamta ML, Bansal Y, Prasert P, Cairns JRK (2011) Structure confirmation of rare conjugate glycosides from *Glycosmis arborea* (Roxb.) with the action of β-glucosidases. Res J Phytochem 5:32–40
8. Murray PR, Baron EJ, Pfaller MA, Tenover FC, Yolke RH (1999) Manual of clinical microbiology, 4th edn. ASM, Washington, p 1527
9. Markham KR (1982) Techniques of flavonoids identification, vol 3. Academic, London, pp 36–51
10. Fang N, Leidig M, Mabry TJ, Munekazu I (1985) Six 2′-hydroxyflavonols from *Gutierrezia microcephala*. Phytochemistry 24:3029–3034
11. Agrawal PK (1989) Carbon-13 NMR of flavonoids. Elsevier Science, Amsterdam
12. Miserez F, Potterat O, Marston A, Mungai GM, Hostettmann K (1996) Flavonol glycosides from *Vernonia galamensis* ssp. *nairobiensis*. Phytochemistry 43:283–286
13. Iheya Y, Sugama K, Maruno M (1994) Chemical constituents from roots of *Polygala japonica*. Chem Pharm Bull 42:2305–2308

6

Chemical characterization, antioxidant and inhibitory effects of some marine sponges against carbohydrate metabolizing enzymes

Mohamed Shaaban[1,2*], Howaida I Abd-Alla[1], Amal Z Hassan[1], Hanan F Aly[3] and Mohamed A Ghani[4]

Abstract

Background: More than 15,000 marine products have been described up to now; Sponges are champion producers, concerning the diversity of products that have been found. Most bioactive compounds from sponges were classified into anti-inflammatory, antitumor, immuno- or neurosurpressive, antiviral, antimalarial, antibiotic, or antifouling. Evaluation of in vitro inhibitory effects of different extracts from four marine sponges versus some antioxidants indices and carbohydrate hydrolyzing enzymes concerned with diabetes mellitus was studied. The chemical characterizations for the extracts of the predominating sponges; SP1 and SP3 were discussed.

Methods: All chemicals served in the biological study were of analytical grade and purchased from Sigma, Merck and Aldrich. All kits were the products of Biosystems (Spain), Sigma Chemical Company (USA), Biodiagnostic (Egypt). Carbohydrate metabolizing enzymes; α-amylase, α-glucosidase, and β-galactosidase (EC3.2.1.1, EC3.2.1.20, and EC3.2.1.23, respectively) were obtained from Sigma Chemical Company (USA).

Results: Four marine sponges; Smenospongia (SP1), Callyspongia (SP2), Niphates (SP3), and Stylissa (SP4), were collected from the Red Sea at Egyptian coasts, and taxonomically characterized. The sponges' extracts exhibited diverse inhibitory effects on oxidative stress indices and carbohydrate hydrolyzing enzymes in linear relationships to some extent with concentration of inhibitors (dose dependant). The extracts of sponges (3, 1, and 2) showed, respectively, potent-reducing power. Purification and Chemical characterization of sponge 1 using NMR and mass spectroscopy, recognized the existence of di-isobutyl phthalate (1), di-n-butyl phthalate (2), linoleic acid (3), β-sitosterol (4), and cholesterol (5). Sponge 3 produced bis-[2-ethyl]-hexyl-phthylester (6) and triglyceride fatty acid ester (7).

Conclusion: Marine sponges are promising sources for delivering of bioactive compounds. Four marine sponges, collected from Red Sea at Egyptian coasts, were identified as Smenospongia (SP1), Callyspongia (SP2), Niphates (SP3), and Stylissa (SP4). The results demonstrated that different sponges extracts exhibited inhibitory effects on oxidative stress indices and carbohydrate hydrolyzing enzymes in linear relationships to some extent with concentration of inhibitors (dose dependant). The extracts of sponges (3, 1, and 2) showed, respectively, potent-reducing power. Chemical characterizations of sponges SP1 and SP3 were discussed. Based on this study, marine sponges are considered as talented sources for production of diverse and multiple biologically active compounds.

Keywords: Sponges, Chemical characterization, α-amylase, α-glucosidase, β-galactosidase, Antioxidants

* Correspondence: mshaaba_99@yahoo.com
[1]Chemistry of Natural Compounds Department, Division of Pharmaceutical Industries, National Research Centre, Dokki, Giza 12622, Egypt
[2]Institute of Organic and Biomolecular Chemistry, University of Göttingen, Tammannstraße 2, Göttingen D-37077, Germany
Full list of author information is available at the end of the article

Background

Pharmaceutical interest in sponges was aroused in the early 1950s by the discovery of a number of unknown nucleosides: spongothymidine and spongouridine in the marine sponge *Cryptotethia crypta* [1,2]. These nucleosides were the basis for the synthesis of Ara-C, the first marine-derived anticancer agent and the antiviral drug Ara-A [3]. Ara-C is currently used in the routine treatment of patients with leukaemia and lymphoma. More than 15,000 marine products have been described up to now [4,5]; Sponges are champion producers, concerning the diversity of products that have been found [6]. They are responsible for more than 5,300 different products and every year hundreds of new compounds are being discovered [4]. Most bioactive compounds from sponges can be classified as anti-inflammatory, antitumor, immuno- or neurosurpressive, antiviral, antimalarial, antibiotic, or antifouling [5-9].

Exogenous chemical and endogenous metabolic processes in the human body or in the digestive system might produce highly reactive free radicals, especially oxygen-derived radicals, which are capable of oxidizing biomolecules, resulting in cell death and tissue damage. Almost all organisms are well protected against free radical damage by anti-oxidative enzymes such as superoxide dismutase and catalase (CAT), or by chemicals such as carotenoids, polyphenols, and glutathione [10]. However, when the process of antioxidant protection becomes unbalanced, deterioration of physiological functions may occur resulting in diseases and accelerated aging. There is an increasing evidence, indicating that reactive oxygen species and free radical-mediated reactions are involved in degenerative or pathological events such as aging, cancer, coronary heart ailments, and Alzheimer's diseases [11]. Moreover, the suppression of the oxidative stress and inflammatory were responded through the inhibition of tumor necrosis factor β-(TNF-β) signaling [12]. Natural triterpenes isolated from different marine sponges inhibited iNOS expression and the activation of NF-β, while polyketides showed antitumoural activity [13]. Most screenings of secondary metabolites of biomedical importance from marine sponge extracts reported an inhibitory effects that turned out to be have strongly cytotoxic effects [14,15].

In this article, evaluation of *in vitro* inhibitory effects of different extracts from four marine sponges *Smenospongia* (SP1), *Callyspongia* (SP2), *Niphates* (SP3), and *Stylissa* (SP4) versus some antioxidants indices and carbohydrate hydrolyzing enzymes concerned with diabetes mellitus. The studied sponges were collected from Red Sea, Hurghada, at Egyptian coasts. Alternatively, the chemical characterizations for two extracts of the predominating sponges; SP1 and SP3 were discussed on the bases of different chromatographic and spectroscopic means. In accordance, di-isobutyl phthalate (**1**), di-*n*-butyl phthalate (**2**), linoleic acid (**3**), β-sitosterol (**4**), and cholesterol (**5**) were obtained from SP1; while SP3 delivered *bis*-[2-ethyl]-hexyl-phthylester (**6**) and triglyceride fatty acid ester (**7**).

Methods

Four marine sponges belonging to the genus *Smenospongia* (SP1), *Callyspongia* (SP2), *Niphates* (SP3) and *Stylissa* (SP4) were collected from Hurghada at El-Gouna and Shaa'b south Giffton island at depth of 5–8 m. Morphologically, the sponges were characterized and specimens of them were deposited at Red Sea Marine parks, P.O. Box 363-Hurgada, Red Sea, Egypt.

The four sponges were individually extracted by DCM–MeOH (2:1), followed by filtration, and the afforded DCM layers were extracted and evaporated *in vacuo* to dryness. Extracts of sponges were applied to a series of chromatographic purifications including Flash chromatography on silica gel (230–400 mesh), Size exclusion chromatography was done on Sephadex LH-20, and PTLC to isolate their produced bioactive compounds in pure forms. Purity of the yielded compounds were monitored by R_f values were measured on Polygram SIL G/UV$_{254}$ TLC cards. This lead to isolate the following compounds; Linoleic acid; (9Z,12Z)-9, 12-octadecanoic acid (**3**), β-sitosterol (**4**), Cholesterol (**5**), Di-(2-ethyl-hexyl)phthalate(DEHP)(**6**), and Triglyceride fatty acids mixture (**7**) were assigned with the aid of different spectroscopic means as follows; NMR (^{1}H & ^{13}C NMR) was served using Varian Unity 300 (300.145 MHz; and Varian Inova 600 (150.820 MHz) spectrometers. ESI MS (Thermo Finnigan LCQ with quaternary pump Rheos 4000 (Flux Instrument); Thermo Scientific, USA). EI MS (a Finnigan MAT 95 spectrometer (70 eV); Thermo Scientific, USA. GC-MS was measured on a Trace GC-MS Thermo Finnigan chromatograph, ionization mode EI (70 eV).

The *in vitro* antioxidant study of the sponges extracts were carried out using Carbohydrate metabolizing enzymes; α-amylase, α-glucosidase, and β-galactosidase. The antioxidant scavenging activity was studied using serial concentrations of different sponge extracts (10:1000 µg/mL) versus DPPH-free radical. The NO-free radical scavenging activity of extracts was determined according to the method of Sreejayan and Rao [16].

Results and discussion

Chemical characterization

Extracts of the four marine sponges *Smenospongia* (SP1), *Callyspongia* (SP2), *Niphates* (SP3), and *Stylissa* (SP4) were applied to a series of chromatographic applications, and hence to identify their bioactive constituents

Table 1 DPPH inhibition percent of the four sponges extracts

Concentrations	Extracts of the four sponges			
	SP1	SP2	SP3	SP4
10 µg/mL	10.85 ± 5.42^{c}	47.7 ± 0.84^{e}	26.31 ± 0.50^{d}	16.39 ± 4.63^{d}
50 µg/mL	10.77 ± 2.09^{c}	60.53 ± 0.50^{d}	26.00 ± 1.38^{d}	22.38 ± 1.23^{c}
100 µg/mL	18.09 ± 1.13^{b}	66.45 ± 0.29^{c}	34.04 ± 0.94^{c}	32.54 ± 2.14^{b}
500 µg/mL	22.81 ± 1.81^{b}	69.52 ± 0.97^{b}	37.39 ± 1.10^{b}	35.94 ± 1.42^{ab}
1000 µg/mL	30.64 ± 0.60^{a}	72.19 ± 0.69^{a}	40.17 ± 0.9^{a}	38.48 ± 0.70^{a}
LSD 5%	5.06	1.26	1.83	4.46

DPPH is expressed %; Data are mean ± SD of 3 replicates; Statistical analysis is carried out using one way analysis of variance (ANOVA) using CoStat: computer program; unshared superscript letters between treatments are significance values at $P < 0.001$.

chemically using diverse spectroscopic means. Both sponges, SP1 and SP3, were intensively studied. Five compounds were revealed from SP1; di-isobutyl phthalate (**1**), di-*n*-butyl phthalate (**2**), linoleic acid (**3**), *β*-sitosterol (**4**), and cholesterol (**5**). The first two esters, di-isobutyl phthalate (**1**, RT: 13.79, 100%) and di-*n*-butyl phthalate (**2**, RT: 14.84, 12%), were established by GC-MS analysis together with further unknown components of RT 19.03 (17%) and 20.01 (78%). Purification of sponge 3 (SP3) afforded *bis*-[2-ethyl]-hexyl-phthylester (**6**) and triglyceride fatty acid ester (**7**). In contrast, working up and purification of the extracts obtained from the remaining two sponges SP2 and SP4 delivered multimetabolites, however, with insufficient amounts for analysis.

Based on their chromatographic properties, spectroscopic means (NMR and MS), and comparison with authentic samples and literatures, the obtained structures were deduced as (9Z,12Z)-9,12-octadecanoic acid (**3**) [17], *β*-sitosterol (**4**) [18,19], cholesterol (**5**) [20-24],

phthalic acid *bis*-[2-ethyl-hexyl] ester (**6**) [25] and triglyceride fatty acid mixture (**7**) [26].

Biological study

The present results demonstrate the inhibitory effect of different extracts of marine sponges, on antioxidant indices and carbohydrate hydrolyzing enzymes *in vitro*. The 2,2-diphenyl-1-picrylhydrazyl (DPPH)-free radical scavenging effects of different extracts from marine sponge were shown in Table 1 and Figure 1. All the tested extracts showed appreciable free radical scavenging activities. Extract of SP2 has the strongest radical scavenging activity at different concentrations compared to other extracts followed by SP3 and SP4. However, SP1 showed the lowest radical scavenging activity. A dose–response relationship was found in the DPPH radical scavenging activity, at where the activity increased as the increase of extracts concentrations. SP2 extract was able to reduce the stable radical DPPH to the yellow color to give significant inhibitory percent 47.7 ± 0.84, 60.53 ± 0.50,

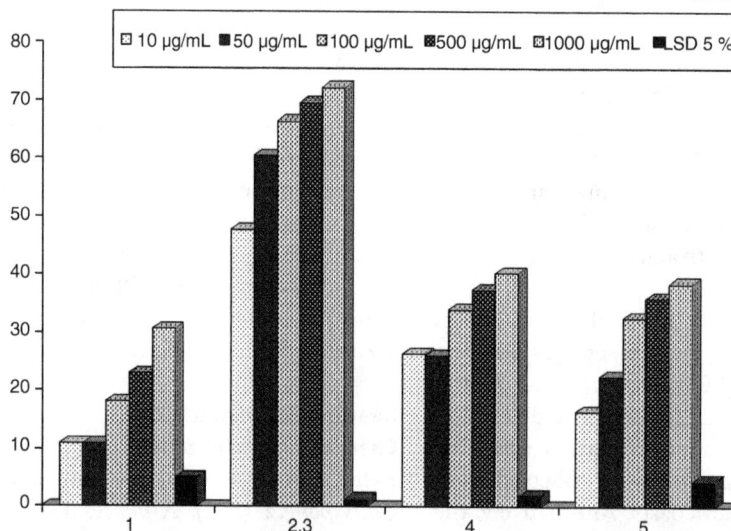

Figure 1 DPPH inhibition percent of the four sponges extracts.

Table 2 Inhibition percent of nitric oxide (NO) of the four sponges extracts

Concentrations	Extracts of the four sponges			
	SP1	SP2	SP3	SP4
10 g/mL	10.30 ± 4.29^c	37.60 ± 1.68^e	15.26 ± 6.94^d	13.50 ± 5.53^d
50 µg/mL	16.92 ± 3.25^c	39.16 ± 9.31^d	24.94 ± 2.89^c	21.41 ± 4.42^c
100 µg/mL	21.95 ± 2.86^b	52.13 ± 6.06^c	33.30 ± 2.65^{bc}	27.80 ± 4.32^{bc}
500 µg/mL	23.59 ± 1.01^b	56.58 ± 3.46^b	36.29 ± 5.18^{ab}	30.32 ± 2.74^b
1000 µg/mL	36.14 ± 2.93^a	53.85 ± 5.12^a	44.64 ± 4.29^a	41.24 ± 3.27^a
LSD 5%	5.06	1.28	8.49	7.59

NO is expressed as%; data are mean ± SD of 3 replicates; statistical analysis is carried out using one way analysis of variance (ANOVA) using CoStat: computer program; unshared superscript letters between treatments are significance values at $P < 0.001$.

66.45 ± 0.29, 69.52 ± 52, and $72.19 \pm 0.69\%$ at concentrations of 10, 50, 100, 500, and 1000 µg/mL, respectively. Alternatively, SP3 showed a reducing inhibitory percent of DPPH amounted 26.31 ± 0.50, 26.00 ± 1.38, 34.04 ± 0.94, 37.39 ± 1.10, and $40.17 \pm 0.9\%$ at the same concentrations of extracts, respectively. Moreover, SP4 showed a significant reducing activity of 16.39 ± 4.63, 22.38 ± 1.23, 32.54 ± 1.42, 35.94 ± 1.42, and $38.48 \pm 0.70\%$, respectively. Contrarily, SP1 exhibited the lowest reducing activity compared with aforementioned sponges extracts. The demonstrated inhibitory activity of the DPPH by the sponges extracts might be mainly attributed to their containing of some terpenoidal analogs [26].

Nitric oxide synthase (NOS) is catalyzing the production of nitric oxide (NO). Inducible NOS (iNOS) is expressed by vascular endothelial cells and smooth muscle cells in response to cytokines, unlike the two other types of NOS, which are constitutive. NO produced by iNOS is implicated in inflammatory diseases [27]. NO-free radicals scavenging capacity of the different marine sponges extracts were illustrated in Table 2 and Figure 2. The most reducing capacity was as well considered for SP2, which showed significant ability to reduce the activity of NO by 37.60 ± 1.68, 39.16 ± 9.13, 52.13 ± 6.06, 56.58 ± 3.46, and $53.85 \pm 5.12\%$ at concentrations of 10–1000 µg/mL. Alternatively, extract of SP3 exhibited lower significant reducing activity of NO (15.26 ± 6.94, 24.94 ± 2.89, 33.30 ± 2.65, 36.29 ± 5.18, and $44.64 \pm 4.29\%$) with lower extent than those of SP2. Based on the percentage scavenging values, it was remarked that SP1 and SP4 exhibited moderate scavenging effects with linear relationships in a dose-dependent manner. Consequently, extracts of SP1 and SP4 recorded potent reducing capability of 41.24 ± 3.27 and $38.17 \pm 3.01\%$, respectively, at a concentration of 1000 µg/mL. Tasi et al. [28] reported that food and phytochemicals exerts NO-suppressing activity via three different pathways: the blocking of iNOS expression, inactivation of iNOS catalytic function, and the scavenging NO. While NO suppressing effect was primarily

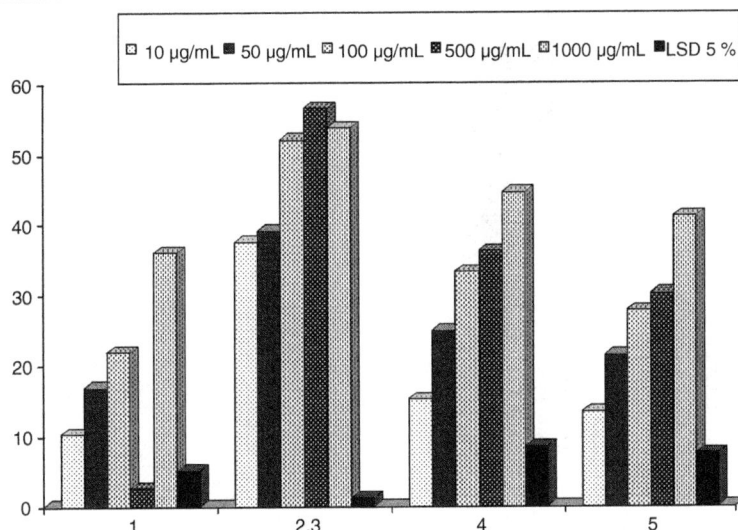

Figure 2 Inhibition percent of NO of the four sponges extracts.

Table 3 α-Amylase inhibition percent of four sponges extracts

Concentrations	Extracts of the four sponges			
	SP1	SP2	SP3	SP4
10 µg/mL	7.41 ± 2.61[e]	92.00 ± 1.21	18.26 ± 3.97[d]	15.44 ± 2.68[e]
50 µg/mL	18.75 ± 2.04[d]	94.35 ± 2.69	24.55 ± 4.03[c]	21.72 ± 3.20[d]
100 µg/mL	24.27 ± 3.07[c]	85.22 ± 4.92	32.56 ± 2.07[b]	27.38 ± 1.73[c]
500 µg/mL	29.05 ± 1.47[b]	89.38 ± 8.22	37.14 ± 0.89[ab]	33.75 ± 2.31[b]
1000 µg/mL	38.13 ± 0.64[a]	88.40 ± 7.29	37.97 ± 1.86[a]	44.59 ± 1.55[a]
LSD 5%	3.9	NS	5.18	4.32

α-amylase is expressed as %; data are mean ± SD of 3 replicates; statistical analysis is carried out using one way analysis of variance (ANOVA) using CoStat: computer program; unshared superscript letters between treatments are significance values at $P < 0.001$.

through regulation of cellular iNOS expression. The extracts' effects on the suppressing activity of NO production might be attributed to their containing of polyphenolic compounds or the triterpenes [29].

In alternative manner, extracts of the four sponges were tested against α-amylase carbohydrate hydrolyzing enzyme activity (Table 3, Figure 3). The four sponges showed potent α-amylase inhibitory activity, which may be potentially useful in control of obesity and diabetes. The inhibition of α-amylase by SP3 and SP4 was remarked to be as dose dependent, exhibiting the highest significant reducing activity 44.59 ± 1.55 and 43.64 ± 1.79%, respectively, at a concentration of 1000 µg/mL. Furthermore, extract of SP2 exhibited the most dramatic inhibiting effect at 10 and 50 µg/mL, displaying insignificant reducing activity 92.00 ± 1.21 and 94.35 ± 2.69%, respectively. In addition, the inhibitory activity of SP2

recorded 88.40 ± 7.29% at 1000 µg/mL. Consequently, SP3 recorded a significant inhibitory percent of 18.26 ± 3.97, 24.55 ± 4.03, 32.56 ± 2.07, 37.14 ± 0.89, and 37.97 ± 1.86% in a dose-dependent manner at 10, 50, 500, and 1000 µg/mL, respectively. The anti-amylase inhibitory activity may be due to the ability of phenolic compounds to interact with and/or inhibit proteins enzymes [30].

One therapeutic approach for treating diabetes is to decrease the post-prandial hyperglycemia. This is done by retarding the absorption of glucose through the inhibition of the carbohydrate hydrolyzing enzymes α-amylase, α-glucosidase, and β-galactosidase in the digestive tract. Inhibition of these enzymes delay carbohydrate digestion and prolong overall carbohydrate digestion time, causing a reduction in the rate of glucose absorption and consequently blunting the post-prandial plasma glucose rise [31]. Many natural resources have been

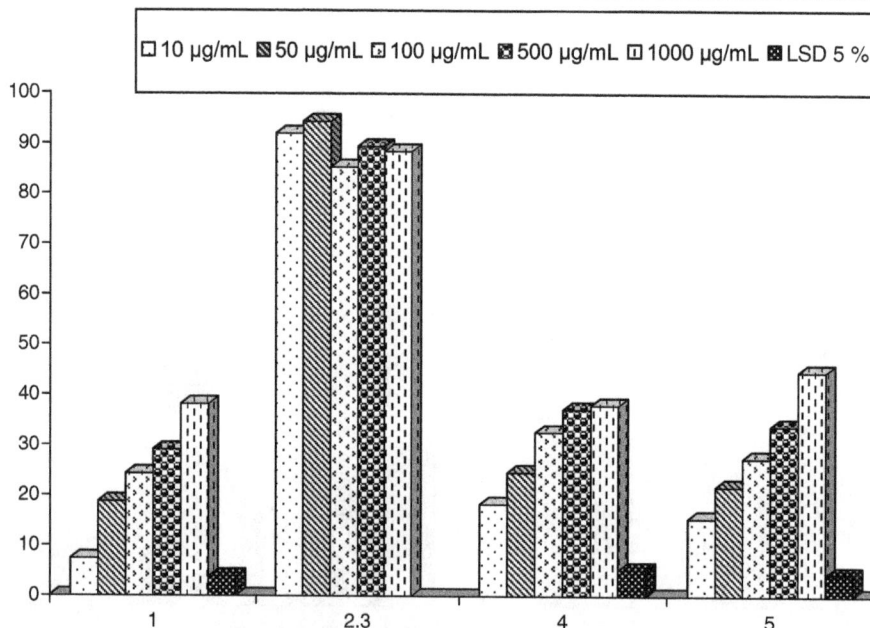

Figure 3 α-Amylase inhibition percent of four sponges extracts.

Table 4 α-Glucosidase inhibition percent of the four sponges extracts

Concentrations	Extracts of the four sponges			
	SP1	SP2	SP3	SP4
10 μg/mL	8.06 ± 3.51[c]	28.05 ± 1.63[c]	25.45 ± 4.04[c]	23.47 ± 4.56[c]
50 μg/mL	21.08 ± 4.68[b]	37.80 ± 2.55[b]	33.91 ± 3.15[b]	33.49 ± 1.76[b]
100 μg/mL	28.95 ± 1.44[a]	44.21 ± 2.87[a]	40.44 ± 4.34[a]	40.55 ± 3.08[a]
500 μg/mL	27.24 ± 3.45[a]	41.19 ± 1.59[ab]	37.42 ± 1.14[ab]	36.01 ± 1.78[ab]
1000 μg/mL	27.65 ± 2.37[a]	42.5 ± 2.24[a]	39.32 ± 2.60[ab]	38.11 ± 2.70[ab]
LSD 5%	5.97	4.14	5.93	5.93

β-galactosidase is expressed as %; data are mean ± SD of 3 replicates; statistical analysis is carried out using one way analysis of variance (ANOVA) using CoStat computer program; unshared superscript letters between treatments are significance values at $P < 0.001$.

investigated with respect to the antidiabetic and suppression of glucose. The inhibitory effects of the four sponges extracts against α-glucosidase carbohydrate hydrolyzing enzyme activity were further studied as listed in Table 4 and Figure 4. Remarkable greater inhibitory effects of SP2 (40.44 ± 4.34, 39.32 ± 2.60%) and SP3 (40.55 ± 3.08, 38.11 ± 2.70%) than SP1 (32.22 ± 3.96, 29.42 ± 0.62%) and SP4 (28.95 ± 1.44, 27.65 ± 2.37%) were deduced at concentrations of 100 and 1000 μg/mL, respectively. Hence, the inhibition percent was significantly correlated with the increase in concentration of inhibitors. The fact that α-glucosidase and α-amylase showed different inhibition kinetics seemed to be due to structural differences related to the origin of the enzymes [32]. Manosroi et al. [33] attributed the anti-diabetic, anti-inflammatory, anti-tumor, and anti-proliferative effect of many species, to their constituents of mono, sesquiterpenes, phenolic compounds, and flavonoids such as cinnamic acid, caffeic acid, and rosmarinic acid.

β-Galactosidase inhibitory activity was finally studied versus the sponges extracts as summarized in Table 5 and Figure 5. Accordingly, SP2 and SP3 provided additional support for the previous finding by having the strongest reducing activity at various concentrations. Hence, SP2 at 500 and 1000 μg/mL displayed significantly the highest inhibitory percent amounted 67.82 ± 3.94 and 66.86 ± 3.79%, respectively, followed by SP3 (62.63 ± 1.89 and 62.12 ± 4.37%, respectively) and SP4 (54.13 ± 2.44 and 55.08 ± 5.11%, respectively). In contrast, SP1 displayed a comparable insignificant inhibitory activity of 45.89 ± 4.91, 43.77 ± 4.5% at 500 and 1000 μg/mL, respectively. From the manipulated results, it was deduced significant increase in reducing activity with the increase in concentrations of the individual extract (linear relationship).

Experimental

The NMR spectra were measured on Varian Unity 300 (300.145 MHz) and Varian Inova 600 (150.820 MHz) spectrometers. ESI MS was recorded on a Thermo Finnigan LCQ with quaternary pump Rheos 4000 (Flux Instrument); Thermo Scientific, USA). EI mass spectra

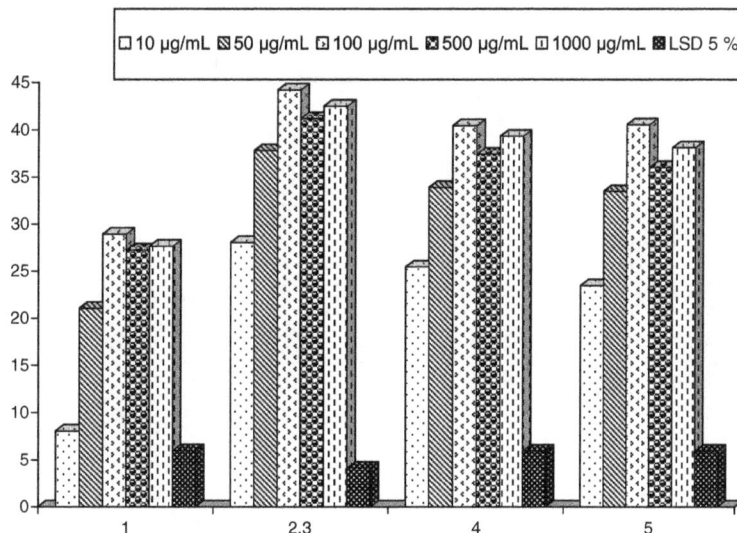

Figure 4 α-Glucosidase inhibition percent of the four sponges extracts.

Table 5 β-galactosidase inhibition percent of four sponges extracts

Concentrations	Extracts of the four sponges			
	SP1	SP2	SP3	SP4
10 µg/mL	11.45 ± 11.54[b]	51.35 ± 5.24[b]	23.09 ± 8.33[b]	17.24 ± 6.39[c]
50 µg/mL	31.58 ± 22.03[ab]	39.62 ± 8.53[bc]	34.78 ± 11.03[b]	35.35 ± 9.72[b]
100 µg/mL	27.37 ± 13.18[ab]	34.49 ± 11.82[c]	36.49 ± 8.35[b]	33.53 ± 11.38[b]
500 µg/mL	46.58 ± 8.22[a]	67.82 ± 3.94[a]	62.63 ± 1.89[a]	54.13 ± 2.44[a]
1000 µg/mL	42.21 ± 5.28[a]	66.86 ± 3.79[a]	62.12 ± 4.37[a]	55.08 ± 5.11[a]
LSD 5%	24.24	13.26	13.7	14.02

β-galactosidase is expressed as%; data are mean ± SD of 3 replicates; statistical analysis is carried out using one way analysis of variance (ANOVA) using CoStat computer program; unshared superscript letters between treatments are significance values at $P < 0.001$.

were recorded on a Finnigan MAT 95 spectrometer (70 eV); Thermo Scientific, USA. GC-MS was measured on a Trace GC-MS Thermo Finnigan chromatograph, ionization mode EI (70 eV), instrument equipped with a capillary column CP-Sil 8 CB for amines (length: 30 m; inside diameter: 0.25 mm; outside diameter: 0.35 mm; film thickness: 0.25 µm); Thermo Scientific., USA. The analysis was carried out at a programmed temperature: initial temperature 40°C (kept for 1 min), then increasing at a rate of 10°C/min and final temperature 280°C (kept for 10 min), injector temperature was 250°C and detector (mode of ionization: EI) temperature at 250°C, He was used as carrier gas at a flow rate of 1 mL/min, total run time 27 min, injection volume 0.2 µL. Flash chromatography was carried out on silica gel (230–400 mesh). R_f values were measured on Polygram SIL G/UV$_{254}$ TLC cards (Macherey-Nagel GmbH & Co. Germany). Size exclusion chromatography was done on Sephadex LH-20 (Lipophilic Sephadex, Amersham Biosciences Ltd. (purchased from Sigma-Aldrich Chemie, Steinheim, Germany). All chemicals served in the biological study

were of analytical grade, which were purchased from Sigma, Merck and Aldrich. All kits were the products of Biosystems (Spain), Sigma Chemical Company (USA), Biodiagnostic (Egypt).

Sponge materials, collection, and taxonomy

Four varieties of sponges belonging to the genus *Smenospongia* (SP1, olieve, 0.75 kg-wet), *Callyspongia* (SP2, faint brown, 0.42 kg-wet), *Niphates* (SP3, faint greenish olieve, 0.15 kg-wet), and *Stylissa* (SP4, orange, 0.16 kg-wet) were collected from two sites at Hurghada-coasts, Red Sea, Egypt. The first site located north Hurghada at El-Gouna, latitude N 27° 24ı 06.72ʺE 33° 41ı 13.52ʺ and the second site is Shaa'b south Giffton island latitude N 27° 10ı 04.61ʺ E 33° 57ı 04.87ʺ (Figure 6). The sponge samples were collected at depth of 5–8 m in September of 2010 (Figure 7) and stored in a freezer until extraction. The four species were morphologically characterized by Mohamed A Ghani, and specimens of them were deposited at Red Sea Marine parks, P.O. Box 363-Hurgada, Red Sea, Egypt.

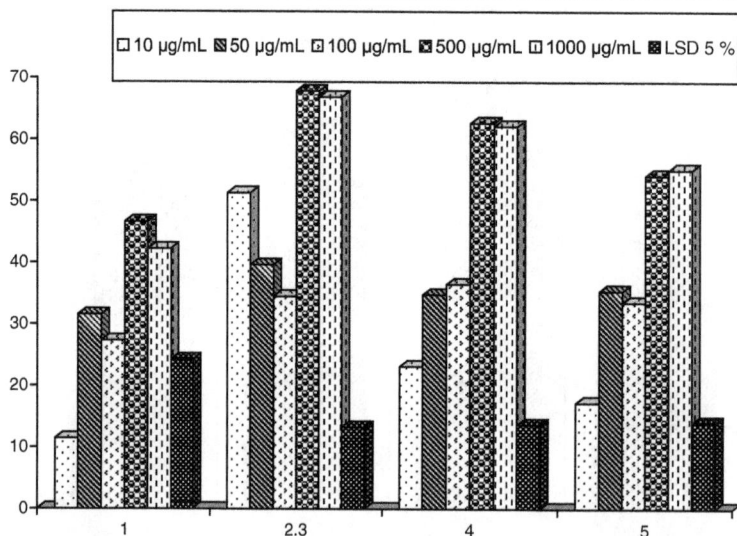

Figure 5 β-Galactosidase inhibition percent of four sponges extracts.

Chemical characterization, antioxidant and inhibitory effects of some marine sponges against...

43

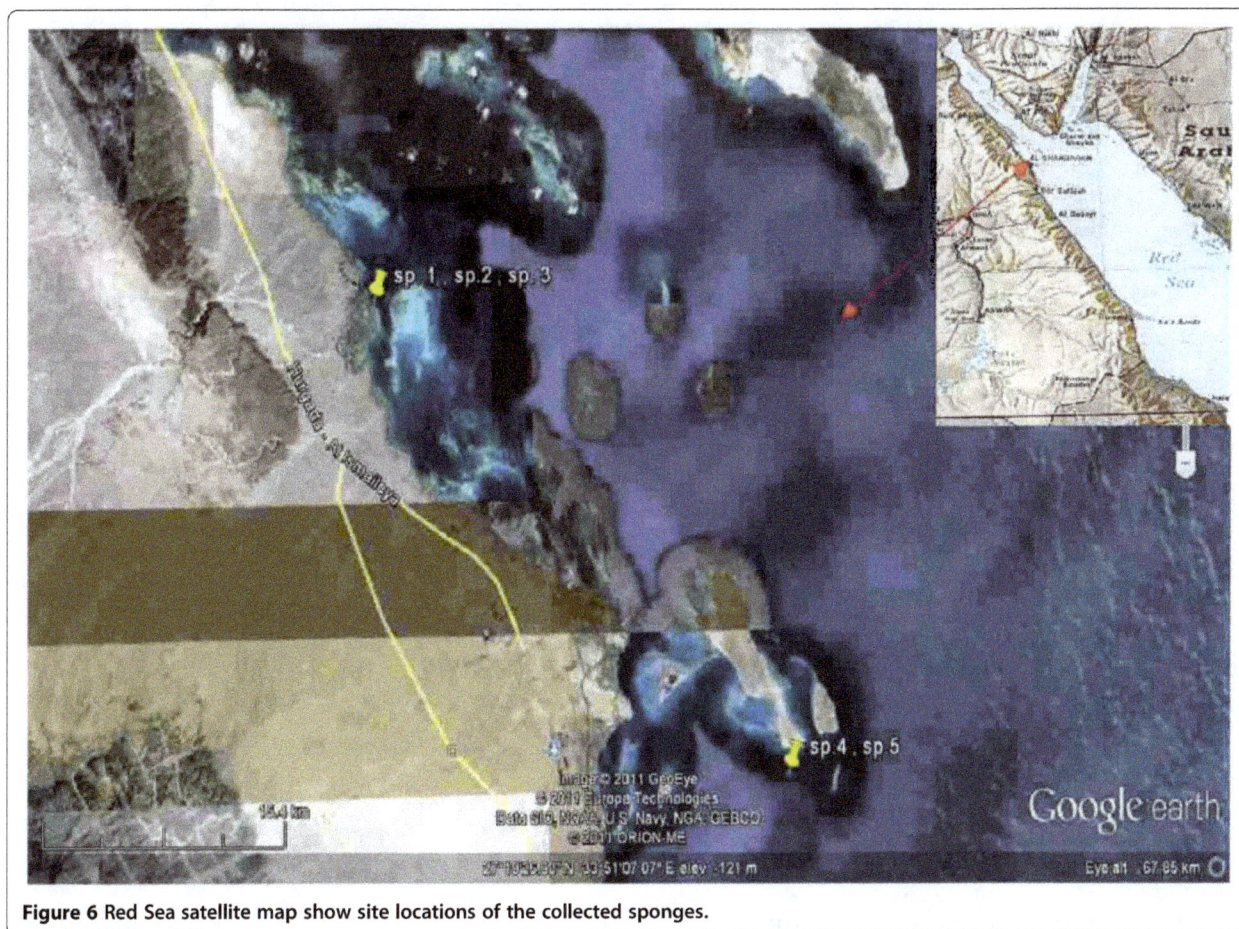

Figure 6 Red Sea satellite map show site locations of the collected sponges.

Taxonomically, the first species (SP1) was belonging to the genus *Smenospongia*, family Thorectidae. Morphologically, the SP1 is Massive with oscular mounds, displaying a bright to dark green coloration. The sponge exuded abundant mucus when handled, exhibiting blunt ends of primary protrude fibers on the surface [34,35]. The second sponge was belonging to the genus *Callyspongia* and family Callyspongiidae [36,37]. Morphologically, it showed bluish to pinkish tubes and sticky massive. Moreover, tissues of the sponge were clear away easily, leaving the clean skeleton. They inhabit as well in the coral reef habitat attached to corals or rocks. The third sponge was belonging to the genus *Niphates* and family Niphatidae. Morphologically, it is massive or encrusting, showing a bluish to purplish grayish cushions and repent branches [36,37]. Finally, the fourth sponge was belonging to the genus *Stylissa* and family Dictyonellidae [36,37]. Morphologically, it is bushy with orange color and tough consistency (Figures 7 and 8).

Extraction and isolation

The four sponges, *Smenospongia* (SP1), *Callyspongia* (SP2), *Niphates* (SP3) and *Stylissa* (SP4), were individually cut into small pieces and homogenized mechanically (Figure 1), treated with DCM–MeOH (2:1) and kept at approximately 5°C for 8 days. After filtration, the DCM layers were extracted and evaporated *in vacuo* to dryness affording 1.59, 0.57, 0.39, and 0.64 g from sponges SP1, SP2, SP3, and SP4, respectively. In contrast with sponges SP1 and SP3, both sponges SP2 and SP4 were applied to a series of chromatographic purifications using silica gel, Sephadex, and PTLC affording no desired and inadequate compounds amounts.

Working up and purification of smenospongia (SP1)

The afforded greenish-brown crude extract of sponge 1 (1.59 g) was subjected to silica gel (column 3×60 cm^2) and eluted with a cyclohexane-hexane/DCM/MeOH gradient. Based on the TLC monitoring, visualized by UV and spraying with anisaldehyde/sulfuric acid, five fractions were obtained: FI (0.1 g), FII (0.2 g), FIII (0.3 g), FIV (0.3 g), and FV (0.4). The fast oil fraction I was applied to GC-MS analysis, displaying a base signal (RT: 25.04 nm, 100%) of unknown component. Fraction II was likely subjected to GC-MS analysis showing four signals representing four components (RT: 13.79, 100%),

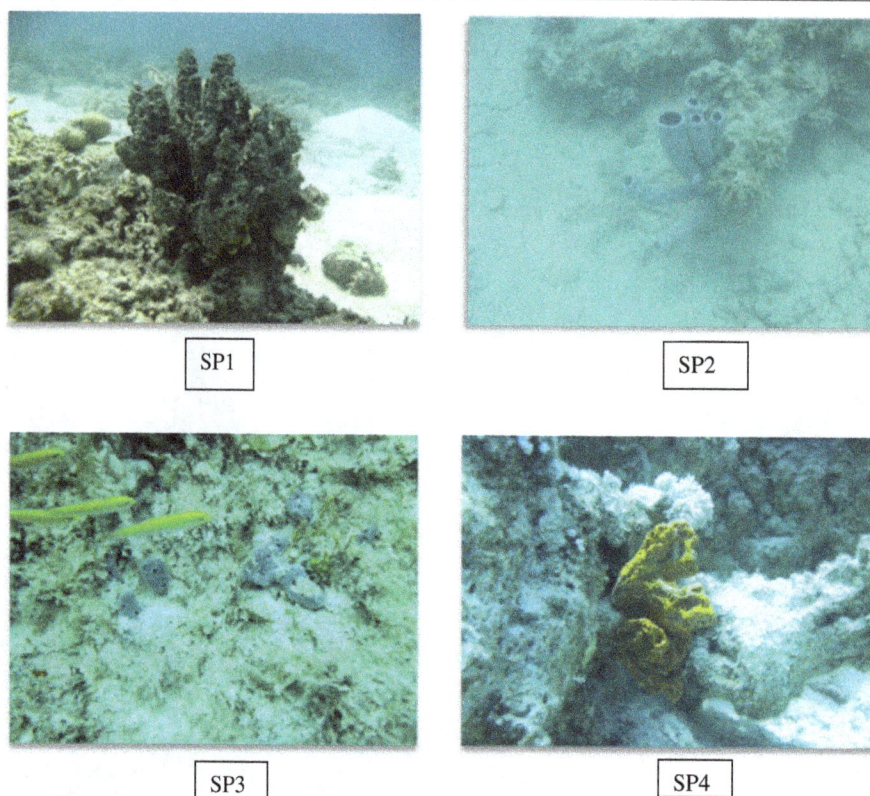

Figure 7 Photos of the collected four sponges (SP1, SP2, SP3, and SP4).

(14.84, 12%), (19.03, 17%), and (20.01, 78%); the first two of them were of unknown structures, while the last two were assigned as di-isobutyl phthalate (**1**) and di-*n*-butyl phthalate (**2**). TLC monitoring of the remaining fractions (III, IV, and V) recognized their similarity, and they were combined therefore (1.0 g). Consequently, the combined fractions were then chromatographed on silica gel using cyclohexane-DCM–MeOH gradient and after monitoring by TLC, six sub-fractions; PIa (80 mg), PIb (35 mg), PIc (70 mg), PId (95 mg), PIe (38 mg), and PIf (27 mg). An application of the sub-fractions to further purification using Sephadex LH-20 (DCM/MeOH, 60:40) was carried out. In accordance, sub-fractions PIa, PIc afforded a colorless semisolid of linoleic acid (**3**, 55 mg), while

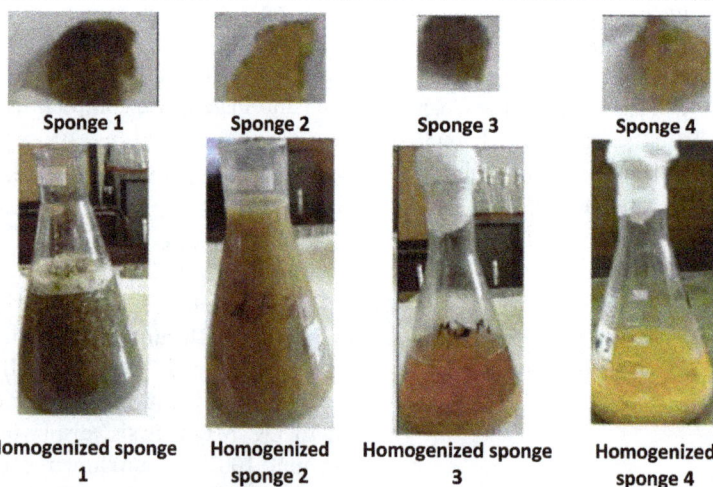

Figure 8 Macerated tissues of the collected four sponges (SP1, SP2, SP3, and SP4).

purification of sub-fraction PIb afforded a colorless solid of β-sitosterol (**4**, 27 mg). Purification of sub-fraction PId afforded a colorless oil of an olefinic fatty acid (23 mg). Similarly, purification sub-fraction PIe yielded a colorless oil of an additional olefinic acid. Finally, an application of the sub-fraction PIf to Sephadex LH-20 (DCM/MeOH, 60:40) resulted in β-sitosterol (**4**, 3 mg) and cholesterol (**5**, 3 mg).

Linoleic acid; (9Z,12Z)-9, 12-octadecanoic acid (3)

Colorless oil (55 mg) was detected as non-polar UV absorbing band at 254 nm and stained to blue when sprayed by anisaldehyde/sulfuric acid and heated. – $C_{18}H_{32}O_2$ (280). – $R_f = 0.90$ (CHCl$_3$/MeOH, 10%). – ^{1}H NMR (CDCl$_3$, 300 MHz): $\delta = 8.98$ (s, br, 1 H, COOH), 5.43–5.28 (m, 4 H, 9,10,12,13-CH), 2.78 (t, $^3J = 6.0$ Hz, 2 H, 11-CH$_2$), 2.38 (t, $^3J = 7.2$ Hz, 2 H, 2-CH$_2$), 2.08 (m, 4 H, 8,14-CH$_2$), 1.63 (m, 2 H, 3-CH$_2$), 1.42–1.23 (m, 14 H, 4,5,6,7,16,17-CH$_2$), 0.85 (m, 3 H, 18-CH$_3$). – ^{13}C/APT NMR (CDCl$_3$, 50 MHz): $\delta = 180.1$ (CO, C$_q$), 130.1 (CH-13), 129.9 (CH-9), 128.0 (CH-10), 127.8 (CH-12), 31.5 (CH$_2$-2), 29.6 (CH$_2$-16), 29.6 (CH$_2$-11), 29.5 (CH$_2$-14), 29.3 (CH$_2$-8), 29.1 (CH$_2$-7), 29.0 (CH$_2$-6), 29.0 (CH$_2$-5), 27.1 (CH$_2$-4), 25.6 (CH$_2$-3), 24.7 (CH$_2$-15), 22.5 (CH$_2$-17) 14.0 (CH$_2$-18). – EI MS (70 eV): m/z (%) = 280 (80), 264 (28), 137 (10), 124 (15), 110 (28), 95 (60), 81 (84), 67 (100), 55 (92), 41 (92).

β-sitosterol (4)

Colorless solid, UV non-absorbing, turned blue on spraying with anisaldehyde/sulfuric. – $C_{29}H_{50}O$ (414). – $R_f = 0.51$(CH$_2$Cl$_2$/CH$_3$OH 9: 0.5). – ^{1}H NMR (CDCl$_3$, 300 MHz): $\delta = 5.36$ (d, $J = 4.7$ Hz, 1 H, H-6), 3.53 (m, 1 H, H-3), 2.36–2.21 (m, 4 H, H$_2$-1, H$_2$-4), 2.01–1.93 (m, 2 H, H$_2$-6), 1.85–1.75 (m, 4 H), 1.58–1.43 (m, 5 H), 1.21–1.03 (m, 14 H), 0.99 (s, 3 H, CH$_3$-19), 0.94 (d, 3 H, $J = 6.1$ Hz, CH$_3$-21), 0.86 (d, 3 H, $J = 6.2$ Hz, CH$_3$-26), 0.84 (d, 3 H, $J = 6.2$ Hz, CH$_3$-27), 0.79 (t, 3 H, $J = 6.7$, CH$_3$-29), 0.67 (s, 3 H, CH$_3$-18). – EI-MS (70 eV): m/z (%) = 414 ([M]$^+$, 100), 396 ([M-H$_2$O]$^+$, 37), 381 (21), 329 (34), 303 (41), 283 (16), 259 (10), 241 (22), 227 (9), 206 (11), 189 (18), 173 (22), 151 (13), 135 (25), 123 (21), 109 (18), 83 (13), 43 (15).

Cholesterol (5)

Colorless solid, UV non-absorbing, turned blue on spraying with anisaldehyde/sulfuric. – $C_{27}H_{46}O$ (386). – $R_f = 0.47$(CH$_2$Cl$_2$/CH$_3$OH 9:0.5). – ^{1}H NMR (CDCl$_3$, 300 MHz): $\delta = 5.37$ (d, $J = 4.7$ Hz, 1 H, H-6), 3.51 (m, 1 H, H-3), 2.35–2.19 (m, 4 H, H$_2$-1, H$_2$-4), 2.02–1.94 (m, 2 H, H$_2$-6), 1.85–1.75 (m, 4 H), 1.58–1.43 (m, 6 H), 1.18–1.02 (m, 12 H), 0.99 (s, 3 H, CH$_3$-19), 0.94 (d, 3 H, $J = 6.1$ Hz, CH$_3$-21), 0.86 (d, 3 H, $J = 6.2$ Hz, CH$_3$-26), 0.84 (d, 3 H, $J = 6.2$ Hz, CH$_3$-27), 0.67 (s, 3 H, CH$_3$-18). – ^{13}C NMR

(CDCl$_3$, 75 MHz): $\delta = 42.7$ (C$_q$, C-13), 36.7 (CH, C-1), 140.6 (C$_q$, C-5), 56.4 (CH, C-14), 50.2 (CH, C-9), 31.8 (CH, C-8), 56.3 (CH, C-17) 121.8 (CH, C-6), 40.0 (CH$_2$, C-24), 32.0 (CH$_2$, C-16), 21.0 (CH$_2$, C-11), 24.3 (CH$_2$, C-15), 37.3 (C$_q$, C-10), 28.2 (CH, C-25), 42.3 (C$_q$, C-4), 35.9 (CH$_2$, C-12), 12.1 (CH$_3$, C-18), 31.7 (CH$_2$, C-7), 31.2 (CH$_2$, C-2), 71.5 (CH, C-3), 19.4 (CH$_3$, C-19), 24.0 (CH$_2$, C-23), 36.3 (CH$_2$, C-22), 18.8 (CH$_3$, C-21), 35.8 (CH, C-20), 22.6 (CH$_3$, 26), 22.6 (CH$_3$, 27). – EI-MS (70 eV): m/z (%) = 386 ([M]$^+$, 100), 368 ([M-H$_2$O]$^+$, 36), 353 (20), 301 (32), 275 (40), 255 (18), 231 (12), 213 (21), 199 (8), 178 (12), 161 (16), 145 (21), 133 (12), 107 (24), 95 (20), 81 (17), 55 (14), 43 (16).

Working up and purification of callyspongia (SP3)

The afforded reddish-brown crude extract of sponge 3 (0.39 g) was subjected to silica gel column (2 × 50 cm) and eluted with a cyclohexane-hexane/DCM/MeOH gradient. According to TLC monitoring, visualized by UV and spraying with anisaldehyde/sulfuric acid, three fractions were obtained: FIa (140 mg), FIb (70 mg), and FIc (60 mg). Purification of FIa using Sephadex LH-20 (DCM/MeOH, 60:40) afforded a colorless oil of phthylester (**6**, 80 mg). Purification of FIb by Sephadex LH-20 (DCM/MeOH, 60:40) resulted in a colorless oil of triglyceride fatty acid ester mixture (**7**, 35 mg). An application of fraction FIc to purification with Sephadex LH-20 (DCM/MeOH, 60:40) afforded a colorless solid of cholesterol (**5**, 28 mg).

Di-(2-ethylhexyl)phthalate(DEHP)(6)

UV-absorbing (254 nm) turned intensive violet on spraying with anisaldehyde/sulfuric acid after heating, and changed latter as blue. – $C_{24}H_{38}O_4$ (390). – $R_f = 0.90$; CHCl$_3$. – ^{1}H NMR (CDCl$_3$, 300 MHz): $\delta = 7.70$ (m, 2 H), 7.50 (m, 2 H), 4.25 (d, $^3J = 5$ Hz, 2 H), 1.80–1.20 (br m, 18 H), 1.00–0.75 (br m, 12 H). – ^{13}C NMR (CDCl$_3$, 75 MHz): $\delta = 167.7$ (C$_q$-1′,1″), 132.4 (C$_q$-1,2), 130.9 (CH-3,6), 128.8 (CH-4,5), 68.1 (CH$_2$-2′, 2″), 38.7 (CH-3′,3″), 30.3 (CH$_2$-4′,4″), 28.9 (CH$_2$-5′,5″), 22.9 (CH$_2$-6′,6″), 14.0 (CH$_3$-7′,7″), 23.7 (CH$_2$-8′,8″), 10.9 (CH$_3$-9′,9″). – EI-MS (70 eV): m/z: 390 (3), 279 (20), 149 (64). – CI-MS (NH$_3$): 798 ([2 M + NH$_4$]$^+$, 62 %), 408 ([M + NH$_4$]$^+$, 100), 391 ([M + H]$^+$, 65).

Triglyceride fatty acids mixture (7)

Colorless oil, turned violet by anisaldehyde/sulfuric acid; – $R_f = 0.78$ (CH$_2$Cl$_2$). – ^{1}H NMR (300 MHz, CDCl$_3$): $\delta = 5.37$ (m, 2 H), 5.34 (m 2 H), 5.27 (m, 1 H), 4.30 (dd, 2 H, $J = 11.9$, 4.3 Hz), 4.14 (dd, 2 H, $J = 11.9$, 6.0 Hz), 2.81 (m, 2 H), 2.31 (m, 2 H), 2.02 (m, 4 H), 1.61 (m, 2 H), 1.40–1.20 (m, 22 H), and 0.88 (t, 9 H, $J = 6.9$ Hz). – ^{13}C NMR (75 MHz, CDCl$_3$): $\delta = 172.9$ (2C$_q$, CO), 172.5 (C$_q$, CO), 129.5 (2CH), 129.1 (2CH), 132–127 (further mCH), 68.8

(CH), 62.5 (2CH$_2$), 34.0 (CH$_2$), 31.9 (CH$_2$), 29.8 (CH$_2$), 29.7 (CH$_2$) 29.6 (CH$_2$) 29.5 (CH$_2$) 29.4 (CH$_2$) 29.3 (CH$_2$) 29.2 (CH$_2$) 29.0 (CH$_2$) 29.1 (CH$_2$), 29.0 (CH$_2$), 27.2 (CH$_2$), 25.6 (CH$_2$), 24.9 (CH$_2$), 22.7 (CH$_2$) and 14.1 (CH$_3$).

In vitro antioxidant study
Purified enzymes
Carbohydrate metabolizing enzymes; α-amylase, α-glucosidase, and β-galactosidase (EC3.2.1.1, EC3.2.1.20, and EC3.2.1.23, respectively) were obtained from Sigma Chemical Company (USA).

The antioxidant scavenging activity
The activity of serial concentrations of different sponge extracts (10:1000 µg/mL) on DPPH-free radical will performed according to the method of McCue et al. [36] and Katsube et al. [37]. The decrease in optical density of DPPH$^-$ is calculated compared with a control substance as follows:

$$\%\text{Inhibition} = A_\text{control} - A_\text{sample} \times 100$$

Determination of NO-free radical scavenging activity
NO-scavenging activity of extracts was determined according to the method of Sreejayan and Rao [16].

Determination of a-amylase
α-Amylase was determined according to the method of Bernfeld [38].

Determination of β-galactosidase activity
β-galactosidase was measured by the method of Sánchez and Hardisson [39].

Estimation of a-glucosidase activity
α-glucosidase activity was determined according to the method of Kapustka et al. [40] and Kim et al. [32].

Conclusions
In conclusion, this study was performed to investigate the effects of the extracts of four marine sponges on some biochemical parameters including antioxidant and three different carbohydrate hydrolyzing enzymes (α-amylase, β-galactosidase, and α-glucosidase). These sponges were collected from Red Sea at Egyptian coasts, which were taxonomically belonged to the genus of *Smenospongia* (SP1), *Callyspongia* (SP2), *Niphates* (SP3), and *Stylissa* (SP4). The results demonstrated that different extracts exhibited inhibitory effects on oxidative stress indices and carbohydrate hydrolyzing enzymes in linear relationships to some extent with concentration of inhibitors (dose dependant). The extracts of sponges (3, 1, and 2) showed, respectively, potent-reducing power. Chemical characterizations of

sponges SP1 and SP3 were discussed, at where di-isobutyl phthalate (**1**), di-*n*-butyl phthalate (**2**), linoleic acid (**3**), β-sitosterol (**4**), and cholesterol (**5**) were obtained from sponge SP1; while sponge SP3 produced *bis*-[2-ethyl]-hexyl-phthylester (**6**) and triglyceride fatty acid ester (**7**).

Competing interests
The authors declare that they have no competing interests.

Authors' contributions
MS is the principle investigator of the research work, who is responsible for points of research in the manuscript. Additionally, he is the responsible investigator for the structural elucidation of the isolated bioactive compounds, in additions to control the whole manuscript research points. HIA-A and AZH are the chemists who mainly made the main work of extraction and isolation of the bioactive constituents obtained from the sponges under study. HFA is the main investigator who studied the whole biological part of the obtained sponges extracts of the research work under study. MAG is the main investigator who collected the sponges under study together with their full taxonomical study. All authors read and approved the final manuscript.

Acknowledgments
The authors are deeply thankful to Prof. H. Laatsch for his Lab facilities and unlimited support. This research work has been financed during German Egyptian Scientific Projects (GESP) No. 7.

Author details
[1]Chemistry of Natural Compounds Department, Division of Pharmaceutical Industries, National Research Centre, Dokki, Giza 12622, Egypt. [2]Institute of Organic and Biomolecular Chemistry, University of Göttingen, Tammannstraße 2, Göttingen D-37077, Germany. [3]Department of Therapeutic Chemistry, National Research Centre, Dokki, Giza 12622, Egypt. [4]Red Sea Marine Parks, P.O. Box 363, Hurghada, Red Sea, Egypt.

References
1. Bergmann W, Feeney RJ: **The isolation of a new thymine pentoside from sponges.** *J Am Chem Soc* 1950, **72**:2809–2810.
2. Bergmann W, Feeney RJ: **Contributions to the study of marine products. XXXII. The nucleosides of sponges. I.** *J Org Chem* 1951, **16**:981–987.
3. Proksch P, Edrada R, Ebel R: **Drugs from the seas-current status and microbiological implications.** *Appl Microbiol Biotechnol* 2002, **59**:125–134.
4. Faulkner DJ: **Marine natural products.** *Nat Prod Rep* 2002, **19**:1–48.
5. Blunt JW, Copp BR, Hu W-P, Munro MHG, Northcote PT, Prinsep MR: **Marine natural products.** *Nat Prod Rep* 2009, **26**:170–244.
6. Gordaliza M: **Review: cytotoxic terpene quinones from marine sponges.** *Mar Drugs* 2010, **8**:2849–2870.
7. Zhu YM, Shen JK, Wang HK, Cosentino LM, Lee KH: **Synthesis and anti-HIV activity of oleanolic acid derivatives.** *Bioorg Med Chem Lett* 2001, **11**:3115–3118.
8. Hsu YL, Kuo PL, Lin CC: **Proliferative inhibition, cell–cycle dysregulation and induction of apoptosis by ursolic acid in human non-small cell lung cancer A549 cell.** *Life Sci* 2004, **75**:2303–2316.
9. Yogeeswari P, Sriram D: **Betulinic acid and its derivatives: a review on their biological properties.** *Curr Med Chem* 2005, **12**:657–666.
10. Gulcin I, Buyukokuroglu ME, Oktay M, Kufrevioglu OI: **On the *in vitro* antioxidative properties of melatonin.** *J Pineal Res* 2002, **33**:167–171.
11. Wang H, Cao G, Prior RL: **Total antioxidant capacity of fruits.** *J Agr Food Chem* 1996, **44**:701–705.
12. Dudhgaonkar S, Thyagarajan A, Sliva D: **Suppression of the inflammatory response by triterpenes isolated from the mushroom *Ganoderma lucidum*.** *Int Immunopharmacol* 2009, **9**:1272–1280.
13. Berrue F, Thomas OP, Laville R, Prado S, Golebiowski J, Fernandezc R, Amadea P: **The marine sponge *Plakortis zyggompha*: a source of original bioactive polyketides.** *Tetrahedron* 2007, **63**:2328–2334.
14. Teeyapant R, Woerdenbag HJ, Kreis P, Hacher J, Wray V: **Antibiotic and cytotoxic activity of K. Cyclostelletamines A-F; pyridine alkaloids which

inhibit brominated compound from marine sponge *Verongia aerobinding* of quinuclidinyl benzilate (QNB) to muscarinic acephoba. *Z Naturforsch* 1993, **48C**:939–945.

15. Bartolotta SA, Scuteri MA, Hick AS, Palermo J, Rodriguez BMF, Hajdu E, Mothes B, Lerner C, Campos M, Carballo MA: **Evaluation of genotoxic biomarkers in extracts of marine sponges from Argentinean South Sea.** *J Exp Mar Biol Ecol* 2009, **369**:144–147.

16. Sreejayan N, Rao MNA: **Nitric oxide scavenging by curcuminoids.** *J Pharm Pharmacol* 1997, **49**:105–107.

17. Khotimchenko S: **V: fatty acids of brown algae from the Russian far east.** *Phytochemistry* 1998, **49**:2363–2369.

18. Viqar Uddin A, Shaheen B: **Isolation of β-sitosterol and ursolic acid from** *Morinda Citrifolia* **Linn.** *J Chem Soc Pak* 1980, **2**:71.

19. Md AM, Tareq SM, Apu AS, Basak D, Islam MS: **Isolation and identification of compounds from the leaf extract of** *Dillenia indica* **Linn.** *Bangladesh Pharm J* 2010, **13**:49–53.

20. Laatsch H: *AntiBase: a data base for rapid dereplication and structure determination of microbial natural products.* Weinheim, Germany: Wiley-VCH; 2010. http://wwwuser.gwdg.de/~ucoc/laatsch/AntiBase.htm.

21. Volkman JK, Farmer CL, Barrett SM, Sikes EL: **Unusual dihydroxysterols as chemotaxonomic markers for microalgae from the order Pavlovales (Haptophyceae).** *J Phycol* 1997, **33**:1016–1023.

22. Subramanian A, Joshi BS, Roy AD, Gupta RRV, Dang RS: **NMR spectroscopic identification of cholesterol esters, plasmalogen and phenolic glycolipids as fingerprint markers of human intracranial tuberculomas.** *NMR Biomed* 2008, **21**:272–288.

23. Ahmad VU, Memon AH, Ali MS, Perveen S, Shameel M: **Somalenone, a C26 sterol from the marine red alga** *Melanothamnus somalensis.* *Phytochemistry* 1996, **42**:1141–1143.

24. Sherif EAB, Shaaban M, Elkholy YM, Helal MH, Hamza AS, Masoud MS, El Safty MM: **Chemical composition and biological activity of ripe pumpkin fruits (*Cucurbita pepo* L.) cultivated in Egyptian habitats.** *Nat Prod Res* 2011, **25**:1524–1539.

25. Sani UM, Pateh UU: **Isolation of 1,2-benzenedicarboxylic acid bis(2-ethylhexyl) ester from methanol extract of the variety minor seeds of** *Ricinus communis* **Linn. (Euphorbiaceae).** *Nig J Pharm Sci* 2009, **8**:107–114.

26. Sato S, Kuramoto M, Ono N: **Ircinamine B, bioactive alkaloid from marine sponge Dactylia sp.** *Tetrahedron Lett* 2006, **47**:7871–7873.

27. Brinker M, Ma J, Lipsky PE, Raskin I: **Medical chemistry and pharmacology of genus** *Tripterygium* **(Celastraceae).** *Phytochemistry* 2007, **68**:732–766.

28. Tasi PJ, Tsai TH, Yu CH, Ho SC: **Evaluation of no-suppressing activity of several Mediterranean culinary spices.** *Food Chem Toxicol* 2007, **45**:440–447.

29. Diouf PN, Stevanovic T, Boutin Y: **The effect of extraction process on polyphenol content, triterpene composition and bioactivity of yellow birch (*Betula alleghaniensis* Britton) extracts.** *Ind Crops Prod* 2009, **30**:297–303.

30. Rohn S, Rawel HM, Kroll J: **Inhibitory effects of plant phenols on the activity of selected enzymes.** *J Agric Food Chem* 2002, **50**:3566–3571.

31. Rhabasa-Lhoret R, Chiasson JL: **Alpha glucosidase inhibitors.** In *International textbook of diabetes mellitus*, 3rd edn, Volume 1. Edited by Defronzo RA, Ferrannini E, Keen H, Zimmet P. UK: John Wiley & Sons Ltd; 2004:901–914.

32. Kim YM, Jeong YK, Wang MH, Lee WY, Rhee HI: **Inhibitory effect of Pine erglycemia.** *Nutrition* 2005, **21**:756–761.

33. Manosroi J, Dhumtanom P, Manosroi A: **Anti-proliferative activity of essential oil extracted from Thai medicinal plants on KB and P388 cell lines.** *Cancer Lett* 2006, **235**:114–120.

34. Pulitzer-Finali G: **A collection of west Indian Demospongiae (Porifera).** In *In appendix, a list of the Demospongiae hitherto recorded from the West Indies.* 86th edition. Gincoma Doria: Annali de1 musco civico di storia naturale; 1986:65–216.

35. John N, Hooper A, Van Soest RWM: *Systema porifera.* A guide to the classification of sponges: Kluwer Academic/Plenum Publishers, New York; 2002.

36. McCue P, Horii A, Shetty K: **Solid-state bioconversion of phenolic antioxidants from defatted soybean powders by** *Rhizopus oligosporus*: **role of carbohydrate-cleaving enzymes.** *J Food Biochem* 2003, **27**:501–514.

37. Katsube T, Tabata H, Ohta Y, Yamasaki Y, Anuurad E, Shiwaku K, Yamane Y: **Screening for the antioxidant activity in edible plant products:** comparison of low-density lipoprotein oxidation assay, DPPH radical scavenging assay, and Folin–Ciocalteu assay. *J Agric Food Chem* 2004, **52**:2391–2396.

38. Bernfeld P: **Amylases, alpha and beta.** *Meth Enzymol* 1955, **1**:149–158.

39. Sánchez J, Hardisson C: **Glucose inhibition of galactose-induced synthesis of β-galactosidase in** *Streptomyces violaceus.* *Arch Crobial* 1979, **125**:111–114.

40. Kapustka LA, Annala AE, Swanson WC: **The peroxidase-glucose oxidase system: a new method to determine glucose liberated by carbohydrate degradino soil enzymes.** *Plant Soil* 1981, **63**:487–490.

7

An anti-inflammatory and anti-microbial flavone glycoside from flowers of *Cleome viscosa*

Musiri Maruthai Senthamilselvi, Devarayan Kesavan and Nagarajan Sulochana[*]

Abstract

Background: Natural products isolated from plant sources have been demonstrated as potential candidates against several ailments. The scientific investigations on the underlying principles of phytotherapy can pave way for the convergence of traditional medicines and modern science and technologies.

Results: Quercetin 3-*O*-(2″-acetyl)-glucoside obtained from ethyl acetate fraction of *Cleome viscosa* is studied against inflammatory of carrageenan-induced rat paw edema (*in vivo*) and microbial activity on (*in vitro*). The structure of the glycoside is confirmed by means of hydrogen-1 nuclear magnetic resonance spectroscopy, carbon nuclear magnetic resonance spectroscopy, attached proton test, and mass spectrum. The flavonoid glycoside showed significant anti-inflammatory activity of on carrageenan-induced rat paw edema (*in vivo*) and anti-microbial activity (*in vitro*) on *Staphylococcus aureus* (gram positive) and *Escherichia coli* (gram negative). The anti-inflammatory effect of the flavonoid glycoside may be due to the inhibition of prostaglandin synthesis. Selective toxicity with flavonoid glycoside towards the gram-positive bacteria was found on *S. aureus*.

Conclusions: The present study reveals the anti-inflammatory and antimicrobial activities of an isolated quercetin 3-*O*-(2″-acetyl)-glucoside from a natural source (*C. viscosa*).

Keywords: Cleome viscosa, Anti-inflammatory, Anti-microbial, Rat paw edema, Flavonoid glycoside

Background

Natural products isolated from plant sources have been demonstrated as potential candidates against several ailments [1,2]. Our research group has been actively involved in exploring the plant sources for isolation of bioactive compounds as well as their medicinal properties [2-7]. *Cleome viscosa* belongs to the Capparidaceae family. They are distributed in tropical regions. In India, the family is represented by seven genera and about 53 species occurring mostly in the western and southern India. This plant is a common weed found all over the plains of India, with bright yellow flowers. Seeds of this plant are carminative and antiseptic. The juice of the leaves has a pungent flavor.

The methanol extract of *C. viscosa* had been reported to show promising analgesic activity [8], psychopharmacological effects [9], and antipyretic activity [10]. The ethanolic extracts of the leaves, flowers, and roots were tested for antimicrobial activity [11]. The aqueous seed extract [12] as well as ethanolic extract of the leaf powder [13] had showed hepatoprotective activity against carbon tetrachloride-induced liver damage in experimental animal. Crude alcohol and aqueous extracts of the seeds of *C. viscosa* Linn. (Capparidaceae) were investigated for their anthelmintic activity against *Pheretima posthuma*. In the present investigation, the flavonoid glucoside responsible for anti-inflammatory and anti-microbial activity of *C. viscosa* had been isolated and its activities were investigated through *in vivo* and *in vitro* studies.

Methods

The extraction of the flavonoid glucoside was performed by means of standard fractional distillation method. The detailed experimental procedure is given under experimental section. UV spectra were obtained from on PerkinElmer UV/Vis Spectrometer 301 (PerkinElmer Inc., Waltham, MA, USA). NMR spectra were recorded on Bruker AMX400 Spectrometer (Bruker Corporation, Billerica, MA, USA) at 400.13 MHz for ^{1}H and 75 MHz for ^{13}C using standard Bruker pulse sequences. Tetramethyl

* Correspondence: n.sulocha@gmail.com
Department of Chemistry, National Institute of Technology, Tiruchirappalli, Tamil Nadu 620 015, India

silane was used as an internal standard. Mass spectra were recorded in Auto spec FAB$^+$ Magnet Bpm: 55 BPI 446544 (AutoSpec Premier, Waters Coporation, MA, USA).

Results and discussion

The fresh yellow flowers of *C. viscosa* have been found to contain quercetin 3-O-(2''-acetyl)-glucoside. The UV spectrum of the glycoside showed two major absorption peaks at 355 (band I) and 257 nm (band II), showing the presence of a flavonol skeleton. Presence of a 4'-OH group is evident from the bathochromic shift of 48 nm in the NaOMe spectrum of the glycoside. A bathochromic shift of 37 and 77 nm respectively, in AlCl$_3$-HCl spectrum and AlCl$_3$ spectrum, was the evidence for the presence of a 5-OH group. In the AlCl$_3$-HCl spectrum of the glycoside and aglycone, three absorption peaks and a shoulder were seen, which was yet another evidence for the presence of a free 5-OH group. A bathochromic shift of 15 nm in band II observed in the NaOAc spectrum of the glycoside and 16 nm in band II of aglycone indicated the presence of a free 7-OH group. The presence of a 7-OH group was further confirmed by the presence of the shoulder at 327 nm in the NaOMe spectrum of both glycoside and aglycone ring which could be further evidenced from the shift of +21 nm noticed in the glycoside and +17 nm noticed in the case of aglycone in the addition of NaOAc-H$_3$BO$_3$. In the case of AlCl$_3$ spectrum of the glycoside, an absorption peak was present at 432 nm (band I), which upon addition of HCl was reduced by 40 nm. This shows the presence of O-dihydroxyl group in the B ring. In the MeOH spectrum of the glycoside, band I was seen at 355 nm and that of the aglycone it was seen at 372 nm, indicating the glycosylation at C-3.

In the hydrogen-1 nuclear magnetic resonance spectroscopy (^{1}H-NMR) spectrum (400 MHz, dimethyl sulfoxide, (DMSO)-d_6, tetramethylsilane, TMS) of the glycoside, the protons at C-6 and C-8 appear as doublets at δ 6.20 and δ 6.40 ppm, respectively. The 5-OH proton appears at δ 12.64 ppm, as a distinct singlet. The C-5' proton appears as doublet due to ortho-coupling with C-6' proton at δ 6.86 ppm. The C-2' and C-6' protons appear at δ 7.58 ppm. The hydrogen of C-1' of the sugar moiety is found at δ 5.5 ppm. The remaining glucosyl protons appear in the range of δ 3.0 to 3.5 ppm. The CH$_3$ protons of the acetyl group appear as a singlet at δ 1.92 ppm.

The supporting evidence for the structure of the glycoside was provided by the analysis of carbon nuclear magnetic resonance spectroscopy (^{13}C-NMR) (75 MHz, DMSO-d_6, TMS) data. The signal positions and their assignments to the different carbons are banded on the attached proton test spectrum (APT). APT values and their assignments are given in Table 1. From the APT

Table 1 APT spectral data and their assignments for the glycoside G1 from the flowers of *C. viscosa*

Chemical shift of carbon atoms (δ, ppm)	Type of APT spectra (Up or down)	Type of carbon atoms	Assignments
156.0	Up	Quaternary[a]	C-2
133.7	Up	Quaternary	C-3
177.1	Up	Quaternary	C-4
160.9	Up	Quaternary	C-5
98.4	Down	CH	C-6
163.8	Up	Quaternary	C-7
93.3	Down	CH	C-8
156.1	Up	Quaternary	C-9
103.8	Up	Quaternary	C-10
121.3	Up	Quaternary	C-1'
115.0	Down	CH	C-2'
144.5	Up	Quaternary	C-3'
148.2	Up	Quaternary	C-4'
116.3	Down	CH	C-5'
121.32	Down	CH	C-6'
100.1	Down	CH	C-1''
76.4	Down	CH	C-2''
73.9	Down	CH	C-3''
69.9	Down	CH	C-4''
77.4	Down	CH	C-5''
61.0	Up	CH$_2$	C-6''
171.1	Up	Quaternary	Carbonyl group
21.8	Down	CH	Methyl group

[a]Quaternary, carbon with no hydrogen.

data, numbers of H atoms attached to each carbon atom were determined. -CH$_3$ and -CH peaks will be down and -CH$_2$ and C with no hydrogen atoms will be up in the APT spectrum [14]. With the help of the APT spectrum, CH$_3$, CH$_2$, CH, and C with no hydrogen (quaternary carbon atom) were identified in ^{13}C spectra. Due to glycosylation, C-3 carbon shows signal at δ 133.7 ppm and ortho carbon atoms C-2 and C-4 show signals at δ156.0 and 177.1 ppm, respectively. Carbonyl carbon of the acetyl group appears at δ 171.1 ppm. Methyl carbon of the acetyl group appears at δ 21.8 ppm.

The structure of the glycoside was further evidenced by mass spectrum. The spectrum of the aglycone had a peak at m/z 302 for M$^+$ ion. The fragmentation pattern following retro-Diels-Alder (RDA), RDA + H and other common fragmentation route [15] is in favor of the identification of the compound. The appearance of a fragment at m/z 137 (RDA) and at 153 (RDA + H) is the evidence for the presence of two hydroxyl groups in ring B and also in ring A. The peak at m/z 165 represented the ion formed from the aglycone through the formation of a five membered ring, which is expected for

3-hydroxy flavones. Peaks at m/z 193 and at m/z 156 are also in favor of the structure of the compound. Based on the above evidences, the glycoside has been characterized at quercetin 3-O-(2''-acetyl)-glucoside (G1) (Figure 1).

Carrageenan-induced inflammation is an acute inflammation. Carrageenan-induced paw edema has been described as biphasic. The initial phase is attributable to the release of histamine, serotonin, and kinin in the first hour after the injection of carrageenan. A more pronounced second phase is related to the release of prostaglandin-like substances in 2 to 3 h. It has been reported that the second phase of edema is sensitive to drugs like phenylbutazone and indomethacin [15]. Table 2 shows that the isolated flavonoid exerted significant anti-inflammatory activity at 100 mg/kg of body weight (BW) during the second phase of inflammation. The significant anti-inflammatory effect of the flavonoid glycoside may be due to the inhibition of prostaglandin synthesis, since it acts in the second phase of inflammation.

Gram-negative bacteria *Escherichia coli* has been inhibited to a lesser extent as compared to the gram-positive bacteria *S. aureus* (Table 3). This suggests that there exists a pattern of selective toxicity with the flavonoid glycoside towards the gram-positive bacteria. This conclusion is in agreement with that of the findings of the earlier researchers that flavonoids of the plant origin could selectively inhibit gram-positive bacteria [16]. The glycoside would have interacted with cell wall

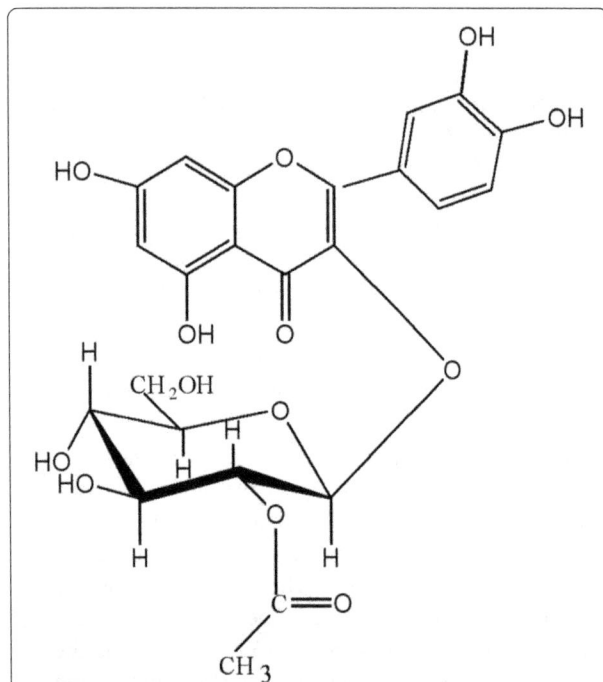

Figure 1 Quercetin 3-O-(2″-acetyl)-glucoside. The chemical structure of quercetin 3-O-(2″-acetyl)-glucoside that was isolated from ethyl acetate fraction of *C. viscose*.

materials causing their lysis. The integrity of the cytoplasmic membrane might have got damaged causing death of the cell. Alteration of protein and nucleic acid molecule is another possibility. Apart from these things, enzyme action, which is the potential target, can be modified with drugs causing serious repair in the cell.

Experimental

Plant material, extraction, and isolation

The fresh flowers of *C. viscosa* (750 g) collected at Musiri of Tiruchirappalli district, India were extracted with 85% methanol (4×500 mL) under reflux. The alcoholic extract was concentrated *in vacuo* and the aqueous extract was fractionated with petroleum ether (60°C–80°C) (3×250 mL), peroxide-free Et_2O (5×250 mL) and ethyl acetate (EtOAc) (4×500 mL). The petroleum ether fraction did not yield any isolable material.

The Et_2O fraction was concentrated *in vacuo* and left in the ice chest for a few days. A yellow solid was separated. It came out as yellow needle (m.p. 317°C–318°C) on crystallization from methanol. It was sparingly soluble in hot water and soluble in organic solvents. It gave a golden yellow color with NH_3 and NaOH and red color with Mg-HCl. It answered Wilson's boric acid test and Molisch's test and responded to Horhammer-Hansel test, Gibb's test, and Wilson's boric acid test. It had λ_{max} MeOH 256, 271, 301sh, 372; +NaOMe 247, 327sh, 413; and + NaOAc 272, 329 nm. It was identified as quercetin.

The residue from EtOAc fraction afforded yellow crystals on crystallization from methanol (m.p. 220°C–221°C). It developed a yellow color when viewed under UV light with and without NH_3. It developed a green color with alcoholic Fe^{3+} and red color with Mg-HCl. It answered Wilson's boric acid test and Molisch's test but did not answer Horhammer-Hansel test. It had λ_{max} MeOH 257, 299, 355; +NaOMe 263, 327sh, 403; and + NaOAc 272, 320sh, and 354 nm. The ^1H, ^{13}C-NMR, and APT spectra were recorded and interpreted.

The glycoside (50 mg) was dissolved in hot aqueous MeOH (5 ml, 50%). An equal volume of H_2SO_4 (7%) was added to it. This mixture was refluxed at 100°C for 2 h. The excess of alcohol was distilled off and the resulting solution was extracted with Et_2O. The residue obtained was studied for the aglycone. It answered Horhammer-Hansel test, Gibb's test and Wilson's boric acid test but did not answer Molisch's test. It had λ_{max} MeOH 253,267,291sh, 335; +NaOMe 266,329sh, 390; and + NaOAc 278, 329sh, 335 nm. A mass spectrum was recorded for aglycone moiety. The filtrate after the aglycone was neutralized with $BaCO_3$. The concentrated filtrate was examined through paper chromatography. The identity was confirmed by comparison with an authentic sample of glucose.

Table 2 Effect of flavonoid glycoside G1 on carrageenan-induced paw edema

Drug	Dose (mg/kg BW)	Paw edema at		Increase in paw volume (mL)	Percentage of inhibition
		(0 h) mL ± SE	(3 h) mL ± SE		
Control	-	0.60 ± 0.01	1.20 ± 0.02	0.60	-
G1	50	0.69 ± 0.01	1.10 ± 0.02	0.41	31.6
	100	0.66 ± 0.01	0.95 ± 0.02	0.29	51.7
	200	0.65 ± 0.01	0.98 ± 0.02	0.33	45.0
Phenylbutazone	100	0.62 ± 0.01	0.80 ± 0.02	0.18	70.0

Anti-inflammatory activity

For the investigation of anti-inflammatory activity of the flavonoid glycoside, rat paw edema was used. This method is based on the inhibition of the swelling induced in rat paw. The quantum of the swelling is measured by determining the thickness of the paw, its weight, and the amount of water or mercury it displaces. Healthy albino rats of either sex weighting between 120 and 200 g were selected for the studies. The right paw of each animal was taken as the comparison and left paw for injecting carrageenan. The flavonoid glycosides were dissolved in sterile water to get the desired concentration. The drugs were injected at doses of 50, 100, and 200 mg/kg BW to different groups of animals. Another group of animals received the standard drug, phenylbutazone (100 mg/kg BW), while the other group served as control. A 0.1 mL of 1% solution of carrageenan was injected into the plantar region of the left hind paw of all the animals. The swelling of the paw was measured at different time intervals. The results were expressed as the increase in foot volume in milliliters over the initial volume.

Antimicrobial activity

In the present study, paper disc agar diffusion method was used to evaluate the antimicrobial activities of the isolated flavonoid glycosides. The bacteria used were *S. aureus* (gram positive) and *E. coli* (gram negative). Nutrient agar was used to cultivate the organism. It comprises of peptone, meat extract, beef extract, and sodium chloride which were properly mixed and heated briefly in the streamer. A 2% agar was added and dissolved by heating. This medium was used for antimicrobial susceptibility testing. Beef infusion, casein acid hydrolysate, starch, and aqueous agar were used. All the above ingredients were mixed in distilled water and dissolved by heating. The mixture was sterilized by autoclaving at

121°C for 15 minutes. The selected stains were subcultured in nutrient broth and these cultivated organisms were used for seeding. The standard drugs used were penicillin and norfloxacin.

The Muller-Hinton agar medium was poured into Petri plates kept on a level surface. The depth of the medium was approximately 4 mm. After the medium got solidified, the plates were allowed to dry for some time by placing them in an incubator about 35°C to 37°C. Pure culture was used for sensitivity testing. Four to five colonies were selected and transferred into a tube containing 5 mL of liquid nutrient medium with the help of a biological loop. The culture was incubated at 35°C to 37°C for 2 to 5 h to obtain moderate turbidity. This was later transferred aseptically into the agar medium and incubated. Filter paper discs (Whatman no.1, Sunrise International (Filter Division), Mumbai, India) with 5.6 mm diameter were punched out. These discs were placed in Petri dishes allowing a distance of 2 to 4 mm between each disc, and the whole was sterilized in a hot air oven at 160°C for 1 h. After allowing the disc to cool, they were impregnated with isolated flavonoid glycoside solution of required concentration. Placing the Petri dishes in a desiccator with lids slightly raised dried the discs. The plate of agar medium was inoculated with the test organism and flavonoid solution. Following incubation, the plates were observed for a zone of inhibition around the drug.

Conclusions

The isolated flavonoid glycoside (quercetin 3-O-(2′′-acetyl)-glucoside) was investigated for its anti-inflammatory activity on carrageenan-induced rat paw edema (*in vivo*) and antimicrobial activity (*in vitro*) on *S. aureus* (gram positive) and *E. coli* (gram negative). The significant anti-inflammatory effect of the flavonoid glycoside

Table 3 Effect of flavonoid glycoside G1 on the growth of bacteria

Drug	Concentration (mg/mL)	Zone of inhibition (mm)		Inhibition (percent)	
		S. aureus	E. coli	S. aureus	E. coli
Penicillin	1	8	-	100	-
Norfloxacin	1	-	16	-	100
G1	1	5	3	62.50	18.75

may be due to the inhibition of prostaglandin synthesis. Selective toxicity with the flavonoid glycoside towards the gram-positive bacteria was found on *S. aureus*.

Abbreviations
APT: Attached proton test; BW: Body weight.

Competing interests
The authors declare that they have no competing interests.

Authors' information
MMS is a professor and head of Department of Chemistry, EVR College Tiruchirappalli, India. Her doctoral work at National Institute of Technology-Tiruchirappalli (NIT-T) was mainly focused on isolation of natural products and their biomedical applications. She is actively working in natural products and green chemistry. DK is a research assistant at Institute of High Polymers Research, Shinshu University, Japan. His master's work at National Institute of Technology, Tiruchirappalli (NIT-T) was mainly focused on electrochemistry of synthetic and natural organic compounds. He is actively working on biopolymers. NS is a professor of the Department of Chemistry at NIT-Tiruchirappalli (on contract). NS is a renowned researcher in the field of phytochemistry/medicinal chemistry and has published more than 130 articles in peer-reviewed international and national journals. Her field of expertise ranges from natural products to electro-organic chemistry.

Acknowledgement
The authors would like to thank the director, NIT-T for supporting our research.

References
1. Bello IA, Ndukwe GI, Audu OT, Habila JD: **A bioactive flavonoid from** *Pavetta crassipes* K. Schum. *Org Med Chem Lett* 2011, **1**:14. doi:10.1186/2191-2858-1-14.
2. Johnmerina A, Kesavan D, Sulochana N: **Isolation and antihyperglycemic activity of flavonoid from flower petals of** *Opuntia stricta*. *Pharm Chem J* 2011, **45**:317. doi:0091-150X/11/4505-0317.
3. Subramanian SS, Nagarajan S, Sulochana N: **Chrysin-7-rutinoside from the leaves of** *Dolichandrone falcata*. *Phytochemistry* 1972, **11**:438–439. doi:10.1016/S0031-9422(00)90041-4.
4. Subramanian SS, Nagarajan S, Sulochana N: **Hydroquinone from the leaves of** *Jacaranda mimosaefolia*. *Phytochemistry* 1973, **12**:220–221. doi:10.1016/S0031-9422(00)84658-0.
5. Subramanian SS, Nagarajan S, Sulochana N: **Flavonoids of the leaves of** *Jatropha gossypifolia*. *Phytochemistry* 1971, **10**:1690. doi:10.1016/0031-9422(71) 85055-0.
6. Subramanian SS, Sulochana N: **Flavonoids of some euphorbiaceous plants.** *Phytochemistry* 1971, **10**:2548–2549. doi:10.1016/S0031-9422(00)89910-0.
7. Senthamilselvi MM, Kesavan D, Sulochana N: **New biflavone glycoside from flowers of** *Asystasia gangetica*. *Chem Nat Compds* 2011, **47**:360–362.
8. Parimaladevi B, Boominathan R, Mandal SC: **Studies on analgesic activity of** *Cleome viscose* in mice. *Fitoterapia* 2003, **74**:262–266. doi:10.1016/S0367-326X(03) 00020-0.
9. Parimaladevi B, Boominathan R, Mandal SC: **Studies on psychopharmacological effects of** *Cleome viscose* Linn. Extract in rats and mice. *Phytother Res* 2004, **18**:169–172. doi:10.1002/ptr.1409.
10. Parimaladevi B, Boominathan R, Mandal SC, Ghosal SK: **Anti-inflammatory evaluation of** *Ionidium suffruticosam* Ging. in rats. *J Ethnopharmacol* 2004, **91**:367–370. doi:10.1016/j.jep.2003.12.019.
11. Sudhakar M, Rao Ch V, Rao PM, Raju DB: **Evaluation of antimicrobial activity of** *Cleome viscosa* and *Gmelina asiatica*. *Fitoterapia* 2006, **77**:47–49. doi:10.1016/j.fitote.2005.08.003.
12. Sengottuvelu S, Duraisamy R, Nandhakumar J, Sivakumar T: **Hepatoprotective activity of** *Cleome viscosa* against carbon tetrachloride induced hepatotoxity in rats. *Pharmacogn Mag* 2007, **3**:120–123.
13. Gupta NK, Dixit VD: **Evaluation of hepatoprotective activity of** *Cleome viscosa* Linn. extract. *Indian J Pharmacol* 2009, **41**:36–40. doi:10.4103/0253-7613.48892.
14. Silverstein RM, Bassler GC, Morrill TC: *Spectrometric identification of organic compounds*. 5th edition. New York: Wiley; 1991.
15. Di Rosa M, Giroud JP, Wiiloughby DA: **Studies of the mediators of the acute inflammatory response induced in rats in different sites by carrageenan and turpentine.** *J Pathol* 1971, **104**:15–29. doi:10.1002/path.1711040103.
16. Wyman JG, Van-Etten HD: **Antibacterial activity of selected isofavonoids.** *Phytopath* 1978, **68**:583–589. doi:00032-949X/78/000.

8

Attenuation of visceral nociception by α-bisabolol in mice: investigation of mechanisms

Gerlânia de Oliveira Leite[1], Cícera Norma Fernandes[1], Irwin Rose Alencar de Menezes[1], José Galberto Martins da Costa[1] and Adriana Rolim Campos[2*]

Abstract

Background: We previously described the visceral antinociceptive property of α-bisabolol (BISA) in mouse models of visceral nociception induced by cyclophosphamide and mustard oil (MO). This study examined the effect of BISA in mouse models of visceral nociception induced by acetic acid, capsaicin, formalin, and the contribution of the nitric oxide system, α_2, K_{ATP}^+, 5-HT$_3$ and TRPV1 receptors to the effect of BISA on MO-evoked nociceptive behaviors. Mice were pretreated orally with BISA (50, 100 and 200 mg/kg) or vehicle, and the pain-related behavioral responses to intraperitoneal administration of acetic acid or intracolonic injection of MO were analyzed.

Results: BISA significantly suppressed the nociceptive behaviors in a dose-unrelated manner. The antinociceptive effect of BISA (50 mg/kg) was show to be glibenclamide resistant, but it was not blocked by pretreatment with the other antagonists tested. In the open-field test that detects sedative or motor abnormality, mice received 50 mg/kg BISA did not show any per se influence in ambulation frequency.

Conclusions: However, their precise antinociceptive mechanisms of action have not been determined.

Keywords: α-bisabolol, Visceral nociception, Mechanisms

Background

Essential oils are natural products that exhibit a variety of biological properties such as analgesic, anticonvulsant, and anxiolytic ones. Such effects are often attributed to the presence of monoterpenes, which are the major chemical components of these oils [1]. Sesquiterpenes, such zerumbone [2], budlein A [3], polygodial [4], and lapidin [5], have been shown to present antinociceptive properties.

Recent studies demonstrated that the sesquiterpene α-bisabolol (BISA) presents antitumor [6], peripheral nervous blocker [7], gastroprotective [8], leishimanicidal [9], antioxidant [10], mutagenic and antimutagenic [11], and wound healing [12] properties. There are also evidences showing that BISA reduced visceral nociceptive pain evoked by intracolonic administration of mustard oil (MO) as well as that induced by intraperitoneal injection of cyclophosphamide, possibly involving the inhibition of sensitization of primary afferent neuron terminals by prostaglandins [13].

* Correspondence: adrirolim@unifor.br
[2]Vice-Reitoria de Pesquisa e Pós-Graduação, Universidade de Fortaleza, Av. Washington Soares, 1321, Fortaleza, Ceará CEP 60811-905, Brazil
Full list of author information is available at the end of the article

However, the mechanisms underlying these antinociceptive properties of BISA are not well understood.

Methods

Animals

Male Swiss albino mice (20–25 g) obtained from the Central Animal House of Regional University of Cariri were used. They were housed in environmentally controlled conditions (22°C, 12-h light–dark cycle), with free access to standard pellet diet (Purina, São Paulo, Brazil) and water. Animals were kept in cages with raised floors to prevent coprophagy. Before the visceral antinociceptive assays, they were fasted over a period of 15 h and were habituated to the test environment for 2 h before the experimentation. The experimental protocols were in accordance with the ethical guidelines of National Institute of Health, Bethesda, USA. The studies were performed in a blinded manner.

Acetic acid-induced visceral nociception

Abdominal constrictions were induced by intraperitoneal injection of acetic acid (0.6%). The animals were pretreated with BISA (50, 100 or 200 mg/kg, p.o.) or vehicle

(2% Tween 80, 10 mL/kg, p.o.) 60-min prior to acetic acid injection. After the challenge, each mouse was placed in a separate glass funnel and the number of contractions of the abdominal muscles, together with stretching, was cumulatively counted over a period of 20 min. Antinociceptive activity was expressed as the reduction in the number of abdominal contractions, comparing the control animals with the mice pre-treated with BISA.

Capsaicin-induced visceral nociception

Male mice divided into groups of eight in each were pre-treated with the vehicle (2% Tween 80 in distilled water, 10 mL/kg, p.o.) or BISA (50, 100 or 200 mg/kg, p.o.). 1 h after oral and 30 min following systemic treatments, capsaicin (0.3% in a solution of PBS:Tween 80:ethanol (8:1:1)) was instilled into the colon (50 μL/animal) using a fine cannula (1.6-mm external diameter), 4-cm far from the anal sphincter. Solid petroleum jelly was applied onto the perianal region to avoid local nerve stimulation. The animals were then observed during a 30-min period for the spontaneous visceral pain-related behaviors (licking the upper abdomen, abdominal contortion and retraction, squashing the abdomen against the floor). A normal group, that received only saline intracolonically, was also included.

Formalin-induced visceral nociception

Male mice divided into groups of eight in each were pre-treated with the vehicle (2% Tween 80 in distilled water, 10 mL/kg, p.o.) or BISA (50, 100 or 200 mg/kg, p.o.). 1 h after oral and 30 min following systemic treatments, formalin (10%) was instilled into the colon (10 μL/animal) using a fine cannula (1.6-mm external diameter), 4-cm far from the anal sphincter. Solid petroleum jelly was applied onto the perianal region to avoid local nerve stimulation. The animals were then observed during a 60-min period for the spontaneous visceral pain-related behaviors (licking the upper abdomen, abdominal contortion and retraction, squashing the abdomen against the floor). A normal group, that received only saline intracolonically, was also included.

MO-induced visceral nociception

To assess the antinociceptive effect of BISA against the MO-induced visceral nociception, mice in groups ($n = 8$) were orally treated with BISA (50, 100 or 200 mg/kg, p.o.) or vehicle (2% Tween 80 in distilled water, 10 mL/kg, p.o.) 1 h before the intracolonic administration of MO (0.75% in saline 0.9%, 50 μL/animal). A group of normal control received a similar dose of saline (10 mL/kg). Immediately following the intracolonic MO or saline administration, the mice were observed for the total number of nociceptive behaviors (licking the upper abdomen, stretching the abdomen, squashing the abdomen against the floor and retraction of the abdomen characterized for an arched position), for a 20-min period.

In order to verify the possible involvement of nitrergic, noradrenergic, K_{ATP}^+, 5-HT$_3$, and TRPV1 receptors in the effect of BISA, the animals were treated with L-NAME (10 mg/kg, i.p), yohimbine (2 mg/kg, i.p), glibenclamide (5 mg/kg, i.p), ondansetron (10 mg/kg, i.p) or ruthenium red (3 mg/kg, s.c.), 30 min before the administration of BISA (50 mg/kg).

Locomotor activity (open-field test)

The open-field area was made of acrylic (transparent walls and black floor: $30 \times 30 \times 15$ cm^2) divided in nine squares of equal area. Four groups of animals ($n = 6$) were used. While groups 1 and 2 were treated, respectively, with vehicle (2% Tween 80, 10 mL/kg, p.o.) and BISA (50 mg/kg, p.o.), groups 3 and 4 received vehicle + MO (0.75%, 50 μL) or BISA (50 mg/kg, p.o.) + MO. The MO was given by an intracolonic route 90 following the vehicle or BISA. The numbers of squares each animal crossed with the four paws were noted during a 4-min period.

Statistical analysis

The results are expressed as mean ± SEM from six or eight mice per group. For statistical analysis, ANOVA followed by Tukey's or Student–Newman–Keul's post hoc test, as appropriate, were used. A $p < 0.05$ was considered statistically significant.

Table 1 Antinociceptive effect of BISA in capsaicin, formalin, MO, and acetic acid-induced visceral nociception in mice

Group	Dose (mg/kg)	Specific behaviors			
		Capsaicin	Formalin	MO	Acetic acid
Normal	-	10.25 ± 6.21**	198.60 ± 47.87**	21.57 ± 7.13***	-
Vehicle	-	84.38 ± 12.99	344.60 ± 50.21	107.80 ± 25.01	48.63 ± 10.81
BISA	50	87.00 ± 19.30	103.00 ± 16.21***	21.67 ± 7.99***	10.50 ± 2.94***
	100	31.00 ± 13.11**	140.40 ± 25.51***	33.83 ± 10.28***	8.50 ± 3.20***
	200	15.33 ± 10.82**	75.13 ± 13.44***	27.17 ± 11.05***	8.43 ± 2.57***

Values represent the mean ± SEM of pain-related behaviors (licking of abdomen, stretching, abdominal retractions). **$p < 0.01$ and ***$p < 0.001$ versus vehicle (ANOVA, Student-Newman-Keul's test).

Table 2 Effect of yohimbine, ondansetron, L-NAME, glibenclamide and ruthenium red against MO-induced visceral pain in mice

Group	Dose (mg/kg)	Specific behaviors
Normal	-	18.14 ± 3.44*
Vehicle	-	44.17 ± 5.59
Yohimbine	2	22.28 ± 3.53*
Ondansetron	0.5	44.75 ± 5.89
L-NAME	20	27.13 ± 3.74
Glibenclamide	5	40.88 ± 8.39
Ruthenium red	0.3	29.25 ± 4.98

Values represent the mean ± SEM of pain-related behaviors (licking of abdomen, stretching, abdominal retractions). *$p < 0.05$ versus vehicle (ANOVA, Student-Newman-Keul's test).

Table 4 Evaluation of involvement of serotonergic, nitrergic, K_{ATP}^+ channels, and TRPV1 receptors in the antinociceptive effect of BISA in MO test

Group	Dose (mg/kg)	Specific behaviors
Normal	-	88.25 ± 18.59**
Vehicle	-	181.90 ± 24.07
BISA	50	115.70 ± 25.33*
BISA + Ondansetron	50 + 0.5	57.13 ± 11.07***
BISA + L-NAME	50 + 20	31.25 ± 8.64***
BISA + glibenclamide	50 + 5	86.57 ± 15.61*
BISA + ruthenium red	50 + 3	61.71 ± 8.41**

Values represent the mean ± SEM of pain-related behaviors (licking of abdomen, stretching, abdominal retractions). *$p < 0.05$, **$p < 0.01$ and ***$p < 0.001$ versus vehicle (ANOVA, Student-Newman-Keul's test).

Results and discussion

Effect of BISA on acetic acid, capsaicin, formalin and MO-induced visceral pain in mice

Table 1 shows the antinociceptive effect of BISA in acetic acid, capsaicin, formalin and MO. Intraperitoneal application of acetic acid (0.6%) provoked a significant increase in abdominal constrictions when compared with saline-treated normal control. In groups pretreated with BISA (50, 100 and 200 mg/kg, p.o.), acetic acid-induced abdominal constrictions were significantly inhibited in a dose-unrelated manner. Intracolonic application of capsaicin (CAP 0.3%), MO (MO 0.75%), or formalin (10%) provoked a significant increase in spontaneous pain-related behaviors when compared with saline-treated normal controls (Table 1). In groups pretreated with BISA, capsaicin, formalin and MO-induced nociceptive behaviors were significantly inhibited. L-NAME, yohimbine, glibenclamide, ondansetron, or ruthenium red failed to revert the antinociceptive effect of BISA (Tables 2, 3 and 4). Table 5 shows the effects of orally administered BISA on behavior in open-field test in mice. At the dose tested (50-mg/kg), BISA showed no significant influence on the number of crossings in open-field test.

In this study, we observed that the acetic acid, capsaicin, formalin, and MO-evoked nociceptive pain behaviors were significantly attenuated in mice pretreated

with BISA, a natural sesquiterpenoid isolated from the different essential oils. It has been well established that many algogenic substances induce nociceptive pain-related behaviors in rodents following intraperitoneal or intracolonic application, and several reports reveal that naturally occurring compounds, like terpenoids, unsaturated dialdehydes and phenolic ketones can suppress these behaviors [14].

Many studies use acetic acid-induced effects as a model of visceral nociception but it lacks specificy [15]. Capsaicin, the pungent ingredient of red peppers applied topically or injected into the skin of humans or experimental animals, is known to stimulate the vanilloid receptor (Transient Receptor Potential cation channel V1 or TRPV1) located on polymodal C-fibers, but also in other tissues and initiates a complex cascade of events, including neuronal excitation and release of pro-inflammatory mediators, desensitization of receptor, and neuronal toxicity [16,17]. The intracolonic instillation of formalin via the anus evokes differentiated behaviors, which reflect visceral nociception. All types of behavior were dose dependently inhibited by morphine, indicating that they are pain-related [18]. As shown before, BISA could significantly suppress the nociception-related behaviors against MO-induced visceral nociception [13].

Visceral pain is a prominent form of pain in many clinical conditions [15]. The results obtained in the

Table 3 Effect of α₂-adrenoceptor antagonism on the antinociceptive effect of BISA in MO test

Group	Dose (mg/kg)	Specific behaviors
Normal	-	4.25 ± 1.77***
Vehicle	-	28.50 ± 4.00
BISA	50	1.29 ± 0.75***
BISA + yohimbine	50 + 2	5.75 ± 1.77***

Values represent the mean ± S.E.M. of pain-related behaviors (licking of abdomen, stretching, abdominal retractions). ***$p < 0.001$ vs Vehicle (ANOVA, Student-Newman-Keul's test).

Table 5 Effect of BISA on mouse behavior in open-field test

Group	Number of crossings
Vehicle	23.50 ± 5.04
BISA	13.57 ± 3.22
Vehicle + MO	31.86 ± 5.06
BISA + MO	19.00 ± 5.27

Mice were pre-treated with vehicle (2% Tween 80 in distilled water, p.o.) or BISA 50 mg/kg (p.o.), before intracolonic instillation of saline or MO (0.75%, 50 μL). Data represent mean ± SEM (n = 8). Data represent the mean ± SEM (n = 8). ANOVA, Student-Newman-Keul's test.

acetic acid-, capsaicin-, formalin-, and MO-induced test models of visceral nociception are shown in Table 1. In vehicle-treated control groups of mice, acetic acid-, capsaicin-, formalin-, and MO-induced spontaneous nociception-related behaviors when compared with respective saline-treated control groups. In groups pretreated with BISA, the nociceptive behaviors induced by algogenic substances were significantly inhibited in a dose-independent manner.

In the search of the possible action mechanism of BISA, we used the acute model of visceral nociception induced by intracolonic instillation of MO, which has disease relevancy to human irritable bowel syndrome [18]. The sesquiterpene BISA could significantly suppress the pain-related behaviors against MO-induced visceral nociception, possibly regulating the functioning of primary afferent fibers. Visceral afferents express a wide range of membrane receptors (including vanilloid receptors, TRPV1) to chemical stimuli, which are involved in sensory signaling from the gut to the central nervous system [19]. When animals were pretreated with BISA and ruthenium red (a non-competitive antagonist of TRPV1) in combination, there was additive antinociception in MO test. Also, BISA 50 mg/kg failed to inhibit the visceral nociception induced by capsaicin. These observations suggest that BISA does not act as a TRPV1 agonist but may possibly induce a modulatory influence on vanilloid-receptors, which needs further clarification.

Previous studies have shown that MO can induce acute colitis and BISA has been reported to exert antiinflammatory action [13,20]. Therefore, it is reasonable to assume that BISA suppresses the inflammatory pain. The α2-adrenoceptor agonist has been shown to induce antinociceptive effect in the experimental model of formalin-induced colitis in rats and reduce visceral hypersensitivity in clinical settings [21,22]. Therefore, a possible involvement of α2-adrenoceptors in the antinociceptive effect of BISA in MO-model of visceral pain, using the antagonist yohimbine was investigated. Yohimbine could not reverse the antinociception produced by BISA, suggesting that α2-adrenoceptors play no role.

K_{ATP}^{+} channel openers induce cell hyperpolarization, decrease the intracellular Ca^{2+} level and neurotransmitter release (calcitonin gene-related peptide and substance P), that may account for antinociception [23,24]. To verify such a possibility, we examined the effect of glibenclamide, a blocker of K_{ATP}^{+} channels on BISA antinociception. Pretreatment of mice with glibenclamide in combination with BISA showed no alteration. When mice were pretreated with L-NAME, a nitric oxide synthase inhibitor and the 5-HT$_3$ antagonist, ondansetron, apparently a potentiated/additive response which needs further analysis through an isobolographic study.

Drugs that impair motor activity or induce sedation may give false-positive/negative results in nociceptive tests. We therefore sought to verify such effects of BISA on open-field test that detects motor incoordination [25]. The sesquiterpene failed to alter significantly the ambulation in open-field test. This result indicates that BISA exerts analgesia without causing neurological or muscular deficits.

Conclusions

Although BISA efficient diminished the acetic acid, capsaicin, formalin, and MO-evoked pain-related behaviors, its mechanism is unclear from this study and future studies are needed to verify how the sesquiterpene exerts its antinociceptive action.

Competing interests

The authors declare that they have no competing interest.

Authors' contributions

GOL carried out the antinociceptive studies. CNF carried out the antinociceptive studies . IRAM carried out the antinociceptive studies. JGMC carried out the antinociceptive studies. ARC carried out the antinociceptive studies and draft the manuscript. All authors read and approved the final manuscript.

Acknowledgments

The authors are grateful to CAPES, CNPq, and Funcap for the fellowship awards and financial support by grants.

Author details

[1]Departamento de Química Biológica, Universidade Regional do Cariri, Crato CE 63105-000, Brazil. [2]Vice-Reitoria de Pesquisa e Pós-Graduação, Universidade de Fortaleza, Av. Washington Soares, 1321, Fortaleza, Ceará CEP 60811-905, Brazil.

References

1. Gonçalves JC, Alves Ade M, de Araújo AE, Cruz JS, Araújo DA (2010) Distinct effects of carvone analogues on the isolated nerve of rats. Eur J Pharmacol 645(1–3):108–112
2. Sulaiman MR, Perimal EK, Zakaria ZA, Mokhtar F, Akhtar MN, Lajis NH, Israf DA (2009) Preliminary analysis of the antinociceptive activity of zerumbone. Fitoterapia 80(4):230–232
3. Valério DA, Cunha TM, Arakawa NS, Lemos HP, Da Costa FB, Parada CA, Ferreira SH, Cunha FQ, Verri WA Jr (2007) Anti-inflammatory and analgesic effects of the sesquiterpene lactone budlein A in mice: inhibition of cytokine production-dependent mechanism. Eur J Pharmacol 562(1–2):155–163
4. Mendes GL, Santos AR, Malheiros A, Filho VC, Yunes RA, Calixto JB (2000) Assessment of mechanisms involved in antinociception caused by sesquiterpene polygodial. J Pharmacol Exp Ther 292(1):164–172
5. Valencia E, Feria M, Díaz JG, González A, Bermejo J (1994) Antinociceptive, anti-inflammatory and antipyretic effects of lapidin, a bicyclic sesquiterpene. Planta Med 60(5):395–399
6. da Silva AP, Martini MV, de Oliveira CM, Cunha S, de Carvalho JE, Ruiz AL, da Silva CC (2010) Antitumor activity of (−)-alpha-bisabolol-based thiosemicarbazones against human tumor cell lines. Eur J Med Chem 45(7):2987–2993
7. Alves AM, Gonçalves JC, Cruz JS, Araújo DA (2010) Evaluation of the sesquiterpene (−)-alpha-bisabolol as a novel peripheral nervous blocker. Neurosci Lett 472(1):11–15
8. Bezerra SB, Leal LK, Nogueira NA, Campos AR (2009) Bisabolol-induced gastroprotection against acute gastric lesions: role of prostaglandins, nitric oxide, and KATP+ channels. J Med Food 12(6):1403–1406

9. Morales-Yuste M, Morillas-Márquez F, Martín-Sánchez J, Valero-López A, Navarro-Moll MC (2010) Activity of (−)alpha-bisabolol against *Leishmania infantum* promastigotes. Phytomedicine 17(3–4):279–281

10. Braga PC, Dal Sasso M, Fonti E, Culici M (2009) Antioxidant activity of bisabolol: inhibitory effects on chemiluminescence of human neutrophil bursts and cell-free systems. Pharmacology 83(2):110–115

11. Gomes-Carneiro MR, Dias DM, De-Oliveira AC, Paumgartten FJ (2005) Evaluation of mutagenic and antimutagenic activities of alpha-bisabolol in the Salmonella/microsome assay. Mutat Res 585(1–2):105–112

12. Villegas LF, Marçalo A, Martin J, Fernández ID, Maldonado H, Vaisberg AJ, Hammond GB (2001) (+) epi-Alpha-bisabolol [correction of bisbolol] is the wound-healing principle of Peperomia galioides: investigation of the in vivo wound-healing activity of related terpenoids. J Nat Prod 64(10):1357–1359

13. Leite GO, Leite LH, Sampaio Rde S, Araruna MK, de Menezes IR, da Costa JG, Campos AR (2011) (−)-α-Bisabolol attenuates visceral nociception and inflammation in mice. Fitoterapia 82(2):208–211

14. Oliveira FA, Costa CL, Chaves MH, Almeida FR, Cavalcante IJ, Lima AF, Lima RC Jr, Silva RM, Campos AR, Santos FA, Rao VS (2005) Attenuation of capsaicin-induced acute and visceral nociceptive pain by alpha- and beta-amyrin, a triterpene mixture isolated from *Protium heptaphyllum* resin in mice. Life Sci 77(23):2942–2952

15. Lima-Júnior RC, Oliveira FA, Gurgel LA, Cavalcante IJ, Santos KA, Campos DA, Vale CA, Silva RM, Chaves MH, Rao VS, Santos FA (2006) Attenuation of visceral nociception by alpha- and beta-amyrin, a triterpenoid mixture isolated from the resin of *Protium heptaphyllum*, in mice. Planta Med 72 (1):34–39

16. Szolcsanyi J (1977) A pharmacological approach to elucidation of the role of different nerve fiber receptor endings in mediation of pain. J Physiol 73 (3):251–259

17. Caterina MJ, Leffler A, Malmberg AB, Martin WJ, Trafton J, Petersen-Zeitz KR, Koltzenburg M, Basbaum AI, Julius D (2000) Impaired nociception and pain sensation in mice lacking the capsaicin receptor. Science 288(5464):306–313

18. Laird JM, Martinez-Caro L, Garcia-Nicas E, Cervero F (2001) A new model of visceral pain and referred hyperalgesia in the mouse. Pain 92(3):335–342

19. Wood JN (2004) Recent advances in understanding molecular mechanisms of primary afferent activation. Gut 53(2):ii9–ii12

20. Kimball ES, Palmer JM, D'Andrea MR, Hornby PJ, Wade PR (2005) Acute colitis induction by oil of mustard results in later development of an IBS-like accelerated upper GI transit in mice. Am J Physiol Gastrointest Liver Physiol 288(6):G1266–G1273

21. Miampamba M, Chery-Croze S, Chayvialle JÁ (1992) Spinal and intestinal levels of substance P, calcitonin gene-related peptide and vasoactive intestinal polypeptide following perendoscopic injection of formalin in rat colonic wall. Neuropeptides 22(2):73–80

22. Blackshaw LA, Gebhart GF (2002) The pharmacology of gastrointestinal nociceptive pathways. Curr Opin Pharmacol 2(6):642–649

23. Ocana M, Cendan CM, Cobos EJ, Entrena JM, Baeyens JM (2004) Potassium channels and pain: present realities and future opportunities. Eur J Pharmacol 500:203–219

24. Lohmann AB, Welch SP (1999) ATP-gated K+ channel openers enhance opioid antinociception: indirect evidence for the release of endogenous opioid peptides. Eur J Pharmacol 385:119–127

25. Novas ML, Wolfman C, Medina JH, De Robertis E (1988) Proconvulsant and anxiogenic effects of *n*-butyl-β-carboline-3-carboxylate, on endogenous benzodiazepine binding inhibitor from brain. Pharmacol Biochem Behav 30:331–336

9

Antibacterial activities and antioxidant capacity of *Aloe vera*

Fatemeh Nejatzadeh-Barandozi

Abstract

Background: The aim of this study was to identify, quantify, and compare the phytochemical contents, antioxidant capacities, and antibacterial activities of *Aloe vera* lyophilized leaf gel (LGE) and 95% ethanol leaf gel extracts (ELGE) using GC-MS and spectrophotometric methods.

Results: Analytically, 95% ethanol is less effective than ethyl acetate/diethyl ether or hexane (in the case of fatty acids) extractions in separating phytochemicals for characterization purposes. However, although fewer compounds are extracted in the ELGE, they are approximately 345 times more concentrated as compared to the LGE, hence justifying ELGE use in biological efficacy studies *in vivo*. Individual phytochemicals identified included various phenolic acids/polyphenols, phytosterols, fatty acids, indoles, alkanes, pyrimidines, alkaloids, organic acids, aldehydes, dicarboxylic acids, ketones, and alcohols. Due to the presence of the antioxidant polyphenols, indoles, and alkaloids, the *A. vera* leaf gel shows antioxidant capacity as confirmed by ORAC and FRAP analyses. Both analytical methods used show the non-flavonoid polyphenols to contribute to the majority of the total polyphenol content. Three different solvents such as aqueous, ethanol, and acetone were used to extract the bioactive compounds from the leaves of *A. vera* to screen the antibacterial activity selected human clinical pathogens by agar diffusion method. The maximum antibacterial activities were observed in acetone extracts (12 ± 0.45, 20 ± 0.35, 20 ± 0.57, and 15 ± 0.38 nm) other than aqueous and ethanol extracts.

Conclusion: Due to its phytochemical composition, *A. vera* leaf gel may show promise in alleviating symptoms associated with/or prevention of cardiovascular diseases, cancer, neurodegeneration, and diabetes.

Keywords: *Aloe vera*; Antibacterial activities; Antioxidant capacity; Gas chromatography; Mass spectrometry

Background

Aloe vera (L.) Burm.f. (*Aloe barbadensis* Miller) is a perennial succulent xerophyte, which develops water storage tissue in the leaves to survive in dry areas of low or erratic rainfall. The innermost part of the leaf is a clear, soft, moist, and slippery tissue that consists of large thin-walled parenchyma cells in which water is held in the form of a viscous mucilage [1]. Therefore, the thick fleshy leaves of aloe plants contain not only cell wall carbohydrates such as cellulose and hemicellulose but also storage carbohydrates such as acetylated mannans [2].

A. vera has been used for many centuries for its curative and therapeutic properties, and although over 75 active ingredients from the inner gel have been identified, therapeutic effects have not been correlated well with each individual component [3]. Many of the medicinal effects of aloe leaf extracts have been attributed to the polysaccharides found in the inner leaf parenchymatous tissue [4,5], but it is believed that these biological activities should be assigned to a synergistic action of the compounds contained therein rather than a single chemical substance [6]. *A. vera* is the most commercialized aloe species, and processing of the leaf pulp has become a large worldwide industry. In the food industry, it has been used as a source of functional foods and as an ingredient in other food products, for the production of gel-containing health drinks and beverages. In the cosmetic and toiletry industry, it has been used as base material for the production of creams, lotions, soaps, shampoos, facial cleansers, and other products. In the pharmaceutical industry, it has been used for the manufacture of topical products such as ointments and gel preparations, as well as in the production of tablets and capsules [7,8]. Important

Correspondence: fnejatzadeh@yahoo.com
Department of Horticulture, Faculty of Agriculture, Khoy Branch, Islamic Azad University, P.O. Box 58168–44799, Khoy, Iran

pharmaceutical properties that have recently been discovered for both the *A. vera* gel and whole leaf extract include the ability to improve the bioavailability of co-administered vitamins in human subjects [9]. Due to its absorption enhancing effects, *A. vera* gel may be employed to effectively deliver poorly absorbable drugs through the oral route of drug administration. Furthermore, the dried powder obtained from *A. vera* gel was successfully used to manufacture directly compressible matrix-type tablets. These matrix-type tablets slowly released a model compound over an extended period of time and thereby showing potential to be used as an excipient in modified release dosage forms [10].

Apart from *Aloe* being used extensively in the cosmetic industry, it has been described for centuries for its laxative, anti-inflammatory, immunostimulant, antiseptic [11], wound and burn healing [12], antiulcer [13], antitumor [14], and antidiabetic [15] activities. These treatments are based on anecdotal evidence or research findings done almost exclusively on *A. vera*. Different *Aloe* species would have various phytochemical contents, health benefits, and possible toxicities. Hence, it is of relevance for scientists, industry, and rural communities not only to research the relevant medicinal uses of their indigenous *Aloe* species but also to determine the active components and their individual or combined mechanisms of biological function. The use of 95% ethanol extracts of various *Aloe* species is extensively described in the literature for determining biological activity in the treatment and prevention of a variety of health conditions [16,17], in particular, diabetes [18,19]. In this study, we determined and compared the phytochemical contents and antioxidant capacities, antibacterial activities of *A. vera* lyophilized leaf gel and 95% ethanol leaf gel extracts using gas chromatography–mass spectrometry (GC-MS) and spectrophotometric methods of analysis. This was done not only to describe *A. vera* leaf gel extracts with regard to phytochemical contents and possible health benefits but also to compare various extraction methods for both analytical efficacy and possible biological relevance.

Methods
Samples
Whole, freshly cut, *A. vera* leaves (100 kg) were harvested in the month of September from farms in the National Institute of Genetic Engineering and Biotechnology (NIGEB), Tehran of Iran. The inner leaf gel was removed, homogenized, freeze-dried, and stored at –20°C until analysis. This was termed the leaf gel extract (LGE) for the purpose of this study. Approximately half of the LGE was used for the preparation of a 95% ethanol extract as described previously [19]. This was termed the 95% ethanol leaf gel extract (ELGE).

Material
All analytical standards were purchased from Sigma-Aldrich (St. Louis, MO, USA), and phenol reagent and other reagent chemicals and all of the organic solvents used were of ultrahigh purity which were purchased from Merck (Darmstadt, Germany).

Ethyl acetate/diethyl ether extraction
The internal standard, 3-phenylbutyric acid (25 mg/50 mL), was added to 25 mg of finely ground LGE and ELGE, followed by the addition of 1 mL of sodium acetate buffer (0.125 M). β-Glucuronidase (30 µL) was added, and the sample was vortexed and incubated overnight at 37°C. The sample was extracted with 6 mL of ethyl acetate followed by 3 mL of diethyl ether. The organic phase was collected after each extraction via centrifugation. The organic phase from each extraction was pooled and dried under nitrogen. The dried extract was derivatized with bis(trimethylsilyl) trifluoroacetamide (BSTFA, 100 µL), trimethylchlorosilane (TMCS, 20 µL), and pyridine (20 µL) at 70°C for 30 min. After cooling, 0.1 µL of the extract was injected into the GC-MS via splitless injection.

Fatty acid extraction
Heptadecanoic acid (72 mM), as an internal standard, was added to 25 mg of LGE and ELGE followed by 100 µL of a 45-mM solution of butylated hydroxytoluene and 2 mL of methanolic HCl (3 N). The samples were then vortexed and incubated for 4 h at 90°C. After cooling to room temperature, the sample was extracted twice with 2 mL of hexane, dried under a nitrogen stream, and finally resuspended with 100 µL of hexane, 1 µL of which was injected onto the GC-MS via splitless injection.

Gas chromatography–mass spectrometry
An Agilent 6890 GC ported to a 5973 mass selective detector (Santa Clara, CA, USA) was used for the identification and quantification of individual fatty acids. For the acquisition of an electron ionization mass spectrum, an ion source temperature of 200°C and electron energy of 70 eV were used. The gas chromatograph was equipped with an SE-30 capillary column (Agilent), a split/splitless injection piece (250°C), and direct GC-MS coupling (260°C). Helium (1 mL/min) was used as the carrier gas. The oven temperature program for analyzing the ethyl acetate/diethyl ether extract was an initial oven temperature of 40°C and was maintained for 2 min, followed by a steady climb to 350°C at a rate of 5°C/min. For the fatty acid analysis, an initial oven temperature of 50°C was maintained for 1.5 min and then allowed to increase to 190°C at a rate of 30°C/min. The oven temperature was maintained at 190°C for 5 min and then allowed to increase to 220°C at a rate of 8°C/min. The oven temperature was again maintained for 2 min and finally ramped to 230°C at a

rate of 3°C/min and maintained for 24 min at this temperature.

Total polyphenol assay

The total polyphenol content of the extracts were determined according to the Folin-Ciocalteu procedure [20]. Briefly, 10 mg of finely ground LGE or ELGE was dissolved in 200 µL of H2O in a test tube followed by 1 mL of Folin-Ciocalteu's reagent. This was allowed to stand for 8 min at room temperature. Next, 0.8 mL of sodium carbonate (7.5%, w/v) was added, mixed, and allowed to stand for 30 min. Absorption was measured at 765 nm (Shimadzu UV-1601 spectrophotometer, Kyoto, Japan). The mean total phenolic content (n = 3) was expressed as milligrams of gallic acid (Sigma-Aldrich) equivalents per 100 g of wet and dry mass (mg of GAE/ 100 g) (standard deviation (SD)).

Total flavonoid assay

The total flavonoid content was measured using the AlCl3 colorimetric assay [21] with some modifications. Briefly, 10 mg of LGE or ELGE was dissolved in 1 mL of H2O, to which 60 µL of 5% (w/v) NaNO2 was added. After 5 min, 60 µL of a 10% (w/v) AlCl3 was added. In the sixth minute, 400 µL of 1 M NaOH was added, and the total volume was made up to 2 mL with H2O. The solution was mixed well, and the absorbance was measured at 510 nm against a reagent blank. Concentrations were determined using a catechin (Sigma-Aldrich) solution standard curve. The mean total flavonoid content (n = 3) was expressed as milligrams of catechin equivalents (CE) per 100 g of wet and dry mass (mg of CE/100 g) (SD).

Oxygen radical absorbance capacity

Oxygen radical absorbance capacity (ORAC) analyses of hydrophilic and lipophilic compounds in LGE and ELGE were performed as described previously [22]. The analysis of lipophilic compounds was aided by the addition of randomly methylated β-cyclodextrin as a solubility enhancer as described before [23]. Briefly, in a volume of 200 µL, the reaction contained 56-nM fluorescein (Sigma-Aldrich) as a target for free radical attack by 240-nM 2,2′-azobis(2-amidinopropane)dihydrochloride (Sigma-Aldrich). A BioTEK fluorescence plate reader (FL-600, Winooski, VT, USA) was used, and the decay of fluorescence of fluorescein (excitation, 485 nm; emission, 520 nm) was measured every 5 min for 2 h at 37°C. Costar black opaque (96 well) plates (Thermo Fisher Scientific, Waltham, MA, USA) were used in the assays. Trolox (Sigma-Aldrich) was used as standard at a range between 0 and 20 tM with a polynomial (second order) curve fit analysis. Mean values (n) 3) of antioxidant capacities were expressed as micromoles of Trolox equivalents (TE) per gram of wet and dry mass (SD).

Ferric reducing antioxidant power

Ferric reducing antioxidant power (FRAP) values were determined essentially as described previously [24]. Briefly, the reduction of a Fe^{3+}-2,3,5-triphenyltetrazolium (Sigma-Aldrich) complex in the assay by the antioxidants in the samples was monitored at 593 nm. As a standard, FeSO4 (Sigma-Aldrich) was used, and the FRAP activities of the samples were expressed as the mean (n = 3) micromoles of Fe^{2+} per gram of wet and dry mass (SD).

Antibacterial activity of *Aloe vera*

The antibacterial studies were carried out by disc diffusion technique [20]. The sterile nutrient agar plates and potato dextrose agar plates were prepared. The bacterial test organisms like *Staphylococcus aureus*, *Streptococcus pyogenes*, *Pseudomonas aeruginosa*, and *Escherichia coli* were spread over the nutrient agar plates using separate sterile cotton buds. After the microbial lawn preparation, three different extracts (20 grams of powdered plant materials mixed with 100 ml of various solvents (distilled water, ethanol, and acetone solution)) of plant disc were placed on the organism-inoculated plates with equal distance; control discs were also prepared. All bacterial plates were incubated at 27°C for 24 h. The diameter of the minimum zone of inhibition was measured in millimeter. For each test, three replicates were performed.

Results and discussion

The compounds identified and their quantities in the *A. vera* LGE and ELGE are summarized in Table 1. Of all the compounds identified, the groups of compounds best described for their health benefits are the phenolic acids/ polyphenols, sterols, fatty acids, and indoles. Apart from these, various alkanes, pyrimidines, alkaloids, organic acids, aldehydes, dicarboxylic acids, ketones, and alcohols were also identified. Although the extraction methods used in this study were not selected to target alcohols, a few of these were also identified. One would, however, expect a far larger variety of alcohols to occur in *Aloe* and in far higher concentrations. For better extraction of these, headspace isolation by simultaneous purging should be used as described previously [25]. However, by employing this method, one would extract far less of the other biologically important health-associated compounds. Therefore, to accomplish the aims of our study, alternative extraction procedures were used as described under the 'Methods' section using ethyl acetate/diethyl ether and hexane.

A general comparison of the phytochemical contents of the LGE and ELGE, calculated per LGE dry mass, shows that with the exception of a few compounds, far fewer compounds and at lower concentrations are extracted from 95% ethanol extracts than directly from the LGE using ethyl acetate/diethyl ether or hexane. The occurrence of

Table 1 Concentrations of GC-MS identified compounds from LGE and 95% ELGE

Compound	Concentration (ppm)		
	LGE (per dry mass LGE)	ELGE (per dry mass LGE	ELGE (per dry mass ELGE)
Phenolic acids/polyphenols			
Phenol	14.32	30.12	1.3×10^4
Vanillic	58.60	24.34	8.5×10^3
Homovanillic	18.55	13.26	5.0×10^3
Protocatechuic	163.21	42.33	1.6×10^4
3,4-Dihydroxyphenylacetic	7.54		
5-Methoxyprotocatechuic	2.5		
Syringic	25.54		
Sinapic	32.68		
p-Coumaric	450.87		
Isoferulic	52.90		
Ferulic	88.67	4.2	1.5×10^3
Aloe emodin	87.79		
4-Phenyllactic	11.02		
4-Ethylphenol	10.12	32.21	1.2×10^4
Hydrocinnamic	36.50		
p-Salicylic	186	59.2	1.8×10^4
Benzoic	870.1	5,507	1.9×10^6
Phenylpyruvic		6.50	2.3×10^5
Hydro-p-coumaric	15.31		
Alcohols			
2-Butanol	13.65		
Glycerol	340.9		
Phenylethanol	86.56		
Aldehydes			
Benzaldehyde	56.34	72.5	2.5×10^4
m-Tolualdehyde	18.21		
Organic acids			
Lactic	148	202.1	7.1×10^4
Glycolic	93.1		
Pyruvic		88.1	3.1×10^4
Furoic	57.43		
Phosphoric		341.2	1.2×10^5
Succinic	383	117.6	4.1×10^4
2-Methylsuccinic	62.1		
Picolinic		281	9.7×10^4
Malic	46.7		
Tartaric	18.3		6.3×10^3
Isonicotinic	40.21		
2-Hydroxybutyric		2.1	829.92
Alkanes			
1,3-Dihydroxybutane	10.22	10.56	3.7×10^3

Table 1 Concentrations of GC-MS identified compounds from LGE and 95% ELGE (Continued)

Pyrimidines			
Uracil	697.23		
Thymine	429.76	189.11	6.3×10^4
Fatty acids			
Lauric (C12:0)	0.32		
Myristic (C14:0)	0.74		
Palmitoleic (C16:1)	1.32	0.19	65.70
Linoleic (C18:2 n-6)	102	0.42	143
Indoles			
Indole-3-acetic acid	2.80		
Alkaloids			
Hypoxanthine	27.65		
Ketones			
Acetophenone	8.02		
Sterols			
Cholestanol	24.32	12.99	4.6×10^3
β-Sitosterol	1,604.5		
Dicarboxylic acids			
Azelaic	0.02		
Undecanedioic	0.04		

higher concentrations of a few compounds from the ELGE is most probably due to matrix protein conformation changes and precipitation by the ethanol, hence making extraction of these protein-associated compounds easier [26]. However, when the concentrations are quantified for the individual compounds occurring in the ELGE per dry mass of ELGE, the concentrations for the compounds extracted are approximately 345 times higher than those for the same compounds occurring in the lyophilized LGE. Similarly, higher concentrations of total polyphenols, total flavonoids, and total non-flavonoids, as well as higher antioxidant capacities using ORAC and FRAP analyses (Table 2) are seen in the ELGE extracts. Additionally, these values are again far less when quantified per LGE dry mass. This indicates that from an analytical perspective, 95% ethanol is in general less effective than direct ethyl acetate/ diethyl ether or hexane extractions (in the case of fatty acids) for the phytochemical characterization of *Aloe* species. However, the results also indicate the ELGE allows for effective concentration of a number of biologically

Table 2 Concentrations of total polyphenols, flavonoids, and non-flavonoids as well as antioxidant capacity via ORAC and FRAP analyses

Compound	LGE (dry mass)	LGE (wet mass)	ELGE (expressed as dry mass ELGE)	ELGE (expressed as dry mass LGE)	ELGE (expressed as wet mass LGE)
Total polyphenols (mg of GAE/100 g ± SD)	78.2 ± 4.03	2.70 ± 0.14	413 ± 9.88	26.8 ± 0.63	0.93 ± 0.02
Total flavonoids (mg of CE/100 g ± SD)	5.3 ± 0.38	0.19 ± 0.01	33.6 ± 1.98	2.15 ± 0.13	0.08 ± 0.003
Total non-flavonoids (by calculation)	73.7 ± 0.43	2.55 ± 0.22	378 ± 6.78	24.5 ± 1.5	0.86 ± 0.02
ORAC, hydrophilic (µmol of TE/g)	53 ± 1.1	1.81 ± 0.04	136 ± 2.3	8.83 ± 0.16	0.30 ± 0.006
ORAC, lipophilic (µmol of TE/g)	ND	ND	ND	ND	ND
ORAC, total (µmol of TE/g)	53 ± 1.1	1.81 ± 0.04	136 ± 2.3	8.83 ± 0.16	0.30 ± 0.006
FRAP (µmol/g)	4.9 ± 0.25	0.17 ± 0.07	19.0 ± 0.3	1.21 ± 0.02	0.05 ± 0.001

Concentrations of total polyphenols, flavonoids, and non-flavonoids as well as antioxidant capacity via oxygen radical absorbance capacity (ORAC) and ferric reducing antioxidant power (FRAP) analyses in lyophilized aloe ferox leaf gel (LGE) and 95% ethanol leaf gel extracts (ELGE). ND, not detected.

active ingredients from LGE, confirming its popularity for use for testing biological activity for certain components *in vivo* and *in vitro*. Additionally, polyphenols are generally classified into flavonoids and non-flavonoids [27]. In Table 1, GC-MS analyses indicate the majority of the polyphenol compounds identified in the *A. vera* leaf gel belonging to the non-flavonoid group of polyphenols. This was confirmed by the spectrophotometic analysis of polyphenols summarized in Table 2, indicating the non-flavonoid components to contribute to 93% of the total polyphenols in the LGE and 92% in the ELGE.

Over the past 10 years, there has been a growing interest in the value of polyphenols among researchers and food manufacturers. This is mainly because of their antioxidant properties, their abundance in our diet, and their role in the prevention of various diseases associated with oxidative stress such as cancer, cardiovascular disease, neurodegeneration [28], and diabetes [29]. Polyphenols constitute a large class of molecules containing a number of phenolic hydroxyl groups attached to ring structures allowing for their antioxidant activities. These compounds are multifunctional and can act as reducing agents, hydrogen-donating antioxidants, and singlet oxygen quenchers [27]. All of the individual *A. vera* leaf gel antioxidant polyphenols identified in Table 1 may contribute to the prevention of the above-mentioned diseases to a greater or lesser extent. The individual contributions of these to disease prevention would, however, depend on their concentrations, antioxidant capacities, bioavailabilities, and specific mechanisms of action. Although the individual phenolic acids/polyphenols occurring in the highest concentrations were benzoic acid, *p*-toluic acid, *p*-coumaric acid, *p*-salicylic acid, protocatechuic acid, hydroxyphenylacetic acid, ferulic acid, aloe emodin, and vanillic acid, it is well-known that the protective health benefits of polyphenols are mainly through a combination of additive and/or synergistic effects between the individual compounds [30]. Consequently, those polyphenol/phenolic compounds identified in lower concentrations may also be of value. Due to the fact that the majority of the phenolic acids/polyphenols identified in *A. vera* leaf gel in Table 1 are antioxidants [27] and these compounds as a group occur in the highest concentrations, one would expect these to contribute to the majority of the antioxidant capacity measured in these extracts (Table 2). However, apart from these polyphenols, the indoles [31] and alkaloids identified

[32] are also known to possess antioxidant activities and may consequently also contribute to the ORAC and FRAP values of these extracts. When interpreting the data of this nature, one should keep in mind that using the concentrations of these antioxidant compounds alone is insufficient criteria for making predictions of individual contributions to oxidative stress. As previously described, this is due to the fact that the concentrations of individual polyphenol antioxidants are not the only factor influencing antioxidant capacity; the structural arrangements (number and position of hydroxyl groups, double bonds, and aromatic rings) of these compounds also play a role [27]. Additionally, their individual contributions to ORAC and FRAP may also differ. Due to the FRAP analysis being an indication of the ferric ion reducing power of a compound or mixture and the ORAC analysis indicating the ability of a compound or mixture to scavenge free radicals, the various individual polyphenol components of the mixture may have stronger free radical scavenging abilities than reducing power, or vice versa, dependent on their chemical structures [33]. Phytosterols are another group of compounds that are well-known for their health benefits. Of the four phytosterols identified in Table 1, β-sitosterol occurred in by far the highest concentrations in the LGE, contributing to 93% of the total phytosterols identified.

Antibacterial activity

Antibacterial activity of *A. vera* was analyzed against *S. aureus*, *S. pyogenes*, *P. aeruginosa* and *E. coli*. The maximum antibacterial activities were observed in acetone extract (12 ± 0.45, 20 ± 0.35, 20 ± 0.57, 15 ± 0.38) other than aqueous extract (0.00, 9 ± 0.54, 0.00, 0.00) and ethanol extract (7 ± 0.38, 20 ± 0.36, 15 ± 0.53, 0.00). Among the three bacterial organisms, maximum growth suppression was observed in *S. pyogenes* (20 ± 0.35) and *P. aeroginosa* (20 ± 0.57) when compared with *S. aureus* (12 ± 0.45) and *E. coli* (15 ± 0.38). Results are presented in Table 3. *A. vera* leaf gel can inhibit the growth of the two gram-positive bacteria *Shigella flexneri* and *Streptococcus progenies* [2]. Specific plant compounds such as anthraquinones and dihhydroxyanthraquinones as well as saponins [32] have been proposed to have direct antimicrobial activity.

The ELGE was once again less effective in extracting these compounds, and only cholestanol was identified. However, the levels normalized to dry mass ELGE were

Table 3 Antibacterial activity of *Aloe vera*

Sample number	Extract	Zone of inhibition (mm in diameter; mean ± SD; n = 3)			
		Staphylococcus aureus	*Streptococcus pyogens*	*Pseudomonas aeruginosa*	*Escherichia coli*
1	Aqueous	-	9 ± 0.53	-	-
2	Ethanol	7 ± 0.37	19 ± 0.36	14 ± 0.53	-
3	Acetone	12 ± 0.45	20 ± 0.35	19 ± 0.57	14 ± 0.38

not insignificant. Phytosterols are best described for their total cholesterol and low-density lipid cholesterol (LDL-C) lowering effects, consequently associated with reducing the risk for cardiovascular disease [26]. As summarized by Devaraj and Jialal [31] evidence for this has been observed in hypercholesterolemic, diabetic, and healthy volunteers. The mechanism proposed by which phytosterols accomplish this is by lowering cholesterol absorption due to the structural similarities these compounds share with cholesterol [27,29]. Apart from lowering cardiovascular risk factors associated with diabetes, phytosterols (â-sitosterol in particular) have been shown to positively affect diabetes by directly lowering fasting blood glucose levels by cortisol inhibition [30]. Additionally, phytosterols have been shown to reduce biomarkers for oxidative stress and inflammation [31], as well as to reduce cancer development by enabling antitumor responses by increasing immune recognition of cancer, influencing hormonal-dependent growth of endocrine tumors, and altering sterol biosynthesis due to the structural similarities of the phytosterols with these compounds and their substrates [32]. Phytosterols have also been shown to directly inhibit tumor growth by slowing cell cycle progression, by induction of apoptosis, and by the inhibition of tumor metastasis [32].

Long-chain polyunsaturated fatty acids (PUFAs) also have important biological functions noted to modulate risks of chronic degenerative and inflammatory diseases, of which the essential PUFAs, linolenic (C18:3 n-3) and linoleic (C18:2 n-6) acids, are best described [30,33]. Both of these were present in the *A. vera* leaf gel extracts, with linoleic acid being the major fatty acid present. However, despite this, the concentrations of these are still very low in comparison to the other compounds identified with possible health benefits and were not even detectable in the lipophilic ORAC analysis. These fatty acids may probably be too low for the *A. vera* leaf gel to contribute to health through its fatty acid composition. In conclusion, the results of this study show that from an analytical perspective, 95% ethanol is a less efficient solvent for the extraction of the phytochemical components of *A. vera* leaf gel for descriptive purposes as compared to ethyl acetate/diethyl ether or hexane (in the case of fatty acids). Although the 95% ethanol extracts contain a smaller variety of extracted compounds, their concentrations are, however, approximately 345 times higher than those of the lyophilized *A. vera* leaf gel when quantified as dry mass ELGE extract. This justifies the popularity of the ELGE for applications testing biological efficacy *in vivo* and *in vitro*. For the purpose of determining possible biological application, *A. vera* leaf gel was characterized.

Conclusion

Various phenolic acids/polyphenols, phytosterols, fatty acids, indoles, alkanes, pyrimidines, alkaloids, organic acids, aldehydes, dicarboxylic acids, ketones, and alcohols were identified and quantified. Due to the presence of the antioxidant polyphenols, indoles, and alkaloids, the *A. vera* leaf gel shows antioxidant capacity as confirmed by ORAC and FRAP analyses. Both GC-MS and spectrophotometric analyses show the non-flavonoid polyphenols to contribute to the majority of the total polyphenol content. Due to the occurrence of the polyphenols, phytosterols, and perhaps the indoles present, *A. vera* leaf gel may show promise in alleviating or preventing the symptoms associated with cardiovascular diseases, cancer, neurodegeneration, and diabetes. This may be due to the well-documented lowering effects of these compounds on total cholesterol, LDL-C, and fasting blood glucose. These results support the current use of *A. vera* by both industry and traditional healers for the treatment of the above-mentioned diseases. However, further clinical trials regarding these claims are necessary before accurate conclusions regarding these heath benefits can be made.

Competing interests

The author declare that she has no competing interests.

Acknowledgement

The financial support of the National Institute of Genetic Engineering and Biotechnology (NIGEB), Iran, was greatly appreciated.

References

1. Dabai YU, Muhammad S, Aliyu BS (2007) Antibacterial activity of anthraquinone fraction of Vitex doniana. Pakistan J Biol Sci:1–3

2. Ferro VA, Bradbury F, Cameron P, Shakir E, Rahman SR, Stimson WH (2003) In vitro susceptibilities of Shigella flexneri and Streptococcus phygenes to inner gel of *Aloe barbadensis* Miller. Antimicro Chemother 47(3):1137–1139

3. Hamman JH (2008) Composition and applications of *Aloe vera* leaf gel. Molecules 13:1599–1616

4. Boutagy J, Harvey DJ (1978) Determination of cytosine arabinoside in human plasma by gas chromatography with a nitrogen-sensitive detector and by gas chromatography–mass spectrometry. J Chromatogr 146:283–296

5. Rice-Evans C (2004) Flavonoids and isoflavones: absorption, metabolism, and bioactivity. Free Radical Biol Med 36:827–828

6. Scalbert A, Williamson D (2000) Dietary intake and bioavailability of polyphenols. J Nutr 130:2073S–2085S

7. Liu RH (2000) Supplement quick fix fails to deliver. Food Technol Int 1:71–72

8. Herraiz T, Galisteo J (2004) Endogenous and dietary indoles: a class of antioxidants and radical scavengers in the ABTS assay. Free Radical Res 38:323–331

9. Azam S, Hadi N, Khan NU, Hadi SM (2003) Antioxidant and prooxidant properties of caffeine, theobromine and xanthine. Med Sci Monit 9:325–330

10. Loots D, der Tw V, Jerling FH (2006) Polyphenol composition and antioxidant activity of Kei-apple (Dovyalis caffra) juice. J Agric Food Chem 54:1271–1276

11. Okyar A, Can A, Akev N, Baktir G, Sutlupinar S (2001) Effect of *Aloe vera* leaves on blood glucose level in type I and type II diabetic rat models. Phytother Res 15:157–161

12. Chithra P, Sajithlal GB, Chandrakasan G (1998) Influence of *Aloe vera* on the healing of dermal wounds in diabetic rats. J Ethnopharmacol 59:195–201

13. Koo MWL (1994) *Aloe vera*, antiulcer and antidiabetic effects. Phytother Res 8:461–464

14. Saito H (1993) Purification of active substances of *Aloe arborescens* Miller and their biological and pharmacological activity. Phytother Res 7:S14–S19

15. Bunyapraphatsara N, Yongchaiyudha S, Rungpitarangsi V, Chokechaijaroenporn O (1996) Antidiabetic activity of *Aloe vera* L. juice. II.

Clinical trials in diabetes mellitus patients in combination with glibenclamide. Phytomedicine 3:245–248

16. Reynolds T, Dweck AC (1999) *Aloe vera* leaf gel: a review update. J Ethnopharmacol 68:3–37

17. Choi S, Chung MH (2003) A review on the relationship between *Aloe vera* components and their biologic effects. Semin. Integrative Med 1:53–62

18. al-Shamaony L, al-Khazraji SM, Twaij SA (1994) Hypoglycaemic effect of *Artemisia herba* alba. II. Effect of a valuable extract on some blood parameters in diabetic animals. J Ethnopharmacol 43:167–171

19. Rajasekaran S, Ravi K, Sivagnanam K, Subramanian S (2006) Beneficial effects of *Aloe vera* leaf gel extract on lipid profile status in rats with streptozotocin diabetes. Clin Exp Pharmacol Physiol 33:232–237

20. Singleton VL, Rossi JA (1965) Colorimetry of total phenolics with phospomolybdic-phosphotungstic acid reagents. Am J Enol Vitic 16:144–158

21. Marinova D, Robarova F, Atanassova M (2005) Total phenolics and total flavonoids in bulgarian fruits and vegetables. J UniV Chem Technol Metal 40:255–260

22. Prior RL, Hoang H, Gu L, Wu X, Bacchiocca M, Howard L, Hampsch-Woodill M, Huang D, Ou B, Jacob R (2003) Assays for hydrophilic and lipophilic antioxidant capacity (oxygen radical absorbance capacity (ORAC(FL))) of plasma and other biological and food samples. J Agric Food Chem 51:3273–3279

23. Huang D, Ou B, Hampsch-Woodill M, Flanagan JA, Deemer EK (2002) Development and validation of oxygen radical absorbance capacity assay for lipophilic antioxidants using randomly methylated â-cyclodextrin as the solubility enhancer. J Agric Food Chem 50(7):1815–1821

24. Benzie IF, Strain JJ (1999) Ferric reducing/antioxidant power assay: direct measure of total antioxidant activity of biological fluids and modified version for simultaneous measurement of total antioxidant power and ascorbic acid concentration. Methods Enzymol 299:15–27

25. Umano K, Nakahara K, Shoji A, Shibamoto T (1999) Aroma chemicals isolated and identified from leaves of *Aloe arborescens* Mill. var. Natalensis Berger. J Agric Food Chem 47:3702–3705

26. Patch CS, Tapsell LC, Williams PG, Gordon M (2006) Plant sterols as dietary adjuvants in the reduction of cardiovascular risk: theory and evidence. Vasc Health Risk Manag 2:157–162

27. Lichtenstein AH, Deckelbaum RG (2001) AHA Science Advisory. Stanol/sterol ester-containing foods and blood cholesterol levels. A statement for healthcare professionals from the Nutrition Committee of the Council on Nutrition, Physical Activity, and Metabolism of the American Heart Association. Circulation 103:1177–1179

28. Normen L, Dutta P, Lia A, Andersson H (2000) Soy sterol esters and â-sitostanol ester as inhibitors of cholesterol absorption in human small bowel. Am J Clin Nutr 71:908–913

29. Jones PJ, Ntanios FY, Raeini-Sarjaz M, Vanstone CA (1999) Cholesterol-lowering efficacy of a sitostanol-containing phytosterol mixture with a prudent diet in hyperlipidemic men. Am J Clin Nutr 69:1144–1150

30. McAnuff MA, Harding WW, Omoruyi FO, Jacobs H, Morrison EY, Asemota HN (2005) Hypoglycemic effects of steroidal sapogenins isolated from Jamaican bitter yam, Dioscorea polygonoides. Food Chem Toxicol 43:1667–1672

31. Devaraj S, Jialal I (2006) The role of dietary supplementation with plant sterols and stanols in the prevention of cardiovascular disease. Nutr Re 64:348–354

32. Bradford PG, Awad AB (2007) Phytosterols as anticancer compounds. Mol Nutr Food Res 51:161–170

33. Simopoulos AP (2006) Evolutionary aspects of diet, the omega-6/ omega-3 ratio and genetic variation: nutritional implications for chronic diseases. Biomed Pharmacother 60:502–507

10

Chemical composition and antibacterial activity of the essential oils of *Ferula vesceritensis* Coss et Dur. leaves, endemic in Algeria

Amar Zellagui[1], Noueddine Gherraf[1*] and Salah Rhouati[2]

Abstract

Background: The biological importance of members of genus *Ferula* promoted us to investigate the leaves of *Ferula vesceritensis* Coss et Dur. (endemic plant) previously not investigated. This study presents the chemical composition and antibacterial activities of the hydrodistilled oils.

Results: Volatile components of the leaves of *F. vesceritensis* have been studied by gas chromatography–mass spectrometry to afford 23 compounds. The major components were found to be 5,9-tetradecadiyne (24.72%), germacrene D (24.51%), farnesene (8.57%), and α-bisabolene (8.57%). The antimicrobial activities of the essential oils were evaluated by disk diffusion method and tested against Gram-positive and Gram-negative bacteria. The volatile oil showed a strong antibacterial activity against *Staphylococcus aureus*, *Escherichia coli*, and *Klebsiella pneumonia*.

Conclusions: These results reinforce the previous studies showing that the genus *Ferula* is considered as a good source of essential oils. The results presented here can be considered as the first information on the antimicrobial properties of *F. vesceritensis*.

Keywords: *Ferula vesceritensis*, Volatile oils, GC-MS, Antimicrobial activity

Background

Since the middle ages, essential oils have widely been used for bactericidal, virucidal fungicidal, antiparasitical, insecticidal, medicinal, and cosmetic applications, especially nowadays in pharmaceutical, sanitary, cosmetic, and agricultural and food industries. Because of the mode of extraction, mostly by hydrodistillation from aromatic plants, they contain a variety of volatile molecules such as terpenes and terpenoids, phenol-derived aromatic components, and aliphatic components [1].

The exclusively old-world genus *Ferula*, belonging to the family *Apiaceae*, has some 130 species distributed throughout the Mediterranean area and Central Asia. These plants are often used as spices and in the preparation of local drugs. The resins are reported to be used for stomach disorders such as a febrifuge and carminative agent [2]. Some species are used in traditional medicine for the treatment of skin infections [3] and hysteria [2]. Previous study dealing with members of this genus revealed that the main constituents are sesquiterpenes and sesquiterpene coumarins. More than 70 species have been studied chemically leading to the fact that germacranes, humulanes, carotanes, himachalanes, and guaianes represent the main sesquiterpene constituents of the genus [4-10]. *Ferula* spp. are also known for their toxicity and pharmacology. Daucane esters from *F. communis* and *Ferula arrigonii* showed antiproliferative activity on human colon cancer lines [11] and calcium ionophoretic and apoptotic effects in the human jurkat T-cell line [12].

Ferula vesceritensis belongs to umbelifereae family, which widely spread in north Africa, this plant is abundant in south east of Algeria. The genus *Ferula* represented in Algeria by six species [13].

Ferula vesceritensis is indigenous to Algerian Sahara. According to ethnobotanical investigation, fruit decoction is used in folk medicine to treat headaches, fever, and throat infections, while the livestock avoids grazing it [14].

* Correspondence: ngherraf@yahoo.com
[1]Laboratory of Biomolecules and Plant Breeding, Life Science and Nature Department, Faculty of Exact Science and Life Science and Nature, University of Larbi Ben Mhidi, Oum El Bouaghi, Algeria
Full list of author information is available at the end of the article

Chemical composition and antibacterial activity of the essential oils of Ferula vesceritensis...

67

Our continuation of investigation carried out on *F. vesceritensis* [15-17]. The essential oils of the leaves of *F. vesceritensis* led to the identification of 23 compounds. Moreover, the evaluation of the antibacterial activity of the essential oils revealed a very important effect against some bacteria strains.

Methods

Gas chromatography/mass spectroscopy

GC/MS analysis was carried out on a Thermoquest-Finnigan Trace GC/MS instrument equipped with a DB-1 fused silica column (30 m, 0.25 mm i.d., film thickness 0.25 m). The oven temperature was raised from 60 to 250°C at a rate of 5°C/min then held at 250°C for 10 min; transfer line temperature was adjusted at 250°C. Helium was used as the carrier gas at a flow rate of 1.1 mL/min with a split ratio of 1/50. Identification of the constituents of each oil was achieved by comparison of their mass spectra and retention times (Rt) with those reported in the literature, and those of authentic samples.

Antimicrobial activity

The antibacterial activity test was carried out on essential oils of the leaves of *F. vesceritensis* roots using disk diffusion method (NCCLS) against four human pathogenic bacteria, including Gram positive, Gram-negative bacteria.

Results and discussion

This study focused essentially on the phytochemical and antibacterial screening of *F. vesceritensis*. The specie has been screened for seven chemical groups. The analyses reveal the presence of volatile oils, flavonoids, saponins, tannins, carotenoids, and coumarins (Table 1).

Essential oils from the leaves of *F. vesceritensis* have been studied by GC–MS to afford 23 components. The yield was 1.82% on dry weight basis. In previous studies, the essential oil obtained from the roots of *Ferula ferulaoides* yielded 2.4–3.2% of essential oil from dry roots [18] and average 1,66–3.85% in the fruits of *Ferula gummosa* [19]. The essential oil components identified from *F. vesceritensis* are

listed in Table 2; the major components were found to be 5,9-tetradecadiyne 24.72%, germacrene D (24.51%), farnesene (8.57%), α-bisabolene (8.57%). Some other compounds were only present in minor amounts.

Concerning the chemical composition of the essential oil of other *Ferula* species, Shatar [18] showed that the roots of *F. ferulaoides* growing in Mongolia were dominated by Guaiol (58.76%), and (*E*)-nerolidol (10.16%). In the fruits of *F. gummosa* from Iran, the major components were β-pinene (43.78%), α-pinene (27.27%) [20], also found β-pinene (43.78%), α-pinene (27.27%) of *F. gummosa* growing in Isfahan [19], also reported that the essential oil of the *Ferula latisecta* collected in Iran was characterized by high contents of (Z)-Ocimenone (32.4%), (*E*)-ocimenone (20.3%), and *cis*-pinocarvone (11.4%) [21].

Antibacterial activity

The antimicrobial activities and toxicity of essential oil have been documented, but their modes of action are complex and still in some cases unknown, considering the large number of different groups of chemical compounds present, this activity is due to the presence of active

Table 2 Chemical composition of essential oils from *F. vesceritensis*

Compounds	Rt	%
Ocimene	07.105	0.31
Limonene	10.554	0.12
Fuseloel	13.587	0.11
Nerylacetone	17.852	**4.45**
Dihydrocarvyl acetate	20.183	**6.20**
Z-ocimene	22.290	03.19
α-methyl pentenal	23.193	0.42
5,9-tetradecadiyne	24.851	**24.72**
1,1-methylene-3-(propenylidene)-5-vinylcyclohexane	25.026	0.69
Calarene	25.173	2.59
Farnesene	25.358	2.71
α-bisabolol	26.632	0.89
Dihydrocarveol acetate	26.769	1.59
A-Bisabolene	26.925	0.53
Nerolidol Rep	27.203	1.02
Xanth ou α farnesene	27.402	2.00
citral	27.595	0.89
Cububene	27.902	**8.57**
Germacrene D	28.311	**24.51**
Nerolidol	31.634	1.55
Bisabolol	32.213	**8.57**
linalol	34.691	4.35
Total		**99.98**

Bold entries highlight the major components.

Table 1 Phytochemical screening from *F. vesceritensis*

Chemical groups	Roots	Leaves	Stems	Flowers	Fruits & seeds
Volatile oils	++	+++	++	+++	+++
Carotenoids	+	+	+	+	++
Alkaloids	–	–	–	–	–
Flavone aglycones	+	+	+–	+	+–
Coumarins	+++	+++	+++	+++	+++
Tanins	+	+	+	+	+
Saponins	++	–	–	–	–
Flavone glycosides	–	++	++	++	++

Table 3 Inhibition effect of essential oils from *F. vesceritensis*

Bacteria	250 µg/mL	500 µg/mL	1000 µg/mL	2000 µg/mL	4000 µg/mL	8000 µg/mL
Escherichia coli ATCC 25922	14.5 ± 0.75	19.0 ± 0.95	19.0 ± 0.81	21.5 ± 0.57	22.0 ± 0.57	26 ± 1.25
Klebsiella pneumonia	11.5 ± 0.0	13.5 ± 0.5	15.0 ± 0.95	20.5 ± 0.95	22.5 ± 0.95	24.5 ± 0.57
S. aureous	12.5 ± 0.57	14 ± 0.57	14.5 ± 0.5	17 ± 1.21	19.5 ± 1.29	27 ± 0.81
Pseudomonas aerugenosa ATCC 27853		06.00	7 ± 1.73	11 ± 0.81	13.5 ± 1.15	16 ± 1.41

constituents, mainly attributable to isoprenes such as monoterpenes, sesquiterpenes, and related alcohols, other hydrocarbons and phenols [1].

The diffusion test was applied to four microorganisms including Gram-positive, -negative bacteria. The results summarized in Table 3 showed that the volatile oil from *F. vesceritensis* prevented the growth of all the tested microorganisms and it has been revealed that the medium diameter of inhibition zone increase proportionally with the increase of concentrations.

The obtained inhibition zone varied from 6.00 to 27.00 mm with a highest inhibition zone recorded with *Staphylococcus aureus* at 8 mg mL and with 26 mm at *E. coli* in the same concentration. This results corresponding with those obtained on *F. gummosa* and *F. latisecta* [20]. It should be mentioned that there are no background antibacterial studies on *F. vesceritensis*.

Experimental
Plant material
The leaves of *F. vesceritensis* were collected on May 2010 near Ghardaya Algeria. The plants were identified by Dr. M. Chahma, Faculty of Sciences, University of Ourgla, Algeria, voucher specimens were deposited at the Chemistry Department, University of Mentouri-Constantine under code number (AM#112).

Extraction
Essential oils were obtained by hydrodistillation of 150 g of dried aerial parts using a Clevenger-type apparatus for 3 h. Diethyl ether (10 mL) was used as the collector solvent as reported in literature. After evaporation of the solvent, the oil was dried over anhydrous sodium sulfate and stored in sealed vials protected from the light at –20°C before analyses. Three oil samples were obtained by hydrodistillation and subsequently analyzed by GC-MS.

Antimicrobial activity
Microorganism strains
All of the bacteria; standard strains *E. coli* ATCC 25922, *P. aerugenosa* ATCC 27853 and (clinical stains: *S. aureus, K. pneumonia*) were obtained from Bacteriology Laboratory Constantine Hospital University (C.H.U).

The bacterial strains were first grown on Muller Hinton medium (MHI) at 37°C for 24 h prior to seeding on to the nutrient agar. A sterile 6-mm-diameter filter disk (Whatman paper no. 3) was placed on the infusion agar seeded with bacteria, and each extract suspended in water was dropped on to each paper disk (40 µL per disk) for all of prepared concentrations (8, 4, 2, 1, 0.5, 0.25 mg/mL). The treated Petri dishes were kept at 4°C for 1 h, and incubated at 37°C for 24 h. The antibacterial activity was assessed by measuring the zone of growth inhibition surrounding the disks. Each experiment was carried out in triplicate.

Conclusions
Our study of the Algerian *F. vesceritensis* leaves led to the extraction and characterization of 23 compounds followed by the evaluation of antimicrobial activity for the first time. These results reinforce the previous studies showing that the genus *Ferula* is considered as a good source of essential oils. The results presented here can be considered as the first information on the antimicrobial properties of *F. vesceritensis*.

Competing interests
The authors declare that they have no competing interests.

Author details
[1]Laboratory of Biomolecules and Plant Breeding, Life Science and Nature Department, Faculty of Exact Science and Life Science and Nature, University of Larbi Ben Mhidi, Oum El Bouaghi, Algeria. [2]Laboratory of Natural Products and Organic Synthesis, Department of Chemistry, Faculty of Science, University of Mentouri-Constantine, Constantine, Algeria.

References
1. Bakkali F, Averbeck D, Idaomar MM (2008) Biological effects of essential oils—a review. Food Chem Toxicol 46:446–475
2. Boulus L (1983) Medicinal plants of North Africa. Algonae, MI, p 183
3. Appendino G, Spagliardi P, Cravotto G, Pocock V, Milligan S (2002) Daucane phytoestrogens: a structure–activity study. J Nat Prod 65:1612–1615
4. Gonzalez AG, Barrera JB (1995) Chemistry and the sources of mono and bicyclic sesquiterpenes from *Ferula* species. Progress Chem Org Nat Prod 64:1–92
5. Appendino G, Jakupovic J, Alloatti S, Ballero M (1997) Daucane esters from *Ferula arrigonii*. Phytochemistry 45:1639–1643
6. Kojima K, Isakam K, Ondognii P, Zevgeegiino O, Gombosurengyin P, Davgiin K, Mizukami H, Ogihiara Y (2000) Sesquiterpenoid derivatives from *Ferula feruloides* IV. Chem Pharm Bull 48:353–356
7. Murray RDH (1989) Coumarins. Nat Prod Rep 6:591–624
8. Ahmed AA (1999) Sesquiterpenes coumarins and sesquiterpenes from *ferula senaica*. Phytochemistry 50:109–112
9. Nagatsu A, Isaka K, Kojima K, Ondognii P, Zevgeegiin O, Gombosurengyin P, Davgiin K, Irfan B, Iqubal CM, Ogihara Y (2002) New sesquiterpenes from *Ferula ferulaeoides*. Chem Pharm Bull 50:675–677
10. El-Razek MH, Ohta S, Hirata T (2003) Terpenoid coumarins of the genus *Ferula*. Heterocycles 60:689–716

Chemical composition and antibacterial activity of the essential oils of Ferula vesceritensis...

69

11. Poli F, Appendino G, Sachetti G, Ballero M, Maggiano N, Ranaletti FO (2005) Antiproliferative effects of daucanes esters from *Ferula communis* and *Ferula arrigonii* on human colon cancer cell lines. Phytother Res 19:152–157

12. Macho A, Blanco-Molina M, Spagliardi P, Appendino G, Bremner P, Heinrich M, Fiebich BL, Munoz E (2004) Calcium ionophoretic and apoptotic effects of ferutinin in the human jurkat line. Biochem Pharmacol 68:875–883

13. Quezel P, Santa S (1962) Nouvelle flore d'Algérie et des régions désertiques méridianales. CNRS, Paris, p 672

14. Oughlissi-Dehak K, Lawton P, Michalet CB, Darbour SN, Hadj-Mahammed M, Badjah-Hadj A, Dijoux Franca MG, Guilet D (2008) Sesquiterpenes from aerial parts of *Ferula vesceritensis*. Phytochemistry 69:1933–1938

15. Ahmed AA, Mohamed-Elamir FH, Zellagui A, Rhouati S, Tarik A, Ahmed AM, Sayed MA, Shinji Ohta TH (2007) Ferulsinaic acid, a sesquiterpene coumarin with a rare carbon skeleton from *Ferula species*. Phytochemistry 68:680–686

16. Lahouel M, Zini R, Zellagui A, Rhouati S, Carrupt PA, Morin D (2007) Ferulenol specifically inhibits succinate ubiquinone reductase at the level of the ubiquinone cycle. Biochem Biophys Res Commun 355:252–257

17. Boussenane HN, Kebsa W, Boutabet K, Rouibah H, Benguedouar L, Rhouati S, Alyane M, Zellagui A, Lahouel M (2009) Disruption of mitochondrial membrane potential by ferulenol and restoration by propolis extract. Antiapoptotic role of propolis. Acta Biologica Hungarica 60(4):385–398

18. Shatar S (2005) Essential oil of *Ferula ferulaoides* from Western Mongolia. Chem Nat Compd 41:5

19. Talebi KE, Naghavi MR, Alayhs M (2008) Study of the essential oil variation of *Ferula gummosa* samples from Iran. Chem Nat Compd 44:1

20. Ghasemi Y, Faridi P, Mehregan I, Mohagheghzadeh A (2005) *Ferula gummosa* fruits: an aromatic antimicrobial agent. Chem Nat Compd 41:3

21. Zohreh H, Peyman S, Yousefi M, Hejazi Y, Laleh A, Mozaffarian V, Masoudi S, Rustaiyan A (2006) Chemical composition and antimicrobial activity of the essential oils of *Ferula latisecta* and *Mozaffariania insignis* from Iran. Chem Nat Compd 42:6

11

Bismuth nitrate-induced microwave-assisted expeditious synthesis of vanillin from curcumin

Debasish Bandyopadhyay and Bimal K Banik[*]

Abstract

Background: Curcumin and vanillin are the two useful compounds in food and medicine. Bismuth nitrate pentahydrate is an economical and ecofriendly reagent.

Method: Bismuth nitrate pentahydrate impregnated montmorillonite KSF clay and curcumin were subjected to microwave irradiation.

Results: Microwave-induced bismuth nitrate-promoted synthesis of vanillin from curcumin has been accomplished in good yield under solvent-free condition. Twenty-five different reaction conditions have been studied to optimize the process.

Conclusion: The present procedure for the synthesis of vanillin may find useful application in the area of industrial process development.

Keywords: Curcumin, Vanillin, Microwave, Bismuth nitrate, Fragrance

Background

Curcumin, a polyphenol derived from *Curcuma longa* (commonly known as turmeric) is an ancient spice and therapeutic used in India for centuries to induce color in food and to treat a wide array of diseases. It has been demonstrated that curcumin has many beneficial pharmacological effects, including anti-inflammatory [1], antioxidant [2], antiviral [3], antiangiogenic [4] effects. Most importantly, curcumin possesses immense antitumorigenic effect. It prevents tumor formation in a number of animal models, including models of skin, colon, liver, esophageal, stomach, and breast cancer [5-8]. Curcumin has also demonstrated the ability to improve patient outcomes in Phase I clinical trials [9]. The potential application of curcumin as a chemopreventive agent in both animal and human studies has been demonstrated [10]. Very recently, curcumin has been reported [11] as a protectant against neurodegenerative diseases through chelation with iron. On the other hand, vanillin (4-hydroxy-3-methoxybenzaldehyde) is an important guaiacol derivative which is extremely selective inhibitor of aldehyde oxidase. It has been found that it acts as a substrate of this enzyme, and is metabolized by aldehyde dehydrogenase [12]. Because of the exceptionally widespread utilization of vanillin in the food, cosmetic, pharmaceutical, nutraceutical and fine chemical industries makes this compound as one of the most important aromas. As a result of these crucial properties, considerable attention has been devoted to the improvement of the production processes of vanillin [13]. We report herein an easy and extremely rapid one-step method for the preparation of vanillin from naturally occurring curcumin in the presence of bismuth nitrate under microwave irradiation (Figure 1).

Methods

FT-IR spectra were registered on a Bruker IFS 55 Equinox FTIR spectrophotometer as KBr discs. ^{1}H NMR (300 MHz) and ^{13}C NMR (75 MHz) spectra were obtained at room temperature with JEOL-300 equipment using d_6-DMSO as solvent. Analytical grade chemicals (Sigma-Aldrich Corporation, Milwaukee, USA) were used throughout the project. Deionized water was used for the preparation of all aqueous solutions.

* Correspondence: banik@utpa.edu
Department of Chemistry, The University of Texas-Pan American, 1201 West University Drive, Edinburg, TX 78539, USA

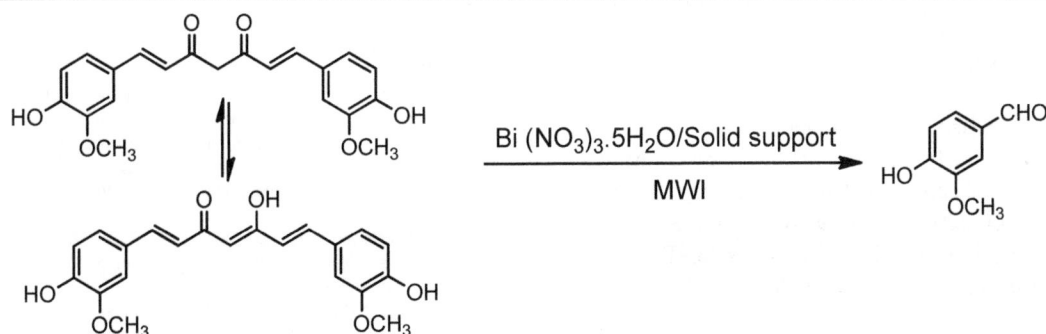

Figure 1 Bismuth nitrate pentahydrate-induced simple synthesis of vanillin from curcumin under microwave irradiation.

Results and discussion

In continuation of our research on environmentally benign reactions, we have been working on methodology development using microwave irradiation for many years. Using microwave irradiation technique, we have successfully developed several new organic methodologies which include stereoselective synthesis of β-lactams [14-16], synthesis of pyrroles [17-20], aza-Michael addition [21], and synthesis of quinoxalines [22]. On the other hand, we have demonstrated the catalytic activity of trivalent bismuth nitrate pentahydrate in a number of occasions. These experiments resulted in various methods that include nitration of aromatic systems [23-25], Michael reaction [26], protection of carbonyl compounds [27], deprotection of oximes and hydrazones [28], Paal-Knorr synthesis of pyrroles [29], hydrolysis of amide [30], electrophilic substitution of indoles [31,32], synthesis of α-aminophosphonates [33], and Biginelli condensation [34]. Our success in the bismuth nitrate-induced reaction has confirmed that this reagent acts as a Lewis acid. Bismuth nitrate pentahydrate is proved to be an effective reagent for the preparation of vanillin. However, $Zn(NO_3)_2$, $Ca(NO_3)_2$, $LaNO_3$, $NaNO_3$, ceric ammonium nitrate, and $Cu(NO_3)_2$ were also studied but without any success. Dry conditions and solvent-free methods along with commercial solvents without any purification were investigated in order to identify the best conditions for this reaction (Table 1). Reactions were performed at high temperature using Dean-Stark water separator, traditional reflux, and conventional kitchen microwave-induced methods. Solid surfaces such as florisil, silica gel, molecular sieves, montmorillonite KSF clay, and neutral alumina were used as solid support in the reaction. It has been found that montmorillonite KSF clay is the best solid surface (entries 4, 9, and 19) among all others.

Experimental

Curcumin (1 mmol), bismuth nitrate pentahydrate (0.75 equivalent), and solid support (500 mg) were mixed in dichloromethane (4 mL) and the solvent was evaporated by rotavapor. The mixture was irradiated in kitchen microwave and the reaction was monitored by TLC. After completion of the reaction (Table 1), the reaction mixture was extracted with dichloromethane and basified with saturated aqueous sodium bicarbonate solution. The organic layer was then washed with brine and

Table 1 Bismuth nitrate pentahydrate-induced simple synthesis of vanillin from curcumin following Figure 1

Entry	Solid surface	Method/solvent	Yield (%)
1	Florisil	Dean-Stark/Benzene	NR[a]
2	Silica gel	Dean-Stark/Benzene	NR
3	Molecular sieves	Dean-Stark/Benzene	NR
4	KSF clay	Dean-Stark/Benzene	10
5	Neutral alumina	Dean-Stark/Benzene	NR
6	Florisil	Reflux/DCM	NR
7	Silica gel	Reflux/DCM	NR
8	Molecular sieves	Reflux/DCM	NR
9	KSF clay	Reflux/DCM	34
10	Neutral alumina	Reflux/DCM	15
11	Florisil	Dry[b]	NR
12	Silica gel	Dry	NR
13	Molecular sieves	Dry	NR
14	KSF clay	Dry	NR
15	Neutral alumina	Dry	NR
16	Florisil	Microwave/solvent free	60
17	Silica gel	Microwave/solvent free	54
18	Molecular sieves	Microwave/solvent free	45
19	KSF clay	Microwave/solvent free	77
20	Neutral alumina	Microwave/solvent free	61
21	Florisil	Reflux/Benzene	NR
22	Silica gel	Reflux/Benzene	NR
23	Molecular sieves	Reflux/Benzene	NR
24	KSF clay	Reflux/Benzene	NR
25	Neutral alumina	Reflux/Benzene	NR

[a]No reaction

[b]Without microwave irradiation, room temperature

water successively, dried with anhydrous sodium sulfate. The pure product (77%) was isolated by flash chromatography over silica gel.

4-hydroxy-3-methoxybenzaldehyde (vanillin)

Light yellow crystals; Mp: 82-83°C, IR (KBr disk, cm^{-1}): 3176, 1679, 1597, 1512, 1426, 1385, 1112, 814, 710; ^{1}H NMR (d$_6$-DMSO, 300 MHz) δ: 9.86 (s, 1 H), 8.09 (m, 2 H), 7.57 (s, 1 H), 3.96 (s, 1 H). ^{13}C NMR (d$_6$-DMSO, 75 MHz) δ: 190.98, 151.33, 148.08, 137.57, 128.28, 121.47, 113.05, and 57.34.

Conclusions

In summary, a new and simple method for the synthesis of vanillin from naturally occurring curcumin has successfully been investigated. Trivalent bismuth nitrate-induced synthesis of vanillin has successfully been carried out under various conditions and the formation of a single product (4-hydroxy-3-methoxybenzaldehyde) has been observed in variable yields. The exploratory results described herein confirm that bismuth nitrate pentahydrate is the reagent of choice for the oxidative cleavage of curcumin to vanillin in the absence of any solvent under microwave-irradiation condition (entry 19). Importantly, no aromatic nitration and rearrangement of curcumin or vanillin has been observed with bismuth nitrate. A selective oxidation of the alkene bond of curcumin to vanillin has taken place. Considering the structure of vanillin and the conditions of the experiments, one can expect further oxidation of the aromatic aldehyde group or nitration of the aromatic system might be other possibilities. However, it is interesting to note that such reactions although feasible, but vanillin is the only isolated product. On the basis of these important and selective observations, this method will find very useful applications in industrial chemistry.

Acknowledgements

We gratefully acknowledge the funding support from the NIH-SCORE (Grant # 2S06M008038-37).

Authors' contributions

DB performed the reactions and structure elucidation of the product. All authors read and approved the final manuscript.

Competing interests

The authors declare that they have no competing interests.

References

1. Srivastava R, Srimal RC (1985) Modification of certain inflammationinduced biochemical changes by curcumin. Ind J Med Res 81:215–223
2. Ruby AJ, Kuttan G, Babu KD, Rajasekharan KN, Kuttan R (1995) Anti-tumour and antioxidant activity of natural curcuminoids. Cancer Lett 94:79–83. doi:10.1016/0304-3835(95)03827-J.
3. Li CJ, Zhang LJ, Dezube BJ, Crumpacker CS, Pardee AB (1993) Three inhibitors of type 1 human immunodeficiency virus long terminal repeat-directed gene expression and virus replication. Proc Natl Acad Sci USA 90:1839–1842. doi:10.1073/pnas.90.5.1839.
4. Aggarwal BB, Kumar A, Bharti AC (2003) Anticancer potential of curcumin: preclinical and clinical studies. Anticancer Res 23:363–398
5. Chuang SE, Kuo ML, Hsu CH, Chen CR, Lin JK, Lai GM, Hsieh CY, Cheng AL (2000) Curcumin-containing diet inhibits diethylnitrosamine-induced murine hepatocarcinogenesis. Carcinogenesis 21:331–335. doi:10.1093/carcin/21.2.331.
6. Ushida J, Sugie S, Kawabata K, Pham QV, Tanaka T, Fujii K, Takeuchi H, Ito Y, Mori H (2000) Chemopreventive effect of curcumin on N-nitrosomethylbenzylamine-induced esophageal carcinogenesis in rats. Jpn J Cancer Res 91:893–898. doi:10.1111/j.1349-7006.2000.tb01031.x.
7. Kawamori T, Lubet R, Steele VE, Kelloff GJ, Kaskey RB, Rao CV, Reddy BS (1999) Chemopreventive effect of curcumin, a naturally occurring anti-inflammatory agent, during the promotion/progression stages of colon cancer. Cancer Res 59:597–601
8. Huang MT, Newmark HL, Frenkel K (1997) Inhibitory effects of curcumin on tumorigenesis in mice. J Cell Biochem Suppl 27:26–34
9. Cheng AL, Hsu CH, Lin JK, Hsu MM, Ho YF, Shen TS, Ko JY, Lin JT, Lin BR, Ming-Shiang W, Yu HS, Jee SH, Chen GS, Chen TM, Chen CA, Lai MK, Pu YS, Pan MH, Wang YJ, Tsai CC, Hsieh CY (2001) Phase I clinical trial of curcumin, a chemopreventive agent, in patients with high-risk or pre-malignant lesions. Anticancer Res 21:2895–2900
10. Jiao Y, Wilkinson J, Pietsch EC, Buss JL, Wang W, Planalp R, Torti FM, Torti SV (2006) Iron chelation in the biological activity of curcumin. Free Rad Biol Med 40:1152–1160. doi:10.1016/j.freeradbiomed.2005.11.003.
11. Minear S, O'Donnell AF, Ballew A, Giaever G, Nislow C, Stearns T, Cyert MS (2011) Curcumin inhibits growth of Saccharomyces cerevisiae through iron chelation. Eukaryot Cell 10:1574–1581. doi:10.1128/EC.05163-11.
12. Panoutsopoulos G, Beedham C (2005) Enzymatic oxidation of vanillin, isovanillin and protocatechuic aldehyde with freshly prepared guinea pig liver slices. Cell Physiol Biochem 15:89–98. doi:10.1159/000083641.
13. Korthou H, Verpoorte R (2007) Vanilla, flavours and fragrances, chap 9. Springer, Berlin pp 203–217
14. Bandyopadhyay D, Banik BK (2010) Microwave-induced stereoselectivity of β-lactam formation with dihydrophenanthrenyl imines via Staudinger cycloaddition. Helv Chim Acta 93:298–301. doi:10.1002/hlca.200900212.
15. Bandyopadhyay D, Yanez M, Banik BK (2011) Microwave-induced stereoselectivity of β-lactam formation: effects of solvents. Heterocycl Lett 1(special issue, July):65–67
16. Bandyopadhyay D, Rivera G, Salinas I, Aguilar H, Banik BK (2010) Iodine-catalyzed remarkable synthesis of novel N-polyaromatic β-lactams bearing pyrroles. Molecules 15:1082–1088. doi:10.3390/molecules15021082.
17. Bandyopadhyay D, Mukherjee S, Banik BK (2010) An expeditious synthesis of N-substituted pyrroles via microwave-induced iodine-catalyzed reaction under solventless conditions. Molecules 15:2520–2525. doi:10.3390/molecules15042520.
18. Andoh-Baidoo R, Danso R, Mukherjee S, Bandyopadhyay D, Banik BK (2011) Microwave-induced N-bromosuccinimide-mediated novel synthesis of pyrroles via Paal-Knorr reaction. Heterocycl Lett 1(special issue, July):107–109
19. Bandyopadhyay D, Banik A, Bhatta S, Banik BK (2009) Microwave-assisted ruthenium trichloride catalyzed synthesis of pyrroles fused with indole systems. Heterocycl Commun 15:121–122
20. Abrego D, Bandyopadhyay D, Banik BK (2011) Microwave-induced indium-catalyzed synthesis of pyrrole fused with indolinone in water. Heterocycl Lett 1:94–95
21. Kall A, Bandyopadhyay D, Banik BK (2010) Microwave-induced aza-Michael reaction in water: a remarkable simple procedure. Synth Commun 42:1730–1735
22. Bandyopadhyay D, Mukherjee S, Rodriguez RR, Banik BK (2010) An effective microwave-induced iodine-catalyzed method for the synthesis of quinoxalines via condensation of 1,2-dicarbonyl compounds. Molecules 15:4207–4212. doi:10.3390/molecules15064207.
23. Canales L, Bandyopadhyay D, Banik BK (2011) Bismuth nitrate pentahydrate-induced novel nitration of Eugenol. Org Med Chem Lett 1:9. doi:10.1186/2191-2858-1-9.

24. Banik BK, Samajdar S, Banik I, Ng S, Hann J (2003) Montmorillonite impregnated with bismuth nitrate: microwave-assisted facile nitration of β-lactams. Heterocycles 61:97–100. doi:10.3987/COM-03-S62.
25. Bose A, Sanjoto WP, Villarreal S, Aguilar H, Banik BK (2007) Novel nitration of estrone by metal nitrates. Tetrahedron Lett 48:3945–3947. doi:10.1016/j.tetlet.2007.04.050.
26. Srivastava N, Banik BK (2003) Bismuth nitrate-catalyzed versatile Michael reactions. J Org Chem 68:2109–2114. doi:10.1021/jo026550s.
27. Srivastava N, Dasgupta SK, Banik BK (2003) A remarkable bismuth nitrate-catalyzed protection of carbonyl compounds. Tetrahedron Lett 44:1191–1193. doi:10.1016/S0040-4039(02)02821-6.
28. Banik BK, Adler D, Nguyen P, Srivastava N (2003) A new bismuth nitrate-induced stereospecific glycosylation of alcohols. Heterocycles 61:101–104. doi:10.3987/COM-03-S63.
29. Rivera S, Bandyopadhyay D, Banik BK (2009) Facile synthesis of N-substituted pyrroles via microwave-induced bismuth nitrate-catalyzed reaction under solventless conditions. Tetrahedron Lett 50:5445–5448. doi:10.1016/j.tetlet.2009.06.002.
30. Bandyopadhyay D, Fonseca RS, Banik BK (2011) Microwave-induced bismuth nitrate-mediated selective hydrolysis of amide. Heterocycl Lett 1(special issue, July):75–77
31. Iglesias L, Aguilar C, Bandyopadhyay D, Banik BK (2010) A new bismuth nitrate-catalyzed electrophilic substitution of indoles with carbonyl compounds under solventless conditions. Synth Commun 40:3678–3682. doi:10.1080/00397910903531631.
32. Rivera S, Bandyopadhyay D, Banik BK (2011) Microwave-induced bismuth nitrate-catalyzed electrophilic substitution of 7-aza indole with activated carbonyl compound under solvent-free conditions. Heterocycl Lett 1(special issue, July):43–46
33. Banik A, Bhatta S, Bandyopadhyay D, Banik BK (2010) A highly efficient bismuth salts-catalyzed route for the synthesis of α-aminophosphonates. Molecules 15:8205–8213. doi:10.3390/molecules15118205.
34. Banik BK, Reddy AT, Datta A, Mukhopadhyay C (2007) Microwave-induced bismuth nitrate-catalyzed synthesis of dihydropyrimidones via Biginelli condensation under solventless conditions. Tetrahedron Lett 48:7392–7394. doi:10.1016/j.tetlet.2007.08.007.

12

Synthesis and biological evaluation of benzimidazole-linked 1,2,3-triazole congeners as agents

Karna Ji Harkala[1], Laxminarayana Eppakayala[1*] and Thirumala Chary Maringanti[2]

Abstract

Background: Benzimidazoles and triazoles are useful structures for research and development of new pharmaceutical molecules and have received much attention in the last decade because of their highly potent medicinal activities.

Findings: A simple and efficient synthesis of triazole was carried out by treatment of 2-(4-azidophenyl)-1H-benzo[d] imidazole (**6**) with different types of terminal alkynes in t-BuOH/H_2O, sodium ascorbate, and $Zn(OTf)_2$, screened for cytotoxicity assay and achieved good results. A series of new benzimidazole-linked 1,2,3-triazole (**8a-i**) congeners were synthesized through cyclization of terminal alkynes and azide. These synthesized congeners **8a-i** were evaluated for their cytotoxicity against five human cancer cell lines. These benzimidazole-linked 1,2,3-triazole derivatives have shown promising activity with IC_{50} values ranging from 0.1 to 43 μM. Among them, the compounds (**8a**, **8b**, **8c**, and **8e**) showed comparable cytotoxicity with adriamycin control drug.

Conclusions: In conclusion, we have developed a simple, convenient, and an efficient convergent approach for the synthesis of benzimidazole-linked 1,2,3-triazole congeners as agents.

Keywords: Benzimidazole; Clic reaction; Cytotoxicity

Findings

Cancer is one of the terrible diseases which cause uncontrolled growth of group of cells. It remains a mean threat to human beings and cause death [1,2]. Recently, many researchers developed safe and effective ways of treating this disease and to search for novel chemotherapeutic agents. The benzimidazole nucleus is an important pharmacophore in medicinal chemistry. The synthesis of novel benzimidazole derivatives remains a main focus of modern drug discovery. The versatility of new generation benzimidazole would represent a fruitful pharmacophore for further development of better medicinal agents. Many researchers have been attracted to benzimidazole derivatives because of their wide range of biological activity. Over the past years, there is a considerable interest in the development and pharmacology of benzimidazole. They are of wide interest because of their diverse biological activity and clinical applications [3].

Some of benzimidazole derivatives have also exhibit antimicrobial [4,5], antitumor [6], anti-inflammatory [7], antihypertensive [8], and antiviral [9] activities. Benzimidazole moiety can also be extracted from naturally occurring compounds such as vitamin B_{12} and its derivatives, and it is similar to the structure of purins. Pyrrolo[1,2-a]benzimidazoles represent a new class of antitumour agent exhibiting cytotoxic activity against a variety of cancer cell lines [10]. Benzimidazole containing anticancer agent, [Hoechst-33342], 2′-(4-ethoxyphenyl)-5-(4-methyl-1-piperazinyl)-2,5′-bis-1H-benzimidazole (**1**), has been reported as inhibitor of topoisomerase-I [11,12]. The other derivative of benzimidazole [Hoechst-33258] (**2** Figure 1) [13,14] shows both *in vitro* antitumour activity, as inhibitor of DNA topoisomerase-I [15]. Hoechst 33258 a fluorescent reagent and as initially found to be active against L1210 murine leukemia. During phase I trial in humans, some responses were seen in pancreatic cancer. However, a subsequent phase II trial did not show any objective responses.

* Correspondence: elxnkits@yahoo.co.in
[1]Department of Physics and Chemistry, Mahatma Gandhi Institute of Technology, Chaitanya Bharathi, Gandipet, Hyderabad 500075, India
Full list of author information is available at the end of the article

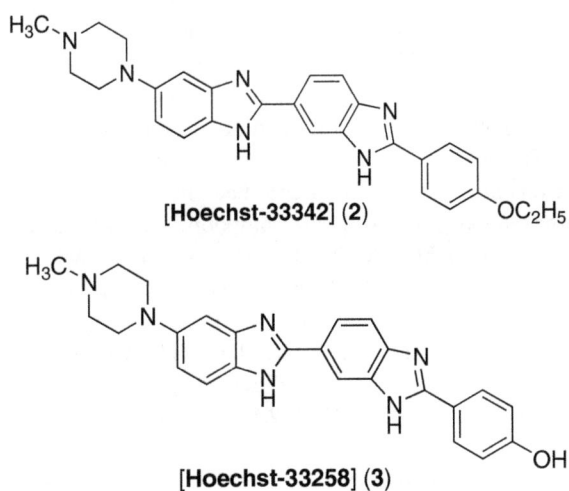

Figure 1 Biologically active benzimidazole derivatives.

In addition, triazoles also display wide spectrum of biological activities and are widely employed as pharmaceuticals and agrochemicals. Triazoles are reported to possess antibacterial, antifungal, and antihelminthic activities [16-21]. They have been regarded as an interesting unit in terms of biological activity [22,23], and some of them have also shown significant anticancer activity in many of the human cell lines [24].

In view of the biological importance of benzimidazole and 1,2,3-triazoles, to know the combined effect of both

benzimidazole and 1,2,3-triazole moieties, it was considered worthwhile to synthesize certain new chemical entities having benzimidazole and 1,2,3-triazole pharmacophores in a single molecular framework, and here we have used Zn (OTf)$_2$ catalyst instead of CuSO$_4$. All of these congeners have been evaluated for their anticancer activity against a panel of five human cancer cell lines (Figure 1).

Experimental section

All chemicals and reagents were obtained from Aldrich (Sigma-Aldrich, St. Louis, MO, USA) and Lancaster (Alfa Aesar, Johnson Matthey Company, Ward Hill, MA, USA) and were used without further purification. Reactions were monitored by TLC and performed on silica gel glass plates containing 60 F-254, and visualization on TLC was achieved by UV light or iodine indicator. ^{1}H and ^{13}C NMR spectra were recorded on Gemini Varian-VXR-unity (Palo Alto, California) (300 and 100 MHz) instrument. Chemical shifts (d) are reported in ppm downfield from internal TMS standard. ESI spectra were recorded on Micromass, Quattro LC (McKinley Scientific, Sparta, NJ, USA) using ESI + software with capillary voltage 3.98 kV and ESI mode positive ion trap detector. Melting points were determined with an electrothermal melting point apparatus and are uncorrected.

Chemistry

The synthesis of novel benzimidazole linked triazole (**8a-i**) derivatives is carried out as shown in Scheme 1. The key intermediate for the preparation of the new analogs is 2-(4-azidophenyl)-1H-benzo[d]imidazole (**6**). The mixture

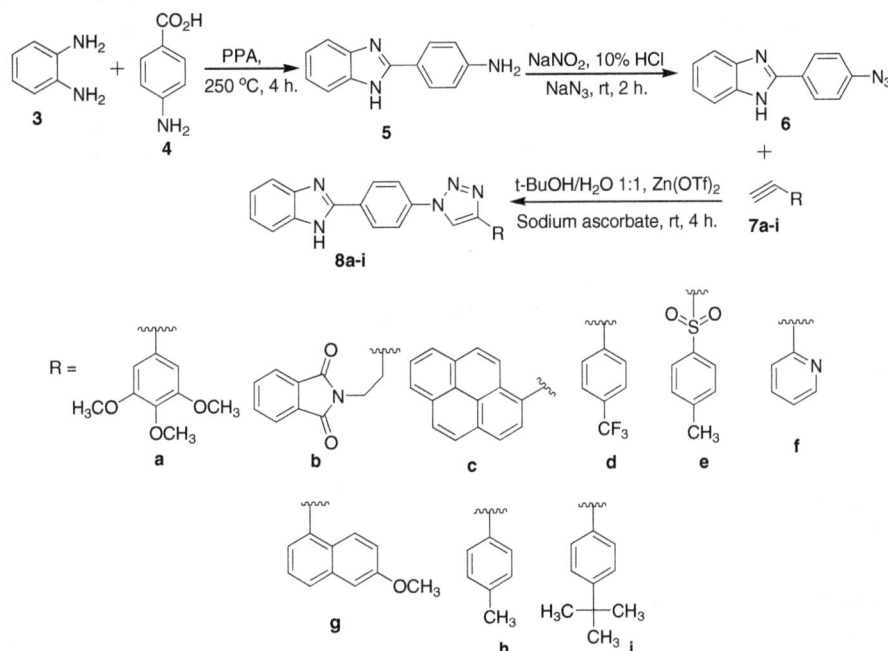

Scheme 1 Synthesis 1,2,3-triazoles.

of O-phenylenediamine (**3**) and 4-aminobenzoic acid (**4**) was mixed with a sufficient quantity of polyphosphoric acid. The resulting solution was stirred at 250°C for 4 h, to afford compound **5**. Compound **5** was diazotized followed by azidation to afford compound **6**. Compound **6** upon treatment with different types of terminal alkynes in t-BuOH/H$_2$O, sodium ascorbate, and Zn(OTf)$_2$ afforded compounds (**8a-i**).

4-(1H-Benzo[d]imidazol-2-yl)benzenamine (5)

A mixture of the O-phenylenediamine (**3**) (500 mg, 3.64 mmol) and the 4-aminobenzoic acid (**4**) (394 mg, 3.64 mmol) was dissolved in sufficient quantity of polyphosphoric acid (PPA). The mixture was heated slowly to 250°C for 4 h, permitted to cool to room temperature, quenched with excess of 10% Na$_2$CO$_3$ solution, and extracted with ethyl acetate. Then, the mixture was dried over anhydrous Na$_2$SO$_4$, and the crude product was purified by column chromatography with ethyl acetate/hexane (6:4) to afford pure compound **5**, 946 mg in 97% yield. Mp: 209°C to 211°C, ^{1}H NMR (300 MHz, DMSO-d$_6$): δ 6.68 (d, 2H, J =7.3 Hz), 7.14 (br s, 2H), 7.50 (br s, 2H), 7.85 (d, 2H, J =7.1 Hz). IR (neat, cm^{-1}): γ_{max} 404.3; 501.4; 537.9; 607.7; 742.3; 833.4; 960.1; 1,009.1; 1,108.6; 1,178.6; 1,225.7; 1,272.2; 1,397.2; 1,444.1; 1,499.2; 1,612.4; 1,701.4; 2,750.1; 2,853.1; 2,921.8; 3,355.4; 3,435.0; MS (ESI): 210 [M + H]$^+$.

2-(4-Azidophenyl)-1H-benzo[d]imidazole (6)

The amine derivative (**5**) (500 mg, 2.39 mmol) was dissolved in 10% aq HCl at room temperature. This reaction mixture upon cooling to 0°C and addition of a solution of NaNO$_2$ (165 mg, 2.39 mmol) was stirred for 10 min at 0°C to 5°C. Sodium azide (186 mg, 2.87 mmol) was added, and the mixture was stirred at room temperature for 2 h. The reaction was worked up by dilution with ethyl acetate. The organic layer was washed with brine and dried over Na$_2$SO$_4$. After evaporation of the solvent, the crude product was purified by column chromatography with ethyl acetate/hexane (3:7) to afford pure compound **6**, 536 mg in 95% yield; Mp: 317°C to 319°C, ^{1}H NMR (300 MHz, DMSO-d$_6$): δ 7.16 to 7.26 (m, 2H), 7.32 (d, 2H, J =9.0 Hz), 7.50 to 7.69 (dd, 2H, J =40.0, 38.5 Hz), 8.22 (d, 2H, J =8.3 Hz), 12.97 (s, 1H). IR (neat, cm^{-1}): γ_{max} 500.6; 541.4; 694.3; 743.3; 838.1; 963.4; 1,011.1; 1,115.8; 1,175.5; 1,283.5; 1,395.2; 1,438.8; 1,485.1; 1,604.6; 1,726.8; 2,120.1; 2,414.9; 2,856.9; 2,918.2; 3,055.5; 3,422.9; MS (ESI): 236 [M + H]$^+$.

2-(4-(4-(3,4,5-Trimethoxyphenyl)-1H-1,2,3-triazol-1-yl)phenyl)-1H-benzo[d]imidazole (8a)

A mixture of the corresponding azide **6** (200 mg, 0.85 mmol) and the corresponding alkyne **7a** (163 mg, 0.85 mmol) was dissolved in t-BuOH/H$_2$O 1:1 (20 mL). Sodium ascorbate (33 mg, 20 mol%) and Zn(OTf)$_2$ (300 mg, 5 mol%) were added. After stirring for 4 h, water/ice (40 mL) was added.

The product was either worked up by filtration, followed by rinsing with aqueous 5% NH$_3$ (×3) and cold ether (×2), or by extraction with dichloromethane (4 × 100 mL). The combined organic layers were washed with aqueous 5% NH$_3$ (3 × 100 mL) and brine (100 mL) and dried over anhydrous MgSO$_4$. The solvent was removed *in vacuo*, and the crude product was purified by column chromatography with ethyl acetate/hexane (3:7) to afford pure compound **8a**, 347 mg in 95% yield. Mp: 270°C to 272°C, ^{1}H NMR (400 MHz, CDCl$_3$): δ 3.71 (s, 3H), 3.89 (s, 6H), 7.24 to 7.28 (m, 4H), 7.63 to 7.66 (m, 2H), 8.17 (d, 2H, J =8.4 Hz), 8.41 (d, 2H, J =8.4 Hz), 9.44 (s, 1H). ^{13}C NMR (100 MHz, CDCl$_3$): δ 57.2, 61.4, 110.2, 114.8, 117.1, 122.1, 123.3, 125.3, 128.4, 129.8, 140.1, 141.8, 143.3, 148.7, 152.4, 154.1; MS (ESI): 428 [M + H]$^+$.

The other derivatives are also prepared according to the same procedure and described in Additional file 1.

Biological evaluation

In vitro cytotoxicity assay

The synthesized compounds **8a-i** were evaluated for their anticancer activity in selected human cancer cell lines of A375, B-16, colon-205, MCF-7, and A-549 by using MTT assay. All the compounds (**8a-i**) exhibited significant anticancer activity with IC$_{50}$ values ranging from 0.1 to 43 µM, while the positive control, adriamycin, demonstrated the IC$_{50}$ in the range of 0.03 to 3.5 µM respectively, in the cell lines employed as shown in Table 1.

Procedure for MTT assay

Toxicity of test compound in cells was determined by MTT assay based on mitochondrial reduction of yellow MTT tetrazolium dye to a highly colored blue formazan product. Cells (1×10^4) (counted by Trypan blue exclusion dye method) in 96-well plates were incubated with compounds with series of concentrations tested for 48 h at 37°C in RPMI/DMEM/MEM with 10% FBS medium. Then, the above media was replaced with 90 µl of fresh serum free media and 10 µl of MTT reagent (5 mg/ml),

Table 1 Cytotoxic activity (IC$_{50}$ µM) of compounds 8a-i

Compound	A375	B-16	Colon-205	MCF-7	A-549
8a	2.7	-	1.3	3.2	0.1
8b	2.3	1.9	3.5	1.7	2.6
8c	1.6	16	0.12	1.9	-
8d	-	4.7	8	-	-
8e	2.1	-	1.3	0.3	1.8
8f	15	3.9	17	-	-
8g	43	-	32	-	26
8h	-	-	-	37	32
8i	27	10	21	-	-
ADR	0.9	1.0	3.5	3.2	0.03

and plates were incubated at 37°C for 4 h, thereafter the above media was replaced with 200 μl of DMSO and incubated at 37°C for 10 min. The absorbance at 570 nm was measured on a spectrophotometer (SpectraMax, Molecular devices, Sunnyvale, CA, USA). IC_{50} values were determined from plot: percent inhibition (from control) versus concentration.

Additional file

Additional file 1: Experimental procedure and characterization data of all new compounds.

Competing interests
The authors declare that they have no competing interests.

Acknowledgements
We thank the management and principal of the Mahatma Gandhi Institute of Technology and the vice-chancellor and the registrar of JNT University Hyderabad for their encouragement.

Author details
[1]Department of Physics and Chemistry, Mahatma Gandhi Institute of Technology, Chaitanya Bharathi, Gandipet, Hyderabad 500075, India. [2]Department of Chemistry, College of Engineering, Jawaharlal Nehru Technological University, Hyderabad, Nachupally, Karimnagar 505501, India.

References
1. El-Azab AS, ElTahir KEH (2012) Design and synthesis of novel 7-aminoquinazoline derivatives: antitumor and anticonvulsant activities Bio Org. Med Chem 22:1879–1885
2. El Azab AS, Al Omar MA, Abdel Aziz AAM, Abdel Aziz NI, El Sayed MAA, Aleisa AM, Sayed Ahmed MM, Abdel Hamide SG (2010) Design, synthesis and biological evaluation of novel quinazoline derivatives as potential antitumor agents: molecular docking study. Eur J Med Chem 45:4188–4198
3. Brunton LL, Lazo JS, Parker KL (2006) The pharmacological basis of therapeutics, 11th edn. Mc Graw-Hill, New York
4. Goker H, Ku C, Boykin DW, Yildiz S, Altanlar N (2002) Synthesis of some new 2-substituted-phenyl-1H-benzimidazole-5-carbonitriles and their potent activity against Candida species. Bioorg Med Chem 10:2589
5. Ozden S, Atabey D, Yildiz S, Goker H (2005) Synthesis and potent antimicrobial activity of some novel methyl or ethyl 1H-benzimidazole-5-carboxylates derivatives carrying amide or amidine groups. Bioorg Med Chem 13:1587
6. Mann J, Baron A, Opoku Boahen Y, Johansoon E, Parkmson G, Kelland LR, Neidle S (2001) A new class of symmetric bisbenzimidazole-based DNA minor groove-binding agents showing antitumor activity. J Med Chem 44:138
7. Achar KS, Hosamani KM, Seetharam HR (2010) Novel benzimidazole derivatives as expected anticancer agents. Eur J Med Chem 45:2048
8. Kumar JR, Jawahar JL, Pathak DP (2006) Synthesis and pharmacological evaluation of benzimidazole derivatives. Eur J Chem 3:278
9. Tewari AK, Mishra A (2006) Synthesis and antiviral activity of N-substituted-2-subastituted benzimidazole derivatives. Ind J Chem Sec B 45:489
10. Schulz WG, Islam I, Skibo EB (1995) Pyrrolo[1,2-a]benzimidazole-based quinones and iminoquinones. The role of the 3-substituent on cytotoxicity. J Med Chem 38:109
11. Chen A, Yu C, Gatto B, Liu LF (1993) Poisoning of human DNA topoisomerase I by ecteinascidin 743, an anticancer drug that selectively alkylates DNA in the minor groove. Proc Natl Acad Sci USA 96:908131
12. Chen AY, Yu C, Bodley AL, Peng LF, Liu LF (1993) Topoisomerase I inhibitors and drug resistance. Cancer Res 53:1332
13. Kraut E, Fleming T, Segal M, Neidhart J, Behrens BC (1999) Hoechst-IR: an Imaging agent that detects necrotic tissue in vivo by binding extracellular DNA. J Invest New Drugs 9:95
14. Tolner B, Hartly JA, Hochhauser D (2001) Transcriptional regulation of topoisomerase II alpha at confluence and pharmacological modulation of expression by bis-benzimidazole drugs. Mol Pharmcol 59:699
15. Beerman TA, McHugh MM, Sigmund R, Lown JW, Rao KE, Bathini Y (1992) Effects of analogs of the DNA. Biochim Biophys Acta 1131:53–61
16. Hardman J, Limbird L, Gilman A (1996) Goodman and Gilman's. The pharmacological basis of therapeutics, 9th edn. McGraw-Hill, New York, p 988
17. Gennaro A, Remington R (1995) A mechanistic analysis of carrier-mediated oral delivery of protein therapeutics. The science and practice of pharmacy. Mack Easton PA II:1327
18. Richardson K, Whittle PJ (1984) 17 human secreted proteins. Eur Pat Appl EP 115:416, Richardson, K.; Whittle, P. (1984) J Chem Abstr 101:230544
19. Ammermann E, Loecher F, Lorenz G, Janseen B, Karbach S, Meyer N (1990) The science and practice of pharmacy. Brighton Crop Prot Conf Pests Dis 2:407
20. Ammermann E, Loecher F, Lorenz G, Janseen B, Karbach S, Meyer N (1991) The science and practice of pharmacy. Chem Abstr 114:223404h
21. Heindel ND, Reid JR (1980) 4-Amino-3-mercapto-4H-1,2,4-triazoles and propargyl aldehydes: a new route to 3-R-8-aryl-1,2,4-triazolo[3,4-b]-1,3,4-thiadiazepines. J Heterocycl Chem 17:1087
22. Dehne H (1994) In: Schumann E (ed) methoden der organischen chemie (Houben-Weyl), 8th edn. Thieme, Stuttgart, p 305
23. Wamhoff H (1984) In: Katritzky AR, Rees CW (eds) In comprehensive heterocyclic chemistry, vol 5. Pergamon, Oxford, p 669
24. De Las Heras FG, Alonso R, Alonso G (1979) Alkylating nucleosides 1. Synthesis and cytostatic activity of N-glycosyl(halomethyl)-1,2,3-triazoles. A new type of alkylating agent. J Med Chem 22:496

13

An expeditious green route toward 2-aryl-4-phenyl-1*H*-imidazoles

Debasish Bandyopadhyay[*], Lauren C Smith, Daniel R Garcia, Ram N Yadav and Bimal K Banik[*]

Abstract

Background: Azaheterocycles are an important class of compounds because of their highly potent medicinal activities, and the imidazole subcategory is of special interest in regard to drug discovery research.

Findings: An expeditious synthetic protocol of 2-aryl-4-phenyl-1*H*-imidazoles has been accomplished by reacting phenylglyoxal monohydrate, ammonium acetate, and aldehyde under sonication. Following this green approach a series of 2-aryl-4-phenyl-1*H*-imidazoles has been synthesized using diversely substituted aldehydes.

Conclusions: A rapid and simple synthetic procedure to synthesize diversely substituted 2-aryl-4-phenyl-1*H*-imidazoles has been reported. Other salient features of this protocol include milder conditions, atom-economy, easy extraction, and minimum wastes. The present procedure may find application in the synthesis of biologically active molecules.

Keywords: Imidazole; Green chemistry; Ultrasound; Heterocycles; Medicinal chemistry; Azaheterocycles

Findings

Global safety of nature is one of the major criteria in modern science and technology, and the concept of 'green chemistry' has been universally adopted to protect human health and environment. Since the last decade of the twentieth century, protection of environment has been considered as one of the major issues by the chemical scientists and R and D experts [1]. The most significant way to fulfill this eco-requirement is to avoid or reduce the use of hazardous solvents and toxic chemicals and to develop new reactions which can minimize unnecessary formation of the by-products (wastes). Development of such methodologies can provide substantial contribution to green chemistry [2,3]. Accordingly, development of greener methods has become a significant and prevalent research topic at present age. In synthetic chemistry, the effort has been made on the development of alternative synthetic routes to undertake the desired chemical conversions with nominal exposure of toxic wastes to the environment. Synthesis of desired molecules by sonication is regarded as a substantial green approach [4,5] to protect the environment by minimizing chemical hazards. Recent research on synthetic organic chemistry indicates that ultrasound can be used

as an important device to achieve a number of chemical reactions in high yield and within a shorter reaction time [6]. On other hand, imidazole pharmacophore is present in several pharmacologically active organic molecules including natural products. For example, imidazole scaffold is present in the benzodiazepine antagonist flumazenil, amino acid histidine, the antiulcerative agent cimetidine, the hypnotic agent etomidate, the proton pump inhibitor omeprazole, and so on [7]. Subsequently, there is a continuous need to develop concise and rapid method for the preparation of biologically important and medicinally active imidazole derivatives.

Results and discussion

Our laboratory is engaged in the green synthesis of novel pharmacophores for many years. To fulfill this goal, we have extensively used automated microwave and ultrasound to induce green technologies in chemical synthesis. We have successfully applied microwave technology to synthesize many novel pharmacophores including, but are not limited to, stereoselective synthesis of β-lactams [8], *N*-polyaromatic pyrroles [9,10], anticancer quinoxalines [11,12], pyrrole-bearing β-lactams [13-16], 1,4-dihydropyridines [17], α-aminophosphonates [18], and so on.

Ultrasound-promoted synthesis of novel anticancer pyrroles has been reported from our laboratory [19]. It has been discovered that ultrasound-assisted aza-Michael reaction

* Correspondence: bandyopad@utpa.edu; banik@utpa.edu
Department of Chemistry, The University of Texas-Pan American, 1201 West University Drive, Edinburg, TX 78539, USA

proceeds much faster in water than in organic solvents or solvent-free condition without using any catalysts or supports [20]. Because of the importance of 2-aryl-4-phenyl-1H-imidazoles in medicinal chemistry, we envisioned the development of an efficient and rapid procedure for the synthesis of 2-aryl-4-phenyl-1H-imidazoles without using any catalyst or support is timely and highly challenging. Following our newly developed procedure, a series of 2-aryl-4-phenyl-1H-imidazoles was prepared (Scheme 1) under ultrasonic irradiation at room temperature without using any catalyst or support.

Our ultrasound-induced reaction (Scheme 1) has been tested with diversely substituted aldehydes. The results have been summarized in Table 1. No catalysts were necessary for the progress of the reaction. All the ultrasound-assisted reactions were very rapid and completed within an hour to give the desired products in moderate to good yields (57% to 73%).

Apparently, the presence of electron-donating or electron-withdrawing substituents has no significant effect on the reaction. It has been reported by Zuliani et al. that the reaction proceeds through hemiacetal formation in the presence of methanol [7]. The introduction of ultrasound (i.e., sound energy with frequencies in the range 15 kHz to 1 MHz) into liquid reaction mixtures is known to cause a variety of chemical transformations. Ultrasonic irradiation of liquid reaction mixtures induces electro hydraulic cavitations by which the radii of preexisting gas cavities in the liquid oscillate in a periodically changing pressure. These oscillations eventually become unstable, forcing violent implosion of the gas bubbles. The rapid implosion of a gaseous cavity is accompanied by adiabatic heating of the vapor phase of the bubble, yielding localized and transient high temperatures and pressures. Thus, the apparent chemical effects in liquid reaction media are either direct or indirect consequences of these extreme conditions [20]. The polar solvent methanol has a permanent dipole moment, which allows the coupling between the oscillating electric field and the molecular tumbling to occur with high efficient heating.

Experimental
General procedure for the synthesis of 2-aryl-4-phenyl-1H-imidazoles
A solution of the aldehyde (1 mmol) and threefold excess of ammonium acetate (3 mmol) in methanol (2 mL)

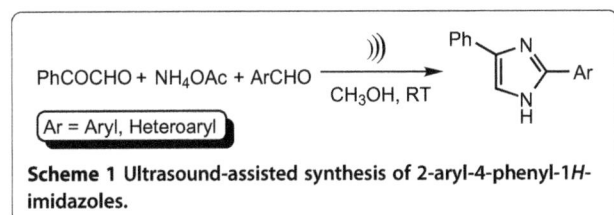

$$PhCOCOCHO + NH_4OAc + ArCHO \xrightarrow[CH_3OH, RT]{))))} \text{(imidazole product)} -Ar$$

Ar = Aryl, Heteroaryl

Scheme 1 Ultrasound-assisted synthesis of 2-aryl-4-phenyl-1H-imidazoles.

Table 1 Ultrasound-mediated synthesis of 2-aryl-4-phenyl-1H-imidazoles

Entry	Product	Time (min)	Yield (%)[a]
1	(2-phenyl)	25	66
2	(2-(4-methoxyphenyl))	35	59
3	(2-(4-methylphenyl))	30	63
4	(2-(4-chlorophenyl))	40	64
5	(2-(4-fluorophenyl))	55	61
6	(2-(4-nitrophenyl))	60	57
7	(2-(furan-2-yl))	35	61
8	(2-(pyridin-3-yl))	25	69
9	(2-(pyridin-2-yl))	30	73

[a]Isolated yield.

was placed in a B5510-DTH (Branson ultrasonic cleaner; Model-5510, frequency 42 KHz with an output power 135 Watts; Branson Ultrasonics, Danbury, CT, USA) sonicator at room temperature. The ultrasonic irradiation was started and a solution of phenylglyoxal monohydrate (1 mmol) in methanol (1 mL) was slowly added drop-wise (by a syringe) to the above solution during a period of 15 min. The resulting mixture was continued to irradiate as specified in Table 1. After completion of the reaction (monitored by TLC with an interval of 5 min), the methanol was evaporated under reduced pressure and the crude mass was extracted with ethyl acetate (2 × 5 mL). The combined organic layer was washed with brine (10 mL) and water (10 mL) successively and dried over anhydrous sodium sulfate. The extract was then concentrated, and the crude product was purified using flash chromatography (neutral alumina, 1% triethylamine in methanol) to afford pure compounds.

Conclusions

In conclusion, the present method demonstrates an operationally simple ultrasound-assisted cleaner procedure for the synthesis of 2-aryl-4-phenyl-1H-imidazoles without using any catalyst/solid support. The present economical method satisfies many green chemistry principles such as cost effectiveness, low toxicity, devoid the use of halogenated solvents, atom economy, and most importantly, time. The moderate to good yields of the desired products within shorter reaction time make this methodology a valid contribution to the existing processes in the same field, and their expeditious synthesis as described herein will find wide applications in drug discovery research.

Competing interests
The authors declare that they have no competing interests.

Authors' information
Lauren C Smith and Daniel R Garcia are undergraduate research participants.

References
1. Anastas PT, Warner JC (1998) Green Chemistry; theory and practice. Oxford University Press, Oxford
2. Polshettiwar V, Varma RS (2008) Aqueous microwave chemistry: a clean and green synthetic tool for rapid drug discovery. Chem Soc Rev 37:1546–1557
3. Tanaka K, Toda F (2000) Solvent-free organic synthesis. Chem Rev 100:1025–1074
4. Xu H, Liao WM, Li HF (2007) A mild and efficient ultrasound-assisted synthesis of diaryl ethers without any catalyst. Ultrason Sonochem 14:779–782
5. Guzen KP, Guarezemini AS, Orfao ATG, Cella R, Pereiraa CMP, Stefani HA (2007) Eco-friendly synthesis of imines by ultrasound irradiation. Tetrahedron Lett 48:1845–1848
6. Bejan V, Moldoveanu C, Mangalagiu II (2009) Ultrasound assisted reactions of steroid analogous of anticipated biological activities. Ultrason Sonochem 16:312–315
7. Zuliani V, Cocconcelli G, Fantini M, Ghiron C, Rivara M (2007) A practical synthesis of 2,4(5)-diarylimidazoles from simple building blocks. J Org Chem 72:4551–4553
8. Bandyopadhyay D, Banik BK (2010) Microwave-induced stereoselectivity of β-lactam formation with dihydrophenanthrenyl imines via Staudinger cycloaddition. Helv Chim Acta 93:298–301
9. Bandyopadhyay D, Mukherjee S, Banik BK (2010) An expeditious synthesis of N-substituted pyrroles via microwave-induced iodine-catalyzed reaction under solventless conditions. Molecules 15:2520–2525
10. Rivera S, Bandyopadhyay D, Banik BK (2009) Facile synthesis of N-substituted pyrroles via microwave-induced bismuth nitrate-catalyzed reaction under solventless conditions. Tetrahedron Lett 50:5445–5448
11. Bandyopadhyay D, Mukherjee S, Rodriguez RR, Banik BK (2010) An effective microwave-induced iodine-catalyzed method for the synthesis of quinoxalines via condensation of 1,2-dicarbonyl compounds. Molecules 15:4207–4212
12. Bandyopadhyay D, Cruz J, Morales LD, Arman HD, Cuate E, Lee YS, Kim DJ, Banik BK (2013) A green approach toward quinoxalines and bis-quinoxalines and their biological evaluation against A431, human skin cancer cell lines. Future Med Chem 5:1377–1390
13. Bandyopadhyay D, Rhodes E, Banik BK (2013) A green, chemoselective, and practical approach toward N-(2-azetidinonyl) 2,5-disubstituted pyrroles. RSC Adv 3:16756–16764
14. Bandyopadhyay D, Cruz J, Banik BK (2012) Novel synthesis of 3-pyrrole substituted β-lactams via microwave-induced bismuth nitrate-catalyzed reaction. Tetrahedron 68:10686–10695
15. Bandyopadhyay D, Cruz J, Yadav RM, Banik BK (2012) An expeditious iodine-catalyzed synthesis of 3-pyrrole-substituted 2-azetidinones. Molecules 17:11570–11584
16. Bandyopadhyay D, Rivera G, Salinas I, Aguilar H, Banik BK (2010) Iodine-catalyzed remarkable synthesis of novel N-polyaromatic β-lactams bearing pyrroles. Molecules 15:1082–1088
17. Bandyopadhyay D, Maldonado S, Banik BK (2012) A microwave-assisted bismuth nitrate-catalyzed unique route toward 1,4-dihydropyridines. Molecules 17:2643–2662
18. Banik A, Bhatta S, Bandyopadhyay D, Banik BK (2010) A highly efficient bismuth salts-catalyzed route for the synthesis of α-aminophosphonates. Molecules 15:8205–8213
19. Bandyopadhyay D, Mukherjee S, Granados JC, Short JD, Banik BK (2012) Ultrasound-assisted bismuth nitrate-induced green synthesis of novel pyrrole derivatives and their biological evaluation as anticancer agents. Eur J Med Chem 50:209–215
20. Bandyopadhyay D, Mukherjee S, Turrubiartes LC, Banik BK (2012) Ultrasound-assisted aza-Michael reaction in water: a green procedure. Ultrason Sonochem 19:969–973

14

Cytotoxic compounds from *Laurencia pacifica*

Diana A Zaleta-Pinet[1], Ian P Holland[1], Mauricio Muñoz-Ochoa[2], J Ivan Murillo-Alvarez[2], Jennette A Sakoff[3], Ian A van Altena[1] and Adam McCluskey[1*]

Abstract

Background: The current investigation sought to explore the nature of the secondary metabolites in the algae, *Laurencia pacifica*.

Results: This report details the first isolation of the sesquiterpenes isoaplysin (1), isolaurenisol (2), debromoisolaurinterol (3), debromoaplysinol (4), laur-11-en-10-ol (5), 10α-hydroxyldebromoepiaplysin (6), and the previously unknown 10-bromo-3,7,11,11-tetramethylspiro[5.5]undeca-1,7-dien-3-ol (7) from the algae, *Laurencia pacifica*. Isoaplysin (1) and debromoaplysinol (4) showed promising levels of growth inhibition against a panel cancer-derived cell lines of colon (HT29), glioblastoma (U87, SJ-G2), breast (MCF-7), ovarian (A2780), lung (H460), skin (A431), prostate (Du145), neuroblastoma (BE2-C), pancreas (MIA), murine glioblastoma (SMA) origin with average GI_{50} values of 23 and 14 μM.

Conclusions: Isoaplysin (1) and debromoaplysinol (4) were up to fourfold more potent in cancer-derived cell populations than in non-tumor-derived normal cells (MCF10A). These analogues are promising candidates for anticancer drug development.

Keywords: *Laurencia pacifica*; Algae; Sesquiterpenes; Anti-cancer; Cytotoxicity

Findings

Introduction

Natural products with their high fraction sp^3 content (Fsp^3) represent a significant proportion of all clinical drugs [1]. Of the 1,355 new entities introduced as therapeutics between 1981 and 2010, 71% were natural products or natural product derived [2]. A high Fsp^3 content imbues natural products with defined three-dimensional geometry that allows for high levels of interaction with a wide range of biological targets. A significant number of natural products adhere to the 'rule of five' and thus present high levels of drug-like character [3,4]. Natural products also afford access to a wide range of novel chemical motifs accessing new chemical space in the drug design and development arena. This has led to the ongoing interest in accessing natural product secondary metabolites (in particular) with their high chemical diversity and biological specificity, making them a favorable source of lead compounds for drug discovery and development [5,6].

Recently, we turned our attention to marine natural products as a potential source for new lead compounds.

In this area, we have identified a small family of cytotoxic steroids from an Australian sponge *Psammoclema* sp. [7], and antimalarial, antialgal, antitubercular, antibacterial, antiphotosynthetic, and antifouling activity of diterpene and diterpene isonitriles from the tropical marine sponge *Cymbastela hooperi* [8]. In this present study, we examined the cytotoxicity of extracts obtained from *Laurencia pacifica* algae collected in the pacific coast of the Baja California Peninsula, Mexico.

The genus *Laurencia* typically inhabits the world's tropical oceans and has been responsible for approximately half of all the reported compounds from red algae. This genus is considered an important producer of halogenated sesquiterpenes, diterpenes, and acetogenins [9-11]. Biological activities of the *Laurencia* family range from antipredatory [12], antifungal [13], antibacterial [14-16], to anticancer [17-19]. Secondary metabolites reported from *L. pacifica* include γ-bisabolene, bromocuparane, laurinterol, debromolauriterol, isolaurinterol, aplysin, debromoaplysin, 10-bromo-α-chamigrene, prepacifenol, pacifenol, pacifidine, and kylinone [10].

Results and discussion

The algae, *L. pacifica* was collected from the Baja California Peninsula, Mexico. The ethanol extracts were examined for

* Correspondence: Adam.McCluskey@newcastle.edu.au
[1]Chemistry, School of Environmental and Life Science, The University of Newcastle, University Drive, Callaghan, NSW 2308, Australia
Full list of author information is available at the end of the article

the potential presence of cytotoxic compounds. Cytotoxicity screening was conducted against a panel of cancer cell lines of colon (HT29), glioblastoma (U87, SJ-G2), breast (MCF-7), ovarian (A2780), lung (H460), skin (A431), prostate (Du145), neuroblastoma (BE2-C), pancreas (MIA), murine glioblastoma (SMA) origin, and a normal line of breast cells (MCF10A) [20]. The preliminary screening showed sufficient promise to embark on an isolation program (data not shown).

Bioassay-guided fractionation (normal phase chromatography) of the *L. pacifica* ethanolic extracts (see Additional file 1) resulted in the isolation of seven sesquiterpenes: isoaplysin (1) [21,22], isolaurenisol (2) [13,22], debromoisolaurinterol (3) [23], debromoaplysinol (4) [10,13,21], laur-11-en-10-ol (5) [13], 10α-hydroxyldebromoepiaplysin (6) [13] (Figure 1) and the previously unreported 10-bromo-1,7-dien-3-ol (7) (Figure 2). Sesquiterpenes 1 to 6 were identified in comparison with their spectroscopic data against literature data [21-23].

Sesquiterpenes 1 to 6 have been found in other *Laurencia* algae: *L. okumurai*, (1, 2, 3, 4, and 6) [21,22], *L. gracilis* (2) [24,25], *L. tristicha* (5) [19], and *L. distichophylla* (3) [26]. This work represents the first identification of these sequiterpenes in *L. pacifica*.

Sesquiterpene 7 was isolated in very small quantities (approximately 100 ng) from 2 kg of algae and was identified through a combination of high resolution mass spectrometry, infrared spectroscopy, and heteronuclear multiple bond correlation (HMBC), heteronuclear single quantum correlation (HSQC), correlated spectroscopy (COSY) NMR (see Additional file 1). The spectral data obtained closely matched reported spectral data of the related 10-bromo-7,8-expoxychamigr-1-en-3-ol (8) (Figure 2) [26], in which the C6 stereochemistry was determined by detailed NMR analysis and was consistent with our data [27-29]. The peak assignment and spectral comparison of 7 and 8 are shown in Table 1. There are three related structures with the C1-C2 double bond, one

of which is supported by crystal structure data and is of the same absolute configuration as shown for 7 and 8. While these data are wholly consistent with our assignment, Suescun et al. have identified another compound with the opposite C6 configuration [29]. We thus consider our absolute configuration assignment as tentative. Notwithstanding this, the spectroscopic data is consistent with the assigned structure and represents a new sesquiterpene from *L. pacifica* (Figure 2).

Sequiterpenes 1 to 5 were isolated in sufficient quantities allowing direct evaluation as pure compounds against a panel of cancer and non-cancer-derived cell lines. Due to the low levels of sesquiterpenes 6 and 7, these were screened as a 1:1 mixture (both were isolated from the same extract fraction as determined by ^{1}H NMR) [30]. Initial cytotoxicity screening was conducted at a single dose of 25 μM, and these data are presented in Table 2.

Analysis of the cytotoxicity data presented in Table 2 highlights the low level of cell death of the 12 cell lines examined on treatment with 2, 3, 5, and 6/7. Isoaplysin (1) and debromoaplysinol (4) displayed promising levels of cell death from 10% to >100% and 31% to >100% at 25 μM drug concentration, respectively. Of the other analogues, only isolaurenisol (2) displayed any growth inhibition at >20% (Du145, prostate cancer cell line). Given the activities of these three analogues, a full dose response evaluation was undertaken across our panel of carcinoma and normal cell lines [20]. These data are presented in Table 3.

As anticipated, isolaurenisol (2) displayed no noteworthy cytotoxicity returning a GI$_{50}$ value > 50 μM across all cell lines examined. Both isoaplysin (1) and debromoaplysinol (4) displayed good to excellent levels of cytotoxicity. Isoaplysin (1) returned an average GI$_{50}$ value of 23 μM (from 15 ± 1.2 μM to 40 ± 0.6 μM against the HT29 and U87 cell lines, respectively), while debromoaplysinol (4) returned an average GI$_{50}$ value of 14 μM (from 6.8 ± 0.3 μM to 26 ± 1.7 μM against the Du145 and U87 cell

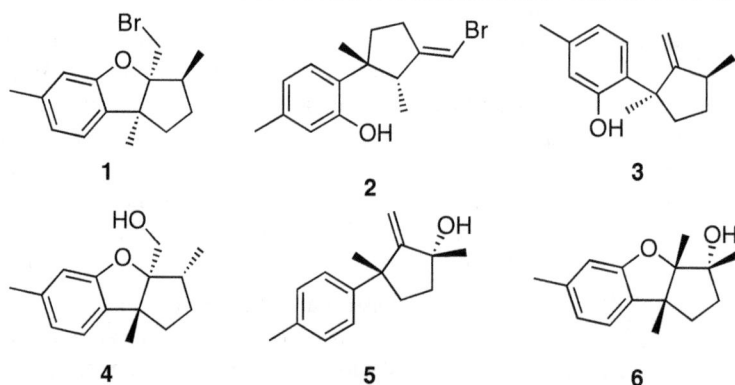

Figure 1 Chemical structures of the known sesquiterpenes isolated from *Laurencia pacifica* in this work. Isoaplysin (1), isolaurenisol (2), debromoisolaurinterol (3), debromoaplysinol (4), laur-11-en-10-ol (5), and 10α-hydroxyldebromoepiaplysin (6).

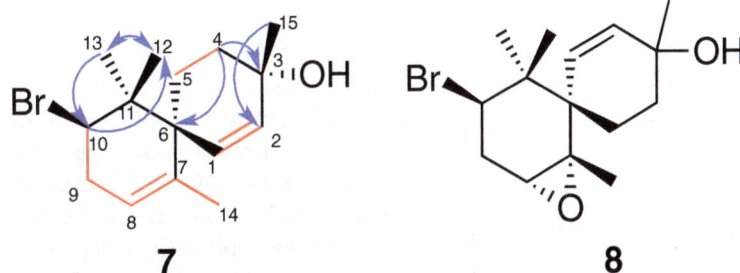

Figure 2 Important HMBC (blue arrows) and COSY (bold bonds) correlations for 7, and the chemical structure of the related 10-bromo-7,8-epoxychamigr-1-en-3-ol (8).

lines, respectively) when screened in cancer-derived cell lines. Both compounds showed the greatest growth inhibitory effect in the prostate cancer-derived cell line Du145 with GI_{50} values of 12 and 6.8 μM, respectively, and the least growth inhibitory effect in the non-cancer-derived normal breast cells with GI_{50} values of 46 and 28 μM, respectively. Indeed, **1** and **4** were up to fourfold more potent in cancer-derived cell populations than normal cells, imbuing them with properties favorable for future development as anti-cancer agents.

Given the structural similarity of the isolated analogues (**1** to **6**), being direct structural homologues or biosynthetically related, the observed differences in cytotoxicity suggest that the presence of the furan moiety and positioning and nature of the pendent substituents was important for cytotoxicity. Analogues **1** and **4** are Br – OH bioisosteres, and **4** and **6** are positional isomers (C3a-OH (**1**) and a C10a-OH (**6**)). The position of the – OH moiety is clearly important with the 3α-hydroxydebromoaplysin (**6**) devoid of cytotoxicity, whereas debromoaplysinol (**4**) displays

Table 1 1D and 2D NMR spectroscopic data (and assignments) obtained from sesquiterpene 7 and 1D NMR data for 10-bromo-7,8-expoxychamigr-1-en-3-ol (8) [26]

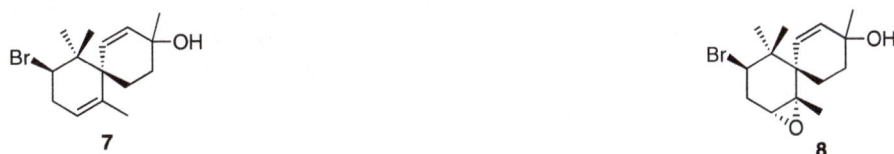

Position	δ_C,[a] type[b]	δ_H (H, multi, J Hz)	^1H-^1H COSY	HMBC	δ_C^c	δ_H (multi, J Hz)
1	136.4, CH	5.84 (1H, d, 10.4)	2	6	136.1	5.84 (dd, 10.4, 1.0)
2	131.1, CH	5.53 (1H, d, 10.4)	1	3, 6, 15	131.3	5.73 (dd, 10.4, 1.6)
3	67.5, qC	-	-	-	66.8	-
4	36.1, CH_2	1.80 (1H, m), 1.73 (1H, m)	5	3	35.0	1.79 (m), 1.81 (m)
5	28.2, CH_2	1.98 (2H, m)	4	3, 6	23.1	1.69 (ddd, 13.2, 11.2, 4.7), 1.94 (d, 13.2)
6	48.0, qC	-	-	-	45.9	-
7	139.0, qC	-	-	-	60.5	-
8	120.2, CH	5.22 (1H, s)	9, 14	-	61.4	2.97 (d, 3.0)
9	35.8, CH_2	2.78 (1H, m), 2.56 (1H, m)	8, 10	-	35.1	2.40 (ddd, 15.4, 11.4, 3.0), 2.69 (dd, 15.4, 5.8)
10	62.0, CH	4.63 (1H, dd, 10.8, 6.3)	9b	12	58.4	4.28 (dd, 11.4, 5.8)
11	41.5, qC	-	-	-	40.0	-
12	17.8, CH_3	1.01 (3H, s)	13	13	18.2	1.08 (s)
13	26.1, CH_3	1.10 (3H, s)	12	6, 10, 12	25.8	0.98 (s)
14	21.7, CH_3	1.55 (3H, s)	9		26.0	1.17 (s)
15	28.6, CH_3	1.29 (3H, bs)	-		29.3	1.33 (s)

[a]Data recorded in $CDCl_3$ calibrated at δH 7.24 ppm an for δc 77.0 for residual solvent; [b]in the case of a diasterotopic pair of hydrogens, 'a' denotes the downfield proton while 'b' denotes the up field proton; [c]chemical shift for the carbons was inferred from HSQC and HMBC data.

Table 2 Percentage growth inhibition by sesquiterpenes (1 to 7)

Cell line	Compound					
	1	2	3	4	5	6/7
HT29[a]	60 ± 3	12 ± 2	12 ± 5	>100	<10	10 ± 5
U87[b]	25 ± 2	13 ± 6	15 ± 7	52 ± 2	12 ± 4	15 ± 6
MCF-7[c]	81 ± 6	<10	<10	>100	<10	<10
A2780[d]	65 ± 5	<10	<10	99 ± 1	<10	<10
H460[e]	11 ± 1	<10	<10	71 ± 1	<10	<10
A431[f]	86 ± 1	<10	<10	>100	<10	<10
Du145[g]	41 ± 1	23 ± 6	18 ± 3	92 ± 2	18 ± 2	17 ± 3
BE2-C[h]	>100	<10	<10	>100	<10	<10
SJ-G2[b]	40 ± 5	<10	10 ± 3	>100	12 ± 3	14 ± 3
MIA[i]	47 ± 2	12 ± 4	17 ± 3	92 ± 2	18 ± 3	19 ± 2
SMA[j]	34 ± 8	<10	<10	95 ± 1	<10	<10
MCF10A[k]	10 ± 6	<10	<10	31 ± 10	<10	<10

Isoaplysin (**1**), isolaurenisol (**2**), debromoisolaurinterol (**3**), debromoaplysinol (**4**), laur-11-en-10-ol (**5**), and a 1:1 mixture of the 3α-hydroxydebromoaplysin (**6**) and 10-bromo-1,7-dien-3-ol (**7**) against a panel of cancer and non-cancer derived cell lines at a single dose (25 μM). Values are measured relative to an untreated control. [a]Colon; [b]glioblastoma; [c]breast; [d]ovarian; [e]lung; [f]skin; [g]prostate; [h]neuroblastoma; [i]pancreas; [j]glioblastoma (murine); [k]breast (normal).

excellent levels of activity (for a potential lead compound) against the HT29 (9.1 μM), A431 (9.6 μM), and Du145 (6.8 μM) cell lines [31]. Isoaplysin (**1**) and debromoaplysinol (**4**) differ only in the presence of the C3a-Br (**1**) and a C3a-OH (**4**) moiety, and **4** displays enhanced specific and broad spectrum cytotoxicity relative to **1**, suggesting that

Table 3 Growth inhibition (GI$_{50}$ μM) of isoaplysin (1), isolaurenisol (2), and debromoaplysinol (4) against a panel of cancer and non-cancer derived cell lines

Cell line	Compound		
	1	2	4
HT29[a]	15 ± 1.2	>50	9.1 ± 1.1
U87[b]	40 ± 0.6	>50	26 ± 1.7
MCF-7[c]	20 ± 1.3	>50	14 ± 1.7
A2780[d]	17 ± 0.6	>50	10 ± 1.7
H460[e]	34 ± 1.2	>50	18 ± 0.3
A431[f]	17 ± 0.6	>50	9.6 ± 0.9
Du145[g]	12 ± 0.3	>50	6.8 ± 0.3
BE2-C[h]	27 ± 2.3	>50	13 ± 0.9
SJ-G2[b]	29 ± 0.7	>50	15 ± 0.7
MIA[i]	23 ± 1.5	>50	16 ± 0.7
SMA[j]	24 ± 3.8	>50	14 ± 1.2
MCF10A[k]	46 ± 3.2	>50	28 ± 1.0

GI$_{50}$ is the concentration of drug that reduces cell growth by 50%. [a]Colon; [b]glioblastoma; [c]breast; [d]ovarian; [e]lung; [f]skin; [g]prostate; [h]neuroblastoma; [i]pancreas; [j]glioblastoma (murine); [k]breast (normal).

the – OH moiety enhances the cytotoxicity of this class of compounds.

Sun et al. isolated and screened the related sesquiterpenes: aplysin-9-ene, epiaplysinol, debromoepiaplysinol, aplysinol, and aplysin isolated from *Laurencia tristicha* in a MTT assay against lung adenocarcinoma (A549), stomach cancer (BGC-823), hepatoma (Bel 7402), colon cancer (HCT-8), and HeLa cell lines [19]. Interestingly, only debromoepiaplysinol (epi-**4**, this work) displayed cytotoxicity with a GI$_{50}$ = 15.5 μM against HeLa cells, where as herein, debromoaplysinol (**4**) displays activity across our panel of 11 cancer cell lines with strong activity in the HT29 (9.1 μM), A431 (9.6 μM), and Du145 (6.8 μM) cells [19]. These findings serve to emphasize the subtle nature of drug-ligand interactions and the role of stereochemistry in eliciting biological activity, c.f. **1**, **4**, and **6**.

Conclusions

Herein, we have identified sesquiterpenes **1** to **6** for the first time in *L. pacifica* and isolated a new sesquiterpene and 10-bromo-1,7-dien-3-ol (**7**). Screening of these analogues against 11 cancer cell lines revealed modest to good levels of cytotoxicity for **1** and **4**, with up to fourfold selectivity towards cancer-derived cell populations compared with normal cells. Given the low molecular weights and high Fsp^3 content, the structure activity data elucidated in this small subset of analogues, we believe that **1** and **4** represent excellent leads for the development of selective and potent anticancer agents [31].

Experimental

General experimental *Solvents.* Solvents used for TLC, speedy column, and centrifugal chromatography were of bulk quality and were distilled from glass prior to use. In the case of HPLC, all of the solvents were HPLC grade and were filtered and degassed prior to their use. The solvent referred as LP (light petroleum), is a mixture of different alkanes with a boiling point 60°C to 80°C.

Collection of the Mexican algae *L. pacifica* algae were collected on the coast of the Baja California Peninsula, Mexico. The algae was cleaned of epiphytes, rinsed with fresh water, and dried in the sun at the collection site. The specimens were stored at –20°C. A voucher specimen of *L. pacifica* was preserved on location in 5% formaldehyde and deposited in a private collection at the Algal Laboratory in the Interdisciplinary Center of Marine Sciences (CICIMAR), La Paz, B.C.S., Mexico, for taxonomical identification and future reference. Subsequently, in the laboratory, 10 g of dry algae was roughly torn or cut to small pieces and then ground with a mortar and pestle. The powdered algae was then submerged in 250 mL of ethanol. The mixture was left for 48 h at 25°C to 35°C.

Afterwards, the mixture was filtered and the residual algal tissue was extracted again under the same conditions. Both filtered extracts were combined and concentrated to dryness under reduced pressure at 40°C to obtain *ca* 30 mg of extract. These extracts were used for biological screening.

Extracts of L. pacifica and its fractionation Crude extract of *L. pacifica* 2 kg of algae was reduced to small pieces of *ca* as before, and then submerged in 1 L of ethanol. The resulting mixture was left for 48 h at 25°C to 35°C. Afterwards, the mixture was filtered and the residual algal tissue was extracted again under the same conditions. Both filtered extracts were combined and concentrated to dryness under reduced pressure at 40°C to obtain 2.2 g of extract. Fractionation of the crude extract was commenced with a speedy column resulting in 18 fractions [32]. All fractions were tested in the colorimetric assay; active fractions were then fractionated in normal phase HPLC until isolation of a pure compound.

NMR Proton and ^{13}C NMR spectra were recorded on a Bruker Ascend 400 or Bruker Ascend 600 (Madison, WI, USA). All NMR spectra were recorded as CDCl$_3$ solutions; the solvent signal was used as internal standard for chemical shifts (^{13}C δ 77.0 ppm, and ^{1}H δ 7.24 ppm for the residual CHCl$_3$ proton). All spectra, including HSQC, HMBC, distortionless enhancement by polarization transfer (DEPT135), distortionless enhancement by polarization transfer with retention of quaternaries (DEPTQ135), and (homonuclear) COSY-utilized standard Bruker pulse programs.

Cell culture and stock solutions Stock solutions were prepared as follows and stored at −20°C: drugs were stored as 20 mM solutions in DMSO. All cell lines were cultured at 37°C, under 5% CO$_2$ in air. All cancer-derived cells lines were maintained in Dulbecco's modified Eagle's medium (Trace Biosciences, Sydney, Australia) supplemented with 10% fetal bovine serum, 10 mM sodium bicarbonate, penicillin (100 IU/mL), streptomycin (100 µg/mL), and glutamine (4 mM). The non-cancer-derived breast cell line MCF10A was maintained in Dulbecco's modified Eagle's medium and Ham's F12 medium (1:1, Trace Biosciences, Sydney, Australia) supplemented with 5% heat inactivated horse serum, HEPES (20 mM), penicillin (100 IU/ml), streptomycin (100 µg/mL), glutamine (2 mM), epidermal growth factor (20 ng/ml), hydrocortisone (500 mg/ml), cholera toxin (100 ng/ml), and insulin (10 µg/mL).

In vitro growth inhibition assay Cells in logarithmic growth were transferred to 96-well plates. Cytotoxicity was determined by plating cells in duplicate in 100 mL

medium at a density of 2,500 to 4,000 cells/well. On day 0, (24 h after plating) when the cells were in logarithmic growth, 100 µL medium with or without the test agent was added to each well. After 72 h, drug exposure growth inhibitory effects were evaluated using the MTT (3-[4,5-dimethyltiazol-2-yl]-2,5-diphenyl-tetrazolium bromide) assay and absorbance read at 540 nm. Percentage growth inhibition was determined at a fixed drug concentration of 25 µM. A value of 100% is indicative of total cell growth inhibition. Those analogues showing appreciable percentage growth inhibition underwent further dose response analysis allowing for the calculation of a GI$_{50}$ value. This value is the drug concentration at which cell growth is 50% inhibited based on the difference between the optical density values on day 0 and those at the end of drug exposure [20].

*Isoaplysin: (3S,3aS,8bS)-3a-(Bromomethyl)-3,6,8b-trimethyl-2,3,3a,8b-tetrahydro-1H-benzo[b]cyclopenta[d]furan (**1**)*

Isolated as a white powder: 1.5 mg; [α] $_{\text{D}}^{20}$ = −5.3° (*c* 0.001, CH$_3$OH); IRv$_{\text{max}}$ 2,927 (C–H), 2,858, 1,620 (C = C), 1,593 (C = C), 1,499, 1,453 (C = C), 1,423, 1,376 (C–H), 1,268 (C–O), 1,135, 946 cm^{-1}; ^{1}H NMR (400 MHz, CDCl$_3$) δ 6.88 (d, *J* = 7.6 Hz, 1H, H-5), 6.66 (dd, *J* = 7.5, 0.7 Hz, 1H, H-4), 6.58 (s, 1H, H-2), 3.66, 3.56 (ABq, *J*$_{\text{AB}}$ = 11.1 Hz, 2H, H-12), 2.27 (s, 3H, H-15), 2.21 to 2.12 (m, 1H, H-10), 1.90 to 1.83 (m, 1H, H-8a), 1.70 to 1.60 (m, 2H, H-8b, H-9a), 1.50 (s, 3H, H-14), 1.20 to 1.13 (m, 1H, H-9b), 1.10 (d, *J* = 6.7 Hz, 3H, H-13). ^{13}C NMR (101 MHz, CDCl$_3$) δ 158.8 (*q*C, C-1), 138.3 (*q*C, C-3), 133.0 (*q*C, C-6), 122.2 (CH, C-5), 121.4 (CH, C-4), 109.3 (CH, C-2), 97.2 (*q*C, C-11), 55.5 (*q*C, C-7), 43.7 (CH, C-10), 42.6 (CH$_2$, C-8), 34.6 (CH$_2$, C-12), 31.5 (CH$_2$, C-9), 22.9 (CH$_3$, C-14), 21.5 (CH$_3$, C-15), 13.8 (CH$_3$, C-13).

*Isolaurenisol: 2-[3-(Bromomethylene)-1,2-dimethylcyclopentyl]-5-methylphenol (**2**)*

Isolated as a white solid: 2.5 mg; [α] $_{\text{D}}^{20}$ = −7.2° (*c* 0.0025, CH$_3$OH); IRv$_{\text{max}}$ 3,513 (O–H), 2,959 (C–H), 2,929, 2,870, 1,616 (C = C), 1,576 (C = C), 1,514, 1,454, 1,412, 1,294 (C–H), 1,254 (C–O), 1,186, 1,123, 809, 787, 653 (C–Br) cm^{-1}; ^{1}H NMR (400 MHz, CDCl$_3$) δ 7.15 (d, *J* = 7.9 Hz, 1H, H-5), 6.68 (dd, *J* = 7.9, 1.0 Hz, 1H, H-4), 6.57 (d, *J* = 1.1 Hz, 1H, H-2), 5.99 (d, *J* = 2.0 Hz, 1H, H-13), 5.06 (s, 1H, OH), 3.05 to 2.95 (m, 1H, H-11), 2.56 (dt, *J* = 12.9, 7.2 Hz, 1H, H-8a), 2.25 (s, 3H, H-15), 2.07 to 1.96 (m, 1H, H-9a), 1.64 to 1.57 (m, 1H, H-8b), 1.45 (s, 3H, H-14), 1.42 to 1.36 (m, 1H, H-9b), 1.22 (d, *J* = 7.2 Hz, 3H, H-12). ^{13}C NMR (101 MHz, CDCl$_3$) δ 160.2 (*q*C, C-10), 153.3 (*q*C, C-1), 138.0 (*q*C, C-3), 128.7 (*q*C, C-6), 128.1 (CH, C-5), 121.3 (CH, C-4), 118.2 (CH, C-2), 101.3 (CH, C-13), 52.0 (*q*C, C-7), 39.2 (CH, C-11), 39.2 (CH$_2$, C-8), 31.0 (CH$_2$, C-9), 26.8 (CH$_3$, H-14), 20.7 (CH$_3$, C-15), 19.1 (CH$_3$, C-12).

*Debromoisolaurinterol: [(1R,3S)-1,3-dimethyl-2-methylenecyclopentyl]-5-methyl-2-phenol (**3**)*

Isolated as a colorless oil: *ca* 1 mg; IRν$_{max}$ 3,458 (O-H), 3,055 (C-H), 2,984 (C-H), 1,641 (C = C), 1,581 (C = C), 1,113 (C-H) cm^{-1}; ^{1}H NMR (400 MHz, CDCl$_3$) δ 7.21 (d, *J* = 8.0 Hz, 1H, H-5), 6.71 (dd, *J* = 8.0, 1.1 Hz, 1H, H-4), 6.65 (d, *J* = 1.4 Hz, 1H, H-2), 5.54 (s, 1H, OH), 5.08 (d, *J* = 2.1 Hz, 1H, H-12a), 4.93 (d, *J* = 2.4 Hz, 1H, H-12b), 2.88 to 2.78 (m, 1H, H-10), 2.26 (s, 3H, H-15), 2.25 to 2.18 (m, 1H, H-8a), 2.07 to 1.98 (m, 1H, H-9a), 1.60 to 1.55 (m, 1H, H-8b, obscured), 1.46 (s, 3H, H-14), 1.41 to 1.36 (m, 1H, H-9b), 1.19 (d, *J* = 7.0 Hz, 3H, H-13).

Debromoaplysinol: 3a-methanol, 1,2,3,8b-Tetrahydro-3,6,8b-trimethylcyclopenta-3H-[b]benzofuran (4)

Isolated as a colorless oil: *ca* 1 mg; [α] $^{20}_D$ = 0° (*c* 0.001, CH$_3$OH); IRν$_{max}$ 3,425 (O-H), 2,940, 2,871, 1,588 (C = C), 1,499, 1,044 (C-O), 860 cm^{-1}; ^{1}H NMR (400 MHz, CDCl$_3$) δ 6.90 (d, *J* = 7.6 Hz, 1H, H-5), 6.66 (dd, *J* = 7.5, 0.7 Hz, 1H, H-4), 6.57 (s, 1H, H-2), 3.84 (dABq, *J* = 12.4$_{(AB)}$, 4.3 Hz, 1H, H-12a), 3.71 (dABq, *J* = 12.4$_{(AB)}$, 8.6 Hz, 1H, H-12b), 2.28 (s, 3H, H-15), 1.88 to 1.78 (m, 2H, H-10, H-8a), 1.72 (dd, *J* = 8.6, 4.3 Hz, 1H, OH), 1.66 to 1.60 (m, 2H, H-8b, H-9a), 1.46 (s, 3H, H-14), 1.16 to 1.11 (m, 1H, H-9b), 1.08 (d, *J* = 6.8 Hz, 3H, H-13). ^{13}C NMR (101 MHz, CDCl$_3$) δ 159.1 (*q*C, C-1), 138.3 (*q*C, C-3), 133.3 (*q*C, C-6), 122.2 (CH, C-5), 121.2 (CH, C-4), 109.0 (CH, C-2), 99.6 (*q*C, C-11), 63.9 (CH$_2$, C-12), 54.2 (*q*C, C-7), 42.3 (CH, C-10), 42.3 (CH$_2$, C-8), 31.5 (CH$_2$, C-9), 22.9 (CH$_3$, C-14), 21.2 (CH$_3$, C-51), 13.7 (CH$_3$, C-13).

Laur-11-en-10-ol. 3-(4'-Methylphenyl)-1,3,dimethyl-2-methylidenecyclopentanol (5)

Isolated as a colorless oil: *ca* 1 mg; ^{1}H NMR (600 MHz, CDCl$_3$) δ 7.21 (d, *J* = 7.9 Hz, 2H, H-1, H-5), 7.07 (d, *J* = 8.1 Hz, 2H, H-2, H-4), 5.44 (s, 1H, H-12a), 4.99 (s, 1H, H-12b), 3.47 (d, *J* = 5.9 Hz, 1H, OH), 2.29 (s, 3H, H-15), 2.08 to 2.04 (m, 1H, H-8a), 1.98 to 1.92 (m, 1H, H-8b), 1.82 to 1.77 (m, 1H, H-9a), 1.67 to 1.62 (m, 1H, H-9b, obscured), 1.48 (s, 3H, H-14), 1.36 (s, 3H, H-13). ^{13}C NMR (151 MHz, CDCl$_3$) δ 166.4 (*q*C, C-11), 145.4 (*q*C, C-6), 135.3 (*q*C, C-3), 129.0 (2 × CH, C-2, C-4), 126.3 (2 × CH, C-1, C-5), 108.6 (CH$_2$, C-12), 79.3 (*q*C, C-10), 50.3 (*q*C, C-7), 39.5 (CH$_2$, C-8), 39.2 (CH$_2$, C-9), 30.8 (CH$_3$, C-14), 28.4 (CH$_3$, C-13), 21.2 (CH$_3$, C-15).

10α-Hydroxyldebromoepiaplysin. (−)-2,3,3a,8b-Tetrahydro-3-hydroxy-3,3a,6,8b-tetramethyl-1H-benzocyclopentafuran (6)

Isolated as a colorless oil: *ca* 1 mg; ^{1}H NMR (600 MHz, CDCl$_3$) δ 6.92 (d, *J* = 7.6 Hz, 1H, H-5), 6.66 (d, *J* = 7.4 Hz, 1H, H-4), 6.49 (s, 1H, H-2), 5.35 (bs, 1H, OH), 2.26 (s, 3H, H-15), 2.01 to 1.96 (m, 1H, H-8a, obscured), 1.76 to 1.71 (m, 1H, H-8b, obscured), 1.61 to 1.57 (m, 2H, H-9, obscured), 1.39 (s, 3H, H-13), 1.38 (s, 3H, H-14), 1.28 (s, 3H, H-12). ^{13}C NMR (151 MHz, CDCl$_3$) δ 158.0 (*q*C, C-1), 138.1 (*q*C, C-3), 133.5 (*q*C, C-6), 122.5 (CH, C-5), 121.0 (CH, C-4), 109.6 (CH, C-2), 100.5 (*q*C, C-11), 82.9 (*q*C,

C-10), 53.6 (*q*C, C-7), 40.8 (CH$_2$, C-8), 37.0 (CH$_2$, C-9), 23.4 (CH$_3$, C-14), 22.2 (CH$_3$, C-13), 21.1 (CH$_3$, C-15), 14.8 (CH$_3$, C-12).

10-Bromo-3,7,11,11-tetramethylspiro[5.5]undeca-1,7-dien-3-ol (7)

Isolated as a colorless oil: *ca* 0.1 mg; ^{1}H NMR (600 MHz, CDCl$_3$) δ 5.84 (d, *J* = 10.4 Hz, 1H, H-4), 5.53 (d, *J* = 10.5 Hz, 1H, H-5), 5.22 (s, 1H, H-8), 4.63 (dd, *J* = 10.8, 6.3 Hz, 1H, H-10), 2.65 to 2.59 (m, 1H, H-9a), 2.57 to 2.50 (m, 1H, H-9b), 2.02 to 1.96 (m, 2H, H-1), 1.82 to 1.77 (m, 1H, H-2a), 1.76 to 1.71 (m, 1H, H-2b, obscured), 1.55 (s, 3H, H-14, obscured), 1.29 (s, 3H, H-15), 1.10 (s, 3H, H-13), 1.01 (s, 3H, H-12). ^{13}C NMR (151 MHz, CDCl$_3$) δ 139.0 (*q*C, C-7), 136.4 (CH, C-4), 131.1 (CH, C-5), 120.7 (CH, C-8), 67.5 (*q*C, C-3), 61.3 (CH, C-10), 47.1 (*q*C, C-6), 41.5 (*q*C, C-11), 36.1 (CH$_2$, C-2), 35.8 (CH$_2$, C-9), 28.6 (CH$_3$, C-15), 28.2 (CH$_2$, C-1), 26.1 (CH$_3$, C-13), 21.7 (CH$_3$, C-14), 17.8 (CH$_3$, C-12).

Additional file

Additional file 1: Structural characterization.

Competing interests

The authors declare that they have no competing interests.

Acknowledgements

DZAP gratefully acknowledges scholarship support from the Mexican government (Nacional Councli of Science and Technology (Consejo Nacional de Ciencia y Technologia, CONCYT)) and the University of Newcastle.

Author details

[1]Chemistry, School of Environmental and Life Science, The University of Newcastle, University Drive, Callaghan, NSW 2308, Australia. [2]Development Technology Department, Interdisciplinary Centre of Marine Sciences, National Technological Institute, La Paz, Mexico. [3]Department of Medical Oncology, Calvary Mater Newcastle Hospital, Waratah, NSW 2298, Australia.

References

1. López-Vallejo F, Giulianotti MA, Houghten RA, Medina-Franco JL (2012) Expanding the medicinally relevant chemical space with compound libraries. Drug Dis Today 17:718–726
2. Newman DJ, Cragg GM (2012) Natural products as sources of new drugs over the 30 years from 1981 to 2010. J Nat Prod 75:311–335
3. Harvey AL (2008) Natural products in drug discovery. Drug Dis Today 13:894–901
4. Lipinski CA, Lombardo F, Dominy BW, Feeney PJ (2001) Experimental and computational approaches to estimate solubility and permeability in drug discovery and development settings. Adv Drug Deliv Rev 46:3–26
5. Koehn FE, Carter GT (2005) The evolving role of natural products in drug discovery. Nat Rev Drug Dis 4:206–220
6. Newman DJ (2008) Natural products as leads to potential drugs: an old process or the new hope for drug discovery? J Med Chem 51:2589–2599
7. Holland IP, McCluskey A, Sakoff JA, Chau N, Robinson PJ, Motti CA, Wright AD, Van Altena IA (2009) New cytotoxic steroids from an Australian sponge *Psammoclema* sp. J Nat Prod 72:102–106
8. Wright AD, McCluskey A, Robertson MJ, MacGregor K, Gordon CP, Guenther J (2011) Anti-malarial, anti-algal, anti-tubercular, anti-bacterial, anti-photosynthetic, and anti-fouling activity of diterpene and diterpene isonitriles from the tropical sponge *Cymbastela hooperi*. Org Biomol Chem 9:400–407

9. Maschek J, Baker B (2008) The chemistry of algal secondary metabolism. In: Maschek J, Baker B (ed) Algal Chemical Ecology. Springer, Germany, pp 1–20. Chapter 1

10. Eickson KL (1983) Constituents of Laurencia. In: Scheuer PJ (ed) Marine Natural Products: Chemical and Biological Perspectives, vol 5. Academic, USA, pp 131–257. Chapter 4

11. Ji N-Y, Xiao-Ming Li X-M, Lia K, Bin-Gui Wang B-G (2009) Halogenated sesquiterpenes from the marine red alga Laurencia saitoi (Rhodomelaceae). Helvet Chim Acta 92:1873–1897

12. Hay ME (2009) Marine chemical ecology: chemical signals and cues structure marine populations, communities, and ecosystems. Annu Rev Mar Sci 1:193–212

13. Shui-Chun M, Yue-Wei G (2010) Sesquiterpenes from Chinese red alga Laurencia okamurai. Chin J Nat Med 8:321–325

14. Crews P, Selover SJ (1986) Comparison the sesquiterpenes from the seaweed Laurencia pacifica and its epiphyte Erythrocystis saccata. Phytochemistry 25:1847–1852

15. Sims JJ, Fenical W, Wing RM, Radlick P (1973) Marine natural products. IV. Prepacifenol, a halogenated epoxy sesquiterpene and precursor to pacifenol from the red alga, Laurencia filiformis. J Am Chem Soc 95:972–972

16. Sims JJ, Donnell MS, Leary JV, Lacy GH (1975) Antimicrobial agents from marine algae. Antimicrob Agents Chemother 7:320–321

17. Dembitsky VM, Gloriozova TA, Poroikov VV (2007) Natural peroxy anticancer agents. Mini-Rev Med Chem 7:571–589

18. Sun J, Shi D, Ma M, Li S, Wang S, Han L, Yang Y, Fan X, Shi J, He L (2005) Sesquiterpenes from the red alga Laurencia tristicha. J Nat Prod 68:915–919

19. Sun J, Shi D, Li S, Wang S, Han L, Fan X, Yang Y, Shi J (2007) Chemical constituents of the red alga Laurencia triticha. J Asian Nat Prod Res 9:725–734

20. Thaqi A, Scott JL, Gilbert J, Sakoff JA, McCluskey A (2010) Synthesis and biological activity of Δ-5,6-norcantharimides: importance of the 5,6-bridge. Eur J Med Chem 45:1717–1723

21. Suzuki M, Kurosawa E (1978) New aromatic sesquiterpenoids from the red alga Laurencia Okamurai yamada. Tetrahedron Lett 28:2503–2506

22. Suziki M, Kurata K, Kurosawa E (1986) The structure of isoaplysin, a brominated rearranged cuparane-type sesquiterpenoid from the red alga Laurencia okamurai Yamada. Bull Chem Soc Jpn 59:3981–3982

23. Harrowven DC, Lucas MC, Howes PD (2001) The synthesis of a natural product family: from debromoisoluaurinterol to the aplysins. Tetrahedron 57:791–804

24. Blunt JW, Lake RJ, Munro MHG (1984) Sesquiterpenes from the marine red alga Laurencia distichophylla. Phytochemistry 23:1951–1954

25. Yamada K, Yazawa H, Uemura D, Toda M, Hirata Y (1969) Total synthesis of (±)aplysin and (±)debromoaplysin. Tetrahedron 25:3509–3520

26. Li X-D, Miao F-P, Li K, Ji N-Y (2012) Sesquiterpenes and acetogenins from the marine red alga Laurencia okamurai. Fitoterapia 83:518–522

27. Davyt D, Fernandez R, Suescun L, Mombrú AW, Saldaña J, Domínguez L, Coll J, Fujii MT, Manta E (2001) New sesquiterpene derivatives from the red alga Laurencia scoparia: isolation, structure determination, and anthelmintic activity. J Nat Prod 64:1552–1555

28. König GM, Wright AD (1997) Laurencia rigida: chemical investigation of its antifouling dichloromethane extract. J Nat Prod 60:967–970

29. Suescun L, Mombrú AW, Mariezcurrena RA, Davyt D, Fernandez R, Manta E (2001) Two natural products from the alga Laurencia scoparia. Acta Cryst Section C C57:286–288

30. Kelman D, Wright AD (2012) The importance of [1]H-nuclear magnetic resonance spectroscopy for reference standard validation in analytical sciences. PLoS One 7:e42061

31. Leeson PD, Springthorpe B (2007) The influence of drug-like concepts on decision-making in medicinal chemistry. Nat Rev Drug Dis 6:881–890

32. Harwood LM (1985) Dry-column flash chromatography. Aldrichimica Acta 18:25–26

15

Effect of nano silver and silver nitrate on seed yield of (*Ocimum basilicum* L.)

Fatemeh Nejatzadeh-Barandozi[1*], Fariborz Darvishzadeh[2] and Ali Aminkhani[3]

Abstract

Background: The aim of this study was to evaluate the effect of nano silver and silver nitrate on yield of seed in basil plant. The study was carried out in a randomized block design with three replications.

Results: Four levels of either silver nitrate (0, 100, 200 and 300 ppm) or nano silver (0, 20, 40, and 60 ppm) were sprayed on basil plant at seed growth stage. The results showed that there was no significant difference between 100 ppm of silver nitrate and 60 ppm concentration of nano silver on the shoot silver concentration. However, increasing the concentration of silver nitrate from 100 to 300 ppm caused a decrease in seed yield. In contrast, a raise in the concentration of nano silver from 20 to 60 ppm has led to an improvement in the seed yield. Additionally, the lowest amount of seed yield was found with control plants.

Conclusions: Finally, with increasing level of silver nitrate, the polyphenol compound content was raised but the enhancing level of nano silver resulting in the reduction of these components. In conclusion, nano silver can be used instead of other compounds of silver.

Keywords: Basil; Nano silver; Silver nitrate; Seed yield; Polyphenol compounds

Background

Basil (*Ocimum basilicum* L.) is aromatic herbs that are used extensively to add a distinctive aroma and flavor to food. The leaves can be used fresh or dried as a spice. Essential oils extracted from fresh leaves and flowers can be used as aroma additives in food, pharmaceuticals, and cosmetics [1-3]. Traditionally, basil has been used as a medicinal plant in the treatment of headaches, coughs, diarrhea, constipation, warts, worms, and kidney malfunction [1]. Phytohormones and environmental stresses are the effective factors in controlling abscission process [4]. It is demonstrated that the ethylene has an important role in initiation of the abscission layer in different plants [5]. Ethylene activates the biosynthesis genes of hydrolytic enzymes, e.g., cellulose and polygalacturonase, which induces separation of plant organs from the main plant [6,7]. In addition, the abscission process could be regulated by the other phytohormones such as auxin (IAA) and abscisic acid (ABA). The later induces the abscission process through stimulation of the ethylene

biosynthesis while auxin is effective in delaying the abscission by reducing the sensitivity of cell to ethylene [4,6,8]. Abscission may be delayed by using some chemical components such as amino isobutyric acid and cobalt ions, (aminooxy) acetic acid, silver thiosulfate (STS), and silver nitrate ($AgNO_3$) [8,9]. Several studies demonstrated that spraying of silver ions decreases the flowers and flower bud abscission in orchid plant [10]. Additionally, it has been reported that silver ions decreased 100% flower abscission of *Alstroemeria* plant as compared to untreated flower within two first days [11]. Moreover, ethylene is involved on senescence of flowers in *Bougainvillea* plant while this process may be postponed by spraying silver thiosulfate [12].

Nano silver solution consisting silver ions in the size range of 10 to 100 nm, and it has more stability in comparison to other solutions. Nano silver particles, also, have more surface area in contact to outer space due to their small size. Thus, the amount of adhesion to the cell surface is increasing which lead to their higher efficacy [13]. Additionally, nano silver may affect the metabolism, respiration, and reproduction of microorganism [14]. For example, the effect of nano silver on extend maintenance period of leaves (from 2 to 21 days) in asparagus plant is

---
* Correspondence: fnejatzadeh@yahoo.com
[1]Department of Horticulture, Faculty of Agriculture, Khoy Branch, Islamic Azad University, P.O. Box 58168–44799, Khoy, Iran
Full list of author information is available at the end of the article

Table 1 Analysis of variance mean square testing traits

SOV	Df	LN	PH	DWP	DWI	LL	LW	SY	WS	PP	TN	SC
R	2	65.95 ns	34.01 ns	5446.50**	1401.62**	1.15 ns	1.85 ns	9.66**	0.060**	0.66*	0.13 ns	282.63*
T	6	315.84**	30.23*	3775.01**	794.02**	0.44 ns	0.23 ns	30.40**	0.044**	0.35*	0.26**	5888.46**
E	12	30.39	10.35	773.46	116.30	0.98	0.56	0.92	0.002	0.103	0.043	65.016
CV		10.20	8.64	9.40	5.70	10.14	14.22	4.63	3.40	11.78	11.7	9.06

* and ** respectively, significant levels of 5% and 1%. LN, leaf number; PH, plant height; DWP, dry weight of plant; DWI, dry weight of inflorescence; LL, leaf length; LW, leaf width; SY, seed yield; WS, weight of 100 seeds; PP, polyphenol; TN, tannin; SC, silver concentration.

reported. Also, during this period, the amount of ascorbate, chlorophyll, and fiber were more in treated leaves [15]. The effect of silver nitrate in delaying the abscission has been studied [15]; however, the influence of nano silver on seed abscission has not been reported. Therefore, this study was carried out to assess the possibility of using nano silver and silver nitrate in delaying the time of seed abscission in basil plant.

Methods

This study was carried out in a completely randomized block design with three replicates in the field research of Islamic Azad University of Khoy (Iran). The data of this study was analyzed by SAS software, and the comparison was done according to least significant difference (LSD) test method. Four levels of either silver nitrate (0, 100, 200, and 300 ppm) or nano silver (0, 20, 40, and 60 ppm) were sprayed with 0.1% Tween 20 (Tween 20, Sigma-Aldrich, St. Louis, MO, USA) on basil plant at seed growth stage (that is 45 days after cultivation) and were repeated after 2 weeks. The nano silver solution with an average particle diameter of 25 nm was obtained from Pars Nano Nasb Company (Pars Nano Nasb Company, Tehran, Iran). Different parameters (that is, leave number, plant height, dry weight of plant, length and width of leaf, dry weight of inflorescence, seed yield, and weight of 100 seeds) were determined; greenness of leaves was measured by a chlorophyll meter. The

biochemical properties included polyphenol and tannin were determined according to [16]. Concentration of silver in the plant shoot was measured by 'inductively coupled plasma' according to the method described by [16]. The principal operating parameters of the instrument were as follows: argon gas flow: auxiliary, 1 L/min, nebulizer (crossflow), 0.8 L/min; sample uptake: 60 s. Measurements were carried out in the axial mode at 328.068 nm.

Results

Using silver (either as nano silver or silver nitrate) had a significant effect on silver concentration in the plant shoot, number of leaves, height of the plant, plant dry weight, inflorescence dry weight, seed yield, weight of 100 seeds, and polyphenol and tannin content in shoot (Table 1). In contrast, the length, width, and greenness of leaves have not affected by silver treatment (Table 1). Silver concentration in shoot was increased by all treatments (either nano silver or silver nitrate) However, the higher concentration of silver in the shoot was obtained by silver nitrate treatment in comparison to others (Figure 1). There was no significant difference between 100 ppm of silver nitrate and 60 ppm concentration of nano silver on the shoot silver concentration (Figure 1).

The highest number of leaves was obtained by spraying 100 ppm of silver nitrate, while the lowest was seen in control plants (Table 2). The number of leaves and plant

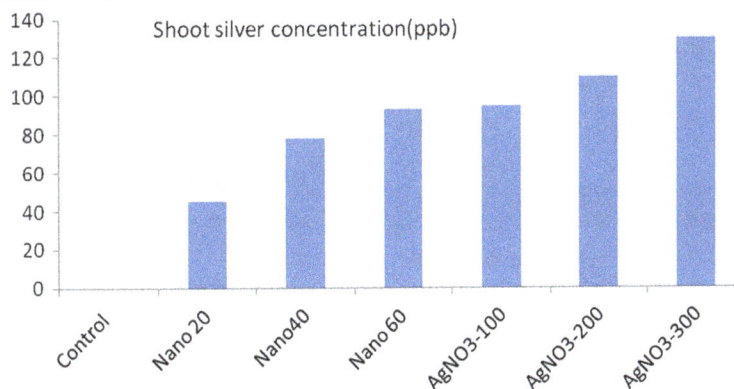

Figure 1 Effect of nano silver and silver nitrate treatments on concentration of silver. In plant tissue (μg/g dry tissue of plant).

Table 2 Comparison mean effect of different concentrations of nano silver and silver nitrate on test traits

Treatment	LN	PH (cm)	DWP (g/m^2)	DWI (g/m^2)	LL (cm)	LW (cm)	SY (g/m^2)	WS (g)	PP	TN
Control	41.530e	30.977c	246.94d	161.90d	8.300a	5.040a	14.62e	2.01e	3.160a	2.220a
NS 20 ppm	46.24de	34.68abc	268.38 dc	174.68 cd	8.324a	5.367a	18.10d	1.860b	2.941ab	1.985ab
NS 40 ppm	50.06cde	38.392ab	301.50abc	188.10bc	8.501a	5.351a	20.41c	1.761bc	2.781abc	1.779bc
NS 60 ppm	53.364 cd	41.445a	347.06a	203.1ab	8.910a	5.701a	22.68b	1.70 cd	2.420ab	1.605 dc
NS 100 ppm	68.130a	39.810ab	325.79ab	210.45a	9.321a	5.725a	24.90a	1.615d	2.208c	1.265d
NS 200 ppm	67.431ab	7.025abc	303.72abc	199.8ab	9.090a	5.110a	23.14b	1.714 cd	2.595abc	1.672bc
NS 300 ppm	57.465bc	33.500bc	278.65bcd	189.30bc	9.920a	5.028a	19.71 cd	1.785bc	3.048a	1.960abc
LSD	9.965	5.750	49.660	19.268	1.765	1.350	1.725	0.105	0.570	0.376

Mean values, followed by the same letters in each column are not significantly different (Duncan's multiple range test at 5%). NS, nano silver; SN, silver nitrate; LN, leaf number; LN, leaf number; PH, plant height; DWP, dry weight of plant; DWI, dry weight of inflorescence; LL, leaf length; LW, leaf width; SY, seed yield; WS, weight of 100 seeds; PP, polyphenol; TN, tannin.

height was improved by increasing the concentration of nano silver while they were reduced by rising in silver nitrate concentration. The longest height of the plant was obtained with the treatment of nano silver 60 ppm, while the lowest amount of this feature was seen with control (Table 2). However, by going up, the concentration of silver nitrate from 100 to 300 ppm caused a decrease in the dry weight of plant and dry weight of inflorescence. In contrast, a raise in the concentration of nano silver from 20 to 60 ppm has led to an improvement in those parameters (Table 2). Raising the concentration of silver nitrate from 100 to 300 ppm caused a decline in the seed yield, but an increase in concentration of nano silver from 20 to

60 ppm leads to arise in the seed yield. The lowest amount of seed yield was found with control samples, and the highest was obtained by silver nitrate 100 ppm treatment. However, seed yield was found to be more than the control sample with different concentrations of nano silver and silver nitrate (Table 2). The highest weight of 100 seeds was observed in the control sample, while this weight was decreased when either nano silver or silver nitrate was applied (Table 2).

The highest content of polyphenol and tannin was observed in control, and the lowest content was observed with silver nitrate 100 ppm (Table 2). The polyphenol and tannin content was raised with the increasing level

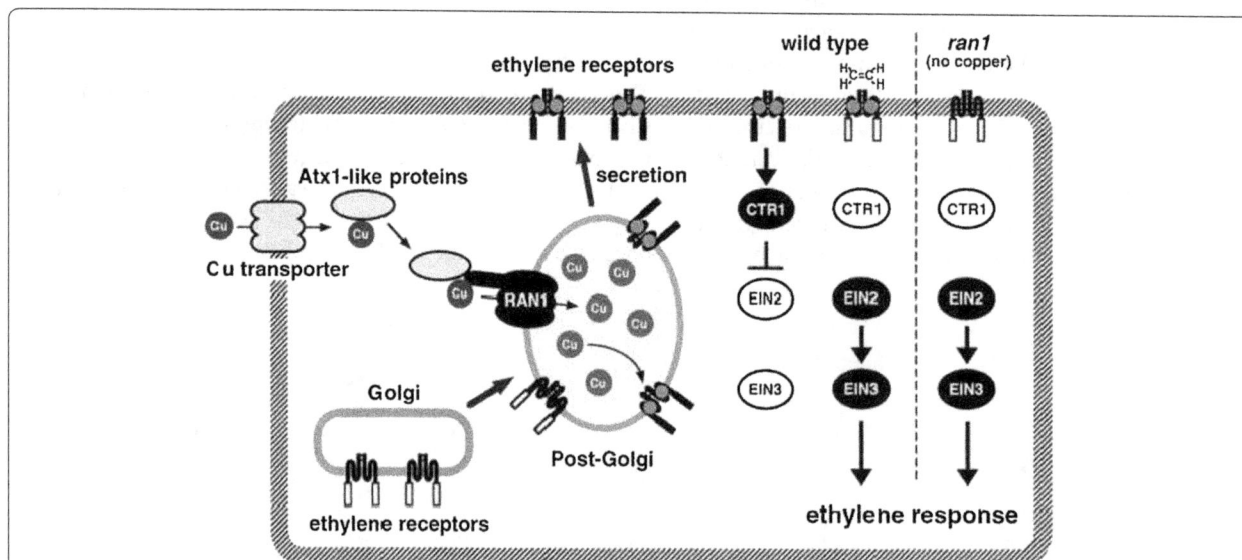

Figure 2 A model for the function of RAN1 in the ethylene signaling pathway. RAN1 is presumed to be localized in the membrane of a post-Golgi compartment. Copper ions received from CCH, a putative copper chaperon, is transported by RAN1 into a post-Golgi compartment, delivering the metal to membrane-targeted ethylene receptor apoproteins that become able to coordinate ethylene after the incorporation of copper ions. In the absence of the hormone, the receptors are active and negatively regulate downstream signaling components, preventing hormone-response phenotypes. Ethylene is expected to inactivate the receptors upon binding, presumably by causing a reduction in histidine kinase/phosphatase activity. This, in turn, results in derepression of downstream signaling components (EIN2, EIN3) and activation of hormone-response phenotypes. The metal-deficient ethylene receptors are nonfunctional, resulting in a constitutively activated signaling pathway.

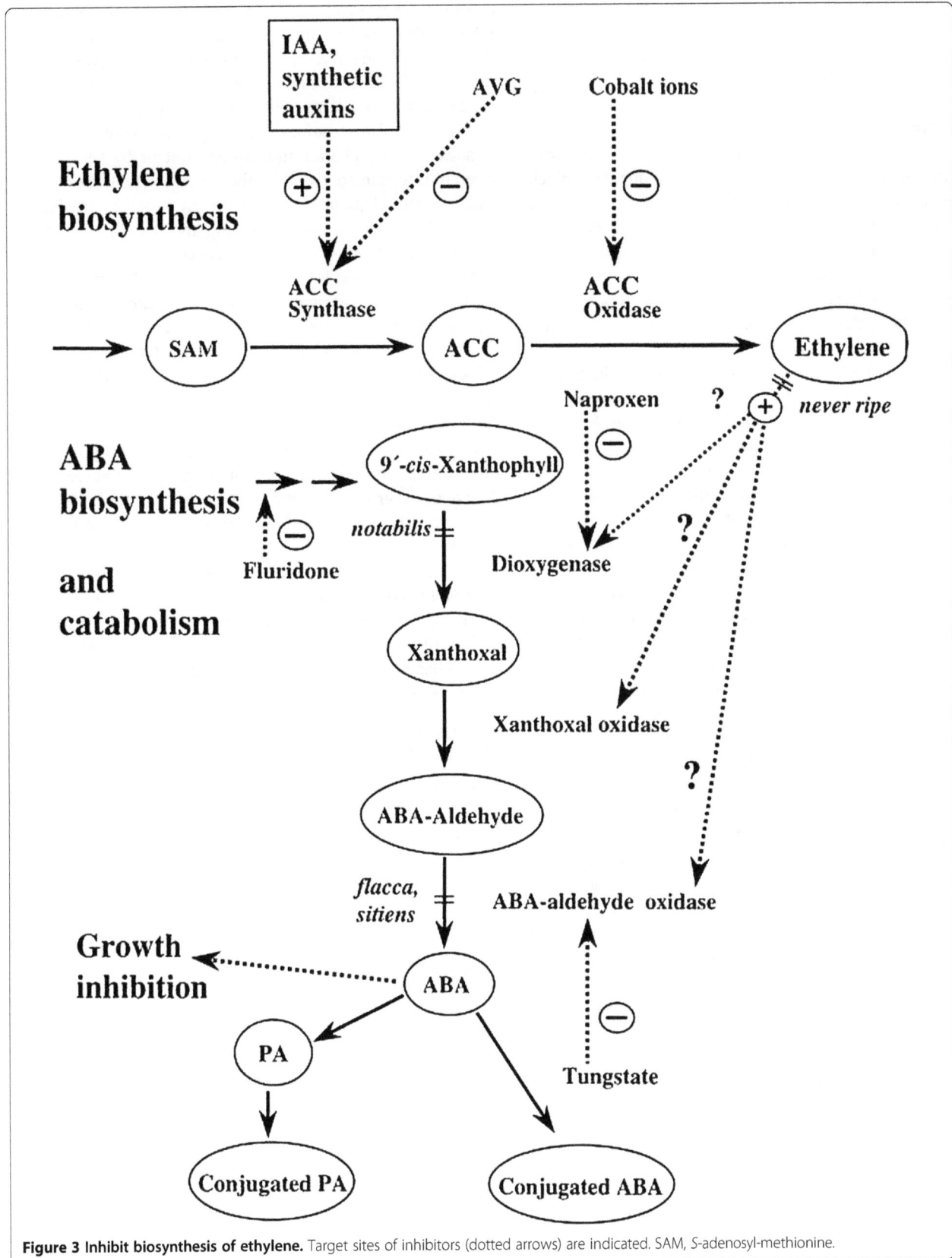

Figure 3 Inhibit biosynthesis of ethylene. Target sites of inhibitors (dotted arrows) are indicated. SAM, *S*-adenosyl-methionine.

of silver nitrate but was decreased with the increase in nano silver. The greenness, length, and width of the leaves were not affected by nano silver and silver nitrate treatments (Table 1).

Discussion

Application of silver ions can displace copper ions from the receptor proteins (Figure 2) consequently, block ethylene perception, since copper ions have a critical role in ethylene binding upon receptors [17-19]. This effect of silver ion on ethylene was reported by several researchers [11,20,21]. Therefore, some results in this study can be referred to the effect of silver in preventing the ethylene action (Figure 3). Decrease of plant's height due to ethylene is proven. For example, mutants of tobacco and *Arabidopsis*, which synthesize a high concentration of ethylene, have lesser height as compared to their wild species [22]. Furthermore, Nichols and Kofranek [23] reported that silver ion causes the increase in stem height of tulips and rose plants. Under the *in vitro* conditions, silver nitrate inhibited biosynthesis of ethylene and caused regeneration of multiple shoots from hypocotyl sections of cotton [24]. Another researcher reported that silver nitrate is effective in increasing wet weight of tobacco [25]. Ethylene caused an increase in enzyme activity of chlorophyllase and destruction of internal membrane of chloroplast, while that 100 ppm of silver nitrate caused decreasing the production of ethylene and destruction of chlorophyll in calamondin fruit [26]. Spraying silver nitrate causes improvement of seed yield in wheat [15]. In the present experiment, foliar application of either nano silver or silver nitrate causes increase in seed yield as compared to control (Table 2). In basil plant, rise in seed yield can be due to increase in the number of inflorescence in unit area, number of seed in the inflorescence, weight of seeds, and decrease in seed abscission. Considering that the seed yield has a significant positive correlation with dry weight of inflorescence ($r = 0.808$, $p < 0.0001$), but it has a significant negative correlation with weight of 100 seeds ($r = -0.835$, $p < 0.0001$). Consequently, it can be concluded that the increase of seed yield in this study is due to the increase of the inflorescence number in unit area and decrease in seed abscission.

Seed abscission is one of the main factors in reducing seed yield in basil plant. It is proven that one of the reasons for plant organ abscission is imbalance between phytohormones. Ethylene is playing an important role in this process. Furthermore, it is proven that silver ions inhibit the ethylene action by preventing its connection to its receptors in plant cells [8, 6, 4]. Thus, the increase in the seed yield was a result of reducing the seed abscission due to the inhibitory effect of silver on ethylene action. These results are confirmed by the results obtained from other studies [10,11,15,20]. There are many reports

about the use of silver nitrate in decreasing the abscission, but this study is the first research which is about nano silver effect on decreasing the abscission of reproductive organs of plants. Increasing silver concentration in aerial organs of sprayed plants with nano silver caused decreasing polyphenol and tannin content. While there was an increased in polyphenol and tannin content by spraying silver nitrate due to rising of the silver concentration in aerial organs of plant. There are many reports available about ethylene effect on increasing the phenol content [27,28]. On the other hand, high concentration of heavy metals (that is silver) in plant tissue causes polymerization of phenol by peroxidase enzyme which chelates the heavy metals [28,29]. Therefore, by increasing the level of silver nitrate more than 100 ppm, phenol and tannin content enhances due to toxicity effect of silver on plant cells.

Conclusions

There was no significant difference between 100 ppm of silver nitrate and 60 ppm concentration of nano silver on the shoot silver concentration. Therefore, permeability of nano silver is far greater than that of silver nitrate. The reason of this matter is the small size of nano particle, which causes more adhesion of nano particles to plant tissues. By considering the lesser use of silver in nano silver, this treatment can be used instead of other combinations of silver. However, the nano silver effect compared with other silver combinations on reducing the ethylene effect needs more researches.

Competing interests
The authors declare that they have no competing interests.

Author details
[1]Department of Horticulture, Faculty of Agriculture, Khoy Branch, Islamic Azad University, P.O. Box 58168–44799, Khoy, Iran. [2]Department of Horticulture, Faculty of Agriculture, Garmsar Branch, Islamic Azad University, P.O. Box 58168-44799 Garmsar, Iran. [3]Department of Chemistry, Khoy Branch, Islamic Azad University, P.O. Box 58168-44799, Khoy, Iran.

References
1. Simon JE, Morales MR, Phippen WB, Vieira RF, Hao Z (1999) A source of aroma compounds and a popular culinary and ornamental herb. In: Janick J (ed) Perspectives on new crops and new uses. ASHS Press, Alexandria, VA, pp 499–505
2. Javanmardi J, Khalighi A, Kashi A, Bais HP, Vivanco JM (2002) Chemical characterization of basil (*Ocimum basilicum* L.) found in local accessions and used in traditional medicines in Iran. J Agri Food Chem 50:5878–5882
3. Senatore F (1996) Influence of harvesting time on yield and composition of the essential oil of a thyme (*Thymus pulegioides* L.) growing wild in Campania (Southern Italy). J Agri Food Chem 44:1327–1332
4. Taylor J, Whitelaw C (2001) 'Singal in abscission' 2001, Tencley review no. 127, USA
5. Macnish AJ, Irvig D, Joyce DC, Vithanage V, Wearing AH (2004) Anatomy of ethylene-induced floral-organ abscission *Chamelaucium uncinatum* (Myrtaceae). University of Florida, Gainesvil, USA
6. Mishra A, Khare S, Trivedi PK, Nath P (2008) Effect of ethylene, 1-MCP, ABA and IAA on break strength, cellulose and polygalacturonase activities during cotton leaf abscission. Afr J Bot 282:6–12

7. Wu Y, Deng Y, Li Y (2008) Change in enzyme activities in abscission zone and berry drop of Kyoho grapes under high O_2 or CO_2 atmospheric storage. LWT 41:175–179

8. Kushad MM, Poovaiah BW (1984) Deferal of senescence and abscission by chemical inhibition of ethylene synthesis and action in bean explants. Plant Physiol 76:293–296

9. Moore TC (2006) Biochemistry and physiology of plant hormones, 2nd edn. Ferdowsi university press, Iran, pp 262–266

10. Uthaichay N, Ketso S, Van doorn WG (2007) 1-MCP pretreatment prevents bud and flower abscission in Dendrobium orchids. Postharvest Boil Technol 43:374–380

11. Wagstaff C, Chanasut U, Harren FJM, Laarhoven LJ, Thomas B, Rogers HJ, Stead AD (2005) Ethylene and flower longevity in Alstroemeria: relationship between tepal senescence, abscission and ethylene biosynthesis. J Exp Bot 56:1007–1016

12. Chang YS, Chen HC (2001) Variability between silver thiosulfate and 1-naphthaleneacetic acid applications in prolonging bract longevity of potted bougainvillea. Scie Hort 87:217–224

13. Shah V, Belozerova I (2008) Influence of metal nanoparticles on the soil microbial community and germination of lettuce seeds. Water Air Soil Pollut 4:9797–9799

14. Lok CN, Ho CM, Chen R, He QY, Yu WY, Sun H, Tam PKH, Chiu JF, Che CM (2007) Silver nanoparticles: partial oxidation and antibacterial activities. Biol Inorg Chem 12:527–534

15. Labraba X, Araus JL (1991) Effect of foliar applications of silver nitrate and ear removal on carbon dioxide assimilation in wheat flag leaves during grain filling. Field Crops Res 28:149–162

16. Makkar HSP (2000) Quantification of tannins in tree foliage. A laboratory manual for the FAO/IAEA co-ordinated research project on use of nuclear and related techiquea to develop simple tannin assays for predicting and improving the safety and efficiency of feeding ruminants on tanniniferous tree foliage, FAO/IAEA Working Document, IAEA, Vienna, Austria

17. Khan NA (2006) Ethylene action in plants', 1st edn. Springer-Verlag Berlin Heidelberg, German

18. Means AR, Malley BWO, Armen LRH, Tashjian JR (2005) Vitamins and hormones. V. 72. Elsevier Inc, USA, pp 395–430

19. Hedden EP, Thomas SG (2006) Annual plant reviews. Blackwell Publishing, Oxford, UK, pp 125–139

20. Eo J, Lee BY (2009) Effects of ethylene, abscisic acid and auxin on fruit abscission in water dropwort (Oenanthe stolonifera DC.). Scie Hort 123:224–227

21. An J, Zhang M, Wang SH, Tang J (2008) Physical, chemical and microbiological change in stored green asparagus spears as affected by coating of silver nanoparticle-pvp. LWT 41:1100–1107

22. Pessarakli M (2001) Handbook of plant and crop physiol, 2nd edn. Marcel Dekker, Inc, USA, pp 35–108

23. Nichols R, Kofranek AM (1982) Reversal of ethylene inhibition of tulip stem elongation by silver thiosulfate. Scie Hort 17:71–79

24. Ouma JP, Young MM, Reichert NA (2004) Optimization of in vitro regeneration of multiple shoots from hypocotyl sections of cotton (Gossypium hirsutum L.). Afr J Biotechnol 3:169–173

25. Tso TC, Sorokin TP, Engelhaupt ME (1973) Effects of some rare elements on nicotine content of the tobacco. Plant Physiol 51:805–806

26. Purvis AC (1980) Sequence of chloroplast degreening in calamondin fruit as influenced by ethylene and $AgNO_3$. Plant Physiol 66:624–627

27. Park HJ, Kim SH, Kim HJ, Choi HS (2006) A new composition of nanosized silica-silver for control of various plant diseases. Plant Pathol 22:295–302

28. Heredia B, Cisneros-zevallos L (2009) The effects of exogenous ethylene and methyl jasmonate on the accumulation of phenolic antioxidants in selected whole and wounded fresh produce. Food Chem 115:1500–1508

29. Elzaawely AA, Xuan TD, Tawata S (2007) Changes in essential oil, kava pyrones and total phenolics of Alpinia zerumbet (Pers.) B.L. Burtt. and R.M. Sm. leaves exposed to copper sulphate. Environ Exper Bot 59:347–353

16

Antioxidant, antimicrobial, and theoretical studies of the thiosemicarbazone derivative Schiff base 2-(2-imino-1-methylimidazolidin-4-ylidene)hydrazinecarbothioamide (IMHC)

Ahmed A Al-Amiery[*], Yasmien K Al-Majedy, Heba H Ibrahim and Ali A Al-Tamimi

Abstract

Background: Adverse antimicrobial activities of thiosemicarbazone (TSC) and Schiff base derivatives have widely been studied by using different kinds of microbes, in addition different methods were used to assay the antioxidant activities using DPPH, peroxids, or ntrosyl methods. However, there are no studies describing the synthesis of TSC derived from creatinine.

Results: In this study, 2-(2-imino-1-methylimidazolidin-4-ylidene)hydrazinecarbothioamide (IMHC) was synthesized by the reaction of creatinine with thiosemicarbazide. The novel molecule was characterized by FT-IR, UV-VIS, and NMR spectra in addition of the elemental analysis. The free radical scavenging ability of the IMHC was determined by it interaction with the stable-free radical 2,2"-diphenyl-1-picrylhydrazyl (or nitric oxide or hydrogen peroxide) and showed encouraging antioxidant activities. Density functional theory calculations of the IMHC performed using molecular structures with optimized geometries. Molecular orbital calculations provide a detailed description of the orbitals, including spatial characteristics, nodal patterns, and the contributions of individual atoms. Highest occupied molecular orbital-lowest unoccupied molecular orbital energies and structures are shown.

Conclusions: IMHC shows considerable antibacterial and antifungal activities. The free radical scavenging activity of synthesized compound was screened for *in vitro* antioxidant activity.

Keywords: antibacterial, antioxidant, antifungal, creatinine, Schiff base, thiosemicarbazone

Background

Schiff-base compounds have been used as fine chemicals and medical substrates [1]. Azomethine group (-C = N-)-containing compounds, typically known as Schiff's bases, have been synthesized via condensation of primary amines with active carbonyls. It is well established that the biological activity of hydrazone compounds is associated with the presence of the active (-CO-NHN = C-) pharmacophore and these compounds form a significant category of compounds in medicinal and pharmaceutical chemistry with several biological applications that include antitumoral [2,3], antifungal [4-9], antibacterial [10,11], antimicrobial [12], and anthelmintic uses

[13]. Schiff's base complexes play an important role in designing metal complexes related to synthetic and natural oxygen carriers [14,15]. Schiff bases (SBs) are important intermediates for the synthesis of some bioactive compounds such as ß-lactams [16-18], and employed as ligands for the complexation of metal ions [19]. SBs and their complexes are largely studied because they interested and important properties such as their ability to bind reversibly oxygen [20] redox systems in biological systems and oxidation of DNA [21].

Antioxidants are extensively studied for their capacity for protect organism and cell from damage that is induced by oxidative stress. Scientists in many different disciplines become more interested in new compounds, either synthesized or obtained from natural sources that

* Correspondence: dr.ahmed1975@gmail.com
Biotechnology Division, Applied Science Department, University of Technology, Baghdad 10066, Iraq

could provide active components to prevent or reduce the impact of oxidative stress on cell [22,23].

The preparation of a 2-(2-imino-1-methylimidazolidin-4-ylidene)hydrazinecarbothioamide (IMHC) from thiosemicarbazide and creatinine is presented in this study. The structure established based on the extensive NMR spectroscopic studies. The microbial activities of IMHC and their *in vitro* antioxidant activities were also investigated. It was envisaged that these two active pharmacological molecules (thiosemicbazide and creatinine) if linked together would generate novel molecular templates, which are likely to exhibit interesting biological properties.

Results and discussion
Chemistry
UV/visible spectra
The UV-VIS of IMHC was recorded. The solution of IMHC in DMF exhibited two peaks at 255 and 322 nm (39215 and 31055 cm^{-1}) which are attributed to $\pi \rightarrow \pi^*$ or $n \rightarrow \pi^*$.

FT-IR spectroscopy
The FT-IR spectra provide valuable information regarding the nature of functional group of IMHC. The appearance of a broad strong band in the IR spectra of IMHC in 3421 cm^{-1} is assigned to N-H stretching vibrations of the primary amine group. The spectrum of IMHC shows two different -C = N bands at 1631 and 1618 cm^{-1}.

Owing to the restricted rotation around the C = N bond, the IMHC may exist into two different geometric isomeric forms. The structure determination of one representative IMHC shows (Scheme 1) that the IMHC exists in thione form and corresponds to structure where the creatinine group is *cis* to the hydrazinic nitrogen across the C = N bond. The existence of the thione form predominantly in the solid state is demonstrated by the presence of two absorption bands at 1273.7 and 3421 cm^{-1} belonging to the C = S and NH groups, respectively, and by absence of SH.

Density functional theory (DFT) studies
DFT calculations of the IMHC (Figure 1) have been done using the optimized geometry molecular structures, Molecular orbital calculations provide a detailed

description of orbitals including spatial characteristics, nodal patterns, and individual atom contributions. The energy of highest occupied molecular orbital (HOMO) of IMHC is -0.150240 Hartree, whereas the energy of lowest unoccupied molecular orbital (LUMO) of IMHC is 0.1102540 Hartree (Table 1). The lower value in the HOMO and LUMO energy gap explains the eventual charge transfer interaction taking place within the molecules.

Pharmacology
Antibacterial activity
The results of antibacterial activity study for IMHC indicated that the new molecule exhibited antibacterial activity against the studied bacteria at low and high concentrations. The increased activity of the synthesized compound can be explained electron delocalization over the whole molecule. This increases the lipophilic character of the molecule and favors its permeation through the lipoid layer of the bacterial membranes. The increased lipophilic character of this molecule seems to be responsible for it enhanced potent antibacterial activity. It may be suggested that this molecule deactivate various cellular enzymes, which play a vital role in various metabolic pathways of these microorganisms (Figure 2).

Antifungal activity
According to Overtone's concept of cell permeability, the lipid membrane that surrounds the cell favors the passage of only lipid-soluble materials, so lipophilicity is an important factor controlling the antifungal activity. Delocalization of π-electrons over the IMHC increased lipophilicity facilitates the penetration of the IMHC into lipid membranes, further restricting proliferation of the microorganisms. Although the exact biochemical mechanism is not completely understood, the mode of action of antimicrobials may involve various targets in the microorganisms.

- Interference with the synthesis of cellular walls, causing damage that can lead to altered cell permeability characteristics or disorganized lipoprotein arrangements, ultimately resulting in cell death.
- Deactivation of various cellular enzymes that play a vital role in the metabolic pathways of these microorganisms.
- Denaturation of one or more cellular proteins, causing the normal cellular processes to be impaired.
- Formation of a hydrogen bond through the azomethine group with the active centers of various cellular constituents, resulting in interference with normal cellular processes [24].

In vitro antifungal screening effects of the investigated compound was tested against some fungal spices

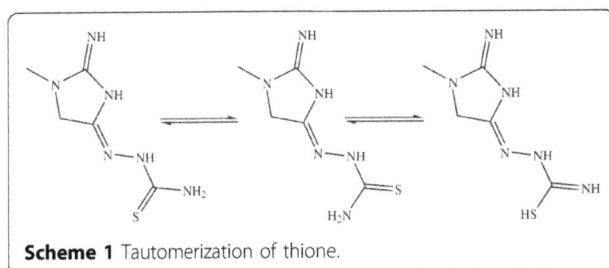

Scheme 1 Tautomerization of thione.

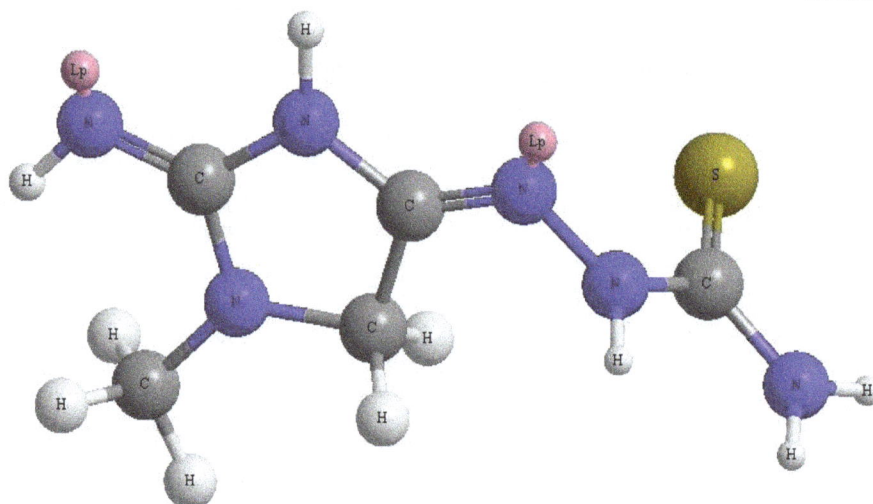

Figure 1 Optimized 3D structure of the IMHC.

(*Aspergillus niger and Candida albicans*). It was found to that the new compound exhibits antifungal activity against *C. albicans* more than *A. niger* (Figure 3).

Antioxidant activity

The role of antioxidant is to remove free radical. One important mechanism through which this is achieved is by donating hydrogen to free radicals in its reduction to an unreactive species. Addition of hydrogen would remove the odd electron feature which is responsible for radical reactivity. The hydrogen-donating activity, measured using DPPH (1,1-diphenyl-2-picrilhydrazyl) radicals as hydrogen acceptor, showed that a significant association could be found between the concentration of novel molecule and percentage of inhibition (Figure 4).

Experiment

Chemistry

Matierials

All chemical used were of reagent grade (supplied by either Merck or Fluka) and used as-received. The FTIR spectra were recorded as KBr disc on FTIR 8300

Shimadzu Spectrophotometer. The UV-Visible spectra were measured using Shimadzu UV-Vis. 160 A spectrophotometer. Proton NMR spectra were recorded on Bruker - DPX 300 MHz spectrometer with TMS as internal standard. Elemental microanalysis was carried out using C.H.N elemental analyzer model 5500-Carlo Erba instrument.

Synthesis of IMHC

This mixture of hot ethanolic solution of thiosemicarbazide (1.82 g, 0.02 mol) and creatinine (2-imino-1-methylimidazolidin-4-one) (2.26 g, 0.02 mol) was refluxed with stirring for 3 h. The completion of the reaction was confirmed by the TLC. The reaction mass was degassed on a rotatory evaporator, over a water bath. Thiosemicarbazone filtered, washed with cold EtOH, and dried under vacuum over P_4O_{10}. Yield, 70; M.P. 153°C; light brown. Proton NMR (1.8(1H) for NH, s. 2.2 (3H) for CH_3, s. 2.7(2H) for CH_2, 8 for NH, 9.1 for NH, 10.9 for NH_2). Element chemical analysis data were C, 32.25(31.91); H, 5.41(5.11); N, 45.13(44.74), and the reaction equation was shown in Scheme 2.

Table 1 HOMO and LUMO energy

-0.150240 Hartree	-0.1102540 Hartree

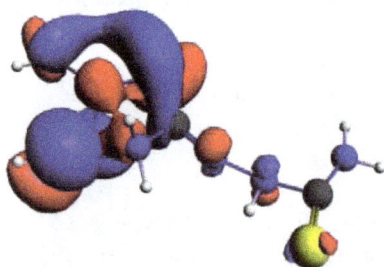

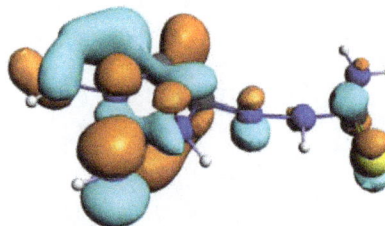

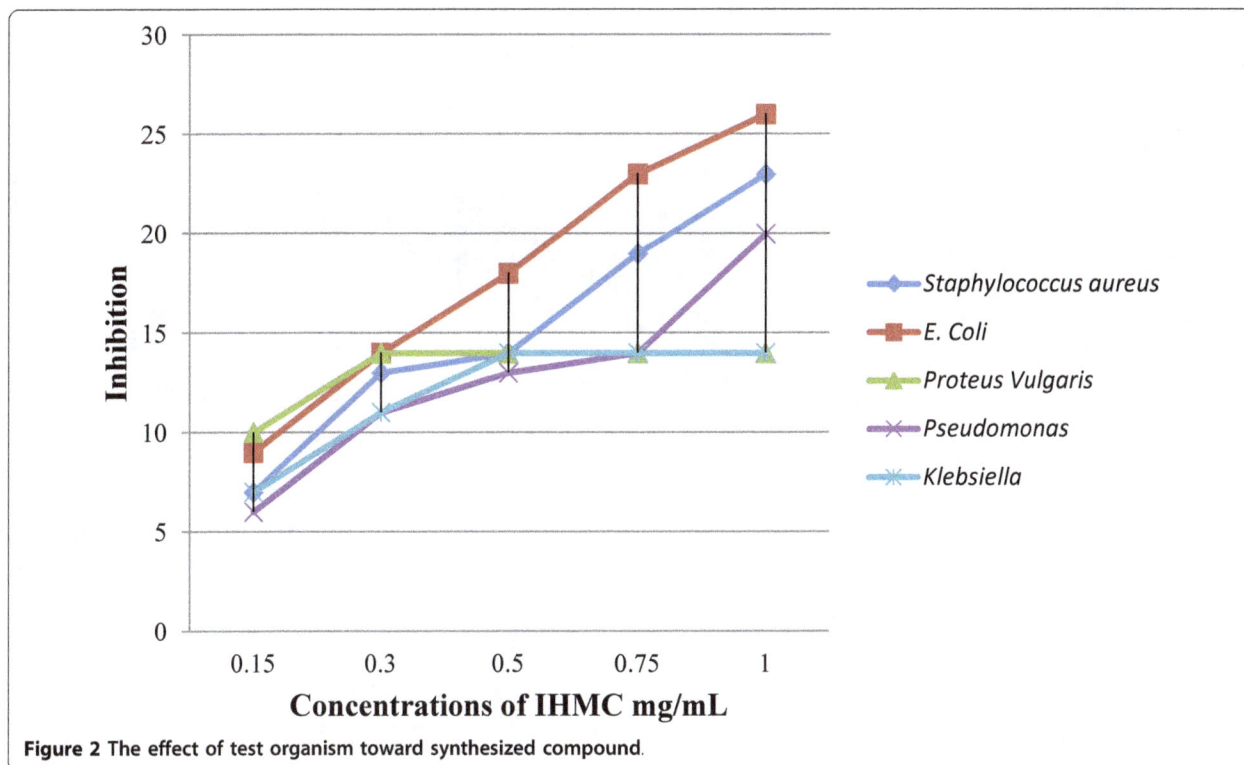

Figure 2 The effect of test organism toward synthesized compound.

Pharmacology

Antimicrobial activities

Antibacterial activity

The biological activity of the new IMHC was studied against selected types of bacteria which included positive bacteria (*Staphylococcus aureus*), and gram negative bacteria (*Escherichia coli, Klebsiella pneumoniae, Proteus vulgaris, Pseudomonas aeruginosa*), in brain hart broth agar media, which is used DMF as a solvent and as a control for the disc sensitivity test [25]. This method

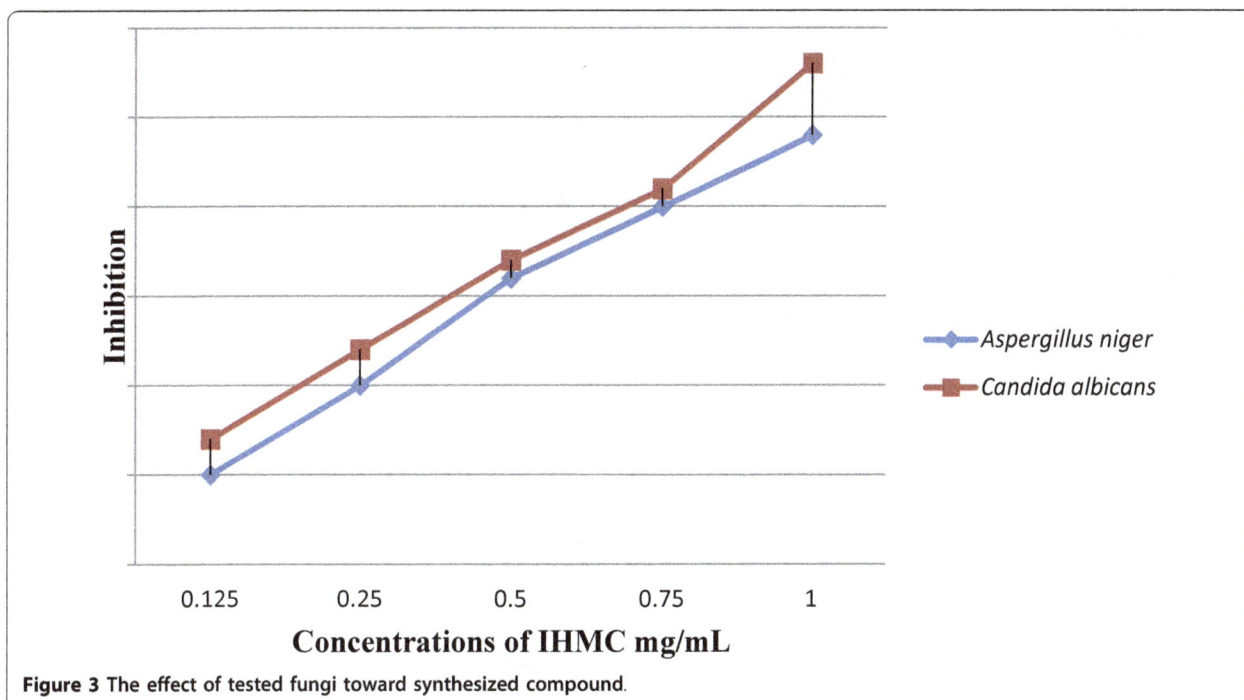

Figure 3 The effect of tested fungi toward synthesized compound.

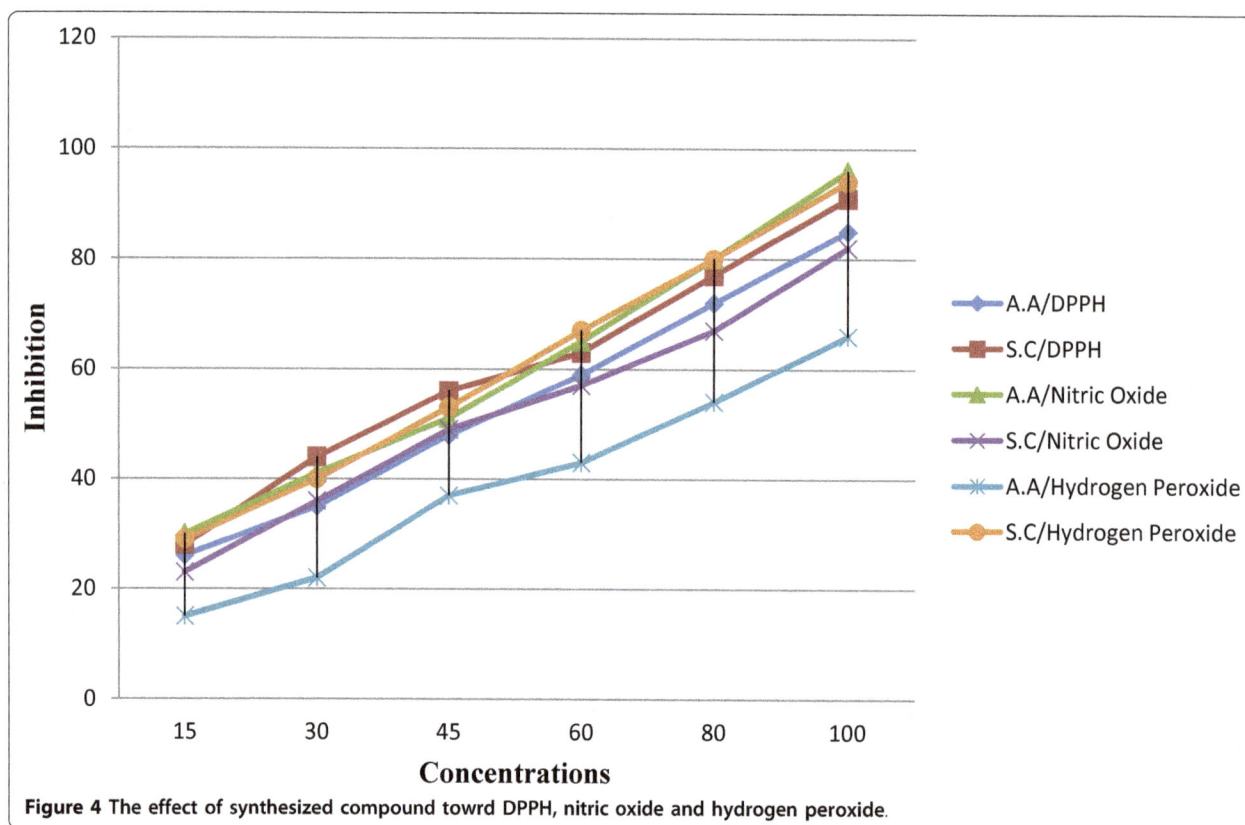

Figure 4 The effect of synthesized compound towrd DPPH, nitric oxide and hydrogen peroxide.

involves the exposure of the zone of inhibition toward the diffusion of microorganism on agar plate. The plates were incubated for 24 h, at 37°C. The antimicrobial activity was recorded as any area of microbial growth inhibition that occurred in the diffusion area.

Antifungal activities

IMHC was screened for it antifungal activity against *A. niger* and *C. albicans* in DMSO by serial plate dilution method using sabourand agar media. Normal saline was used to make a suspension of corresponding species. Twenty milliliters of agar media was poured in each Petri dish. Excess suspension was decanted and the plates were dried by placing in an incubator at 37°C for 1 h [15]. The fungal zone of inhibition values is given in Figure 3. The nutrient broth was inoculated with approximately 1×10^5 cfu/mL. The cultures were incubated for 48 h at 35°C and the growth was monitored.

Hint: Sabourand agar media were prepared by dissolving peptone (1 g), D-glucose (4 g), and agar (2 g) in distilled water (100 mL) and adjusting pH to 5.7.

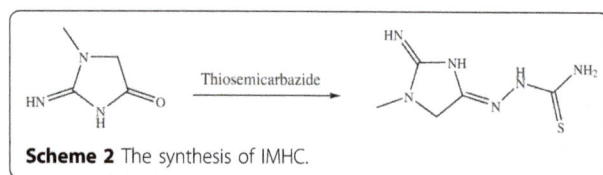

Scheme 2 The synthesis of IMHC.

Antioxidant studies

(2,2-diphenyl-1-picrylhydrazyl) radical scavenging activity The DPPH radical scavenging activities of the test IMHC were evaluated [26]. Initially, 0.1 mL of IMHC at concentration of 250, 500, 750, and 1000 μg/mL was mixed with 1 mL of 0.2 mM DPPH that was dissolved in methanol. The reaction mixture was incubated in the dark for 20 min at 28°C. The control contained all reagents without the sample while methanol was used as blank. The DPPH radical scavenging activity was determined by measuring the absorbance at 517 nm using the UV-Vis spectrophotometer. The DPPH radical scavenging activity of ascorbic acid was also assayed for comparison. The percentage of DPPH radical scavenger was calculated using Equation 1.

$$\text{Scavenging effects}(\%) = \frac{A_0 - A_1}{A_0} \times 100$$

where A_0 is the absorbance of the control reaction and A_1 is the absorbance in the presence of the samples or standards.

Nitric oxide scavenging activity Sodium nitroprusside in aqueous solution at physiological pH generates nitric oxide spontaneously; it interacts with oxygen to produce nitrite ions, which can be estimated by the use of GriessIllosvoy reaction [27,28]. In this investigation,

GriessIllosvoy reagent was modified using naphthylethy-lenediaminedihydrochloride (0.1% w/v) instead of 1-naphthylamine (5%). The reaction mixture (3 mL) containing sodium nitroprusside (10 mM, 2 mL), phosphate buffer saline (0.5 mL), and IMHC (250, 500, 750, and 1000 μg/mL) or standard solution (0.5 mL) was incubated at 25°C for 150 min. After the incubation, 0.5 mL of the reaction mixture containing nitrite was pipetted and mixed with 1 mL of sulfanilic acid reagent (0.33% in 20% glacial acetic acid) and allowed to stand for 5 min for completing diazotization. Then, 1 mL of naphthylethylenediaminedihydrochloride (1%) was added, mixed, and allowed to stand for 30 min. A pink-colored chromophore was formed in diffused light. The absorbance of these solutions was measured at 540 nm against the corresponding blank. Ascorbic acid was used as standard. Nitric oxide percentage scavenging activity was then calculated using Equation 1.

Hydrogen peroxide scavenging activity A solution of hydrogen peroxide (40 mM) was prepared in phosphate buffer (pH 7.4). Different concentrations (250, 500, 750, and 1000 μg/mL) of IMHC (or ascorbic acid) were added to a hydrogen peroxide solution (0.6 mL, 40 mM). Absorbance of hydrogen peroxide at 230 nm was determined after 10 min against a blank solution containing phosphate buffer without hydrogen peroxide [29]. Hydrogen peroxide percentage scavenging activity was then calculated using Equation 1.

DFT

All quantum chemical calculations were performed using the DFT in the methodology. DMol3 model was employed to obtain quantum chemical parameters and optimization of the molecule geometry.

Competing interests

The HOMO-LUMO explain the presence of an isolated state within the electronic structure of the compound, which is responsible for the intense blue-violet emission. It is well-known that orbital energy differences strongly overestimate actual excitation energies, and either configuration interaction or time-dependent treatments are needed to model the energetics of the electronic excitations. Nevertheless, the orbital energies provide a useful qualitative description [29].

References

1. Asiri A, Al-Youbi A, Khan S, Tahir M (2011) N-[(E)-Anthracen-9-ylmethylidene]-3,4-dimethyl-1,2-oxazol-5-amine. Acta Crystallogr Sect E 67(Pt 12):o3487
2. Mladenova R, Ignatova M, Manolova N, Petrova T, Rashkov I (2002) Preparation characterization and biological activity of Schiff base compounds derived from 8-hydroxyquinoline-2-carboxaldehyde and Jeffamines ED. Eur Polym J 38:989–999. doi:10.1016/S0014-3057(01)00260-9.
3. Walsh OM, Meegan MJ, Prendergast RM, Nakib TA (1996) Synthesis of 3-acetoxyazetidin-2-ones and 3-hydroxyazetidin-2-ones with antifugal and antifungal and antibacterial activity. Eur J Med Chem 31:989–1000. doi:10.1016/S0223-5234(97)86178-8.
4. Singh K, Barwa MS, Tyagi P (2006) Synthesis characterization and biological studies of Co(II), Ni(II), Cu(II) ad Zn(II) complexes with bidentate Schiff bases derived by heterocyclic ketone. Eur J Med Chem 41:147–153. doi:10.1016/j.ejmech.2005.06.006.
5. Al-Amiery AA, Al-Majedy Y, Abdulreazak H, Abood H (2011) Synthesis, characterization, theoretical crystal structure and antibacterial activities of some transition metal complexes of the thiosemicarbazone (Z)-2-(pyrrolidin-2-ylidene)hydrazinecarbothioamide. Bioinorg Chem Appl 2011:1–6. Article ID 483101
6. Sengupta AK, Sen S, Srivastava V (1989) Synthesis of coumarin derivatives as possible antifungal and antibacterial agents. J Ind Chem Soc 66:710–716
7. Panneerselvam P, Nair RR, Vijayalakshmi G, Subramanian EH, Sridhar SK (2005) Synthesis of Schiff bases of 4-(4-aminophenyl)-morpholine as potential antimicrobial agents. Eur J Med Chem 40:225–229. doi:10.1016/j.ejmech.2004.09.003.
8. Sridhar SK, Saravan M, Ramesh A (2001) Synthesis and antibacterial screening of hydrazones Schiff and Mannich bases of isatin derivatives. Eur J Med Chem 36:615–623. doi:10.1016/S0223-5234(01)01255-7.
9. Pandeya SN, Sriram D, Nath G, De Clercq E (1999) Synthesis antibacterial antifungal and anti-HIV activities of Schiff and Mannich bases derived from isatin derivatives and N-[4-(4'-chlorophenyl)thiazol-2-yl]thiosemicarbazide. Eur J Pharmacol Sci 9:25–31. doi:10.1016/S0928-0987(99)00038-X.
10. Abu-Hussen AAA (2006) Synthesis and spectroscopic studies on ternary bis-Schiff-base complexes having oxygen and/or nitrogen donors. J Coord Chem 59:157–176. doi:10.1080/00958970500266230.
11. Karthikeyan MS, Prasad DJ, Poojary B, Subramanya Bhat K, Holl BS, Kumari NS (2006) Synthesis and biological activity of Schiff and Mannich bases bearing 2,4-dichloro-5-fluorophenyl moiety. Bioorg Med Chem 14:7482–7489. doi:10.1016/j.bmc.2006.07.015.
12. Sharma BM, Parsania MV, Baxi AJ (2008) Synthesis of some azetidinones wih coumarinyl moiety and their antimicrobial activity. Org Chem 4:304–308
13. Husain MI, Shukla MA, Agarwal SK (1979) Search for potent anthelmintics. Part VII. Hydrazones derived from 4-substituted 7-coumarinyloxyacetic acid hydrazides. J Ind Chem Soc 56:306–307
14. Thangadurai TD, Gowri M, Natarajan K (2002) Synthesis and characterization of ruthenium(III) complexes containing monobasic bidentate Schiff bases and their biological activities. Synth React Inorg Met Org Chem 32:329–343. doi:10.1081/SIM-120003211.
15. Kadhum AH, Mohamad A, Al-Amiery AA, Takriff MS (2011) Antimicrobial and antioxidant activities of new metal complexes derived from 3-aminocoumarin. Molecules 16:6969–6984. doi:10.3390/molecules16086969.
16. Aydogan F, Öcal N, Turgut Z, Yolacan C (2011) Transformations of aldimines derived from pyrrole-2-carbaldehyde and Synthesis of thiazolidino-fused compounds. Bull Korean Chem Soc 22:476–480
17. Park S, Mathur VK, Park RP, Mathur VK, Planalp RP (1998) Syntheses solubilities and oxygen absorption properties of new cobalt(II) Schiff-base complexes. Polyhedron 17:325–330. doi:10.1016/S0277-5387(97)00308-2.
18. Landy LF (ed) (1989) The chemistry of macrocyclic ligand complexes. Cambridge University Press, Cambridge
19. Zaheer M, Akhter Z, Bolte M, Siddiqi HM (2008) N-(3-nitrobenzylidene) aniline. Acta Cryst 64:2381–2382
20. Yang DP, Ji HF, Tang GY, Ren W, Zhang HY (2007) How many drugs are catecholics? Molecules 12:878–884. doi:10.3390/12040878.
21. Berners SJ (2007) Metals in medicine. Keynote Lectures. KL01: the mitochondrial cell death pathway as a target for gold and other metal-based antitumor compounds. J Biol Inorg Chem 12:S7–S52
22. Corona-Bustamante A, Viveros-Paredes J, Flores-Parra A, Peraza-Campos A, Martínez-Martínez J, Sumaya-Martínez M, Ramos-Organillo A (2010) Antioxidant activity of butyl- and phenylstannoxanes derived from 2-, 3- and 4-pyridinecarboxylic acids. Molecules 15:5445–5459. doi:10.3390/molecules15085445.
23. Dharmaraj N, Viswanathamurthi P, Natarajan K (2001) Ru(II) complexes containing bidendate Schiff bases and their antifungal activity. Transition Met Chem 26:105–110. doi:10.1023/A:1007132408648.
24. Al-Amiery AA, Mohammed A, Ibrahim H, Abbas A (2009) Study the biological activities of tribulus terrestris extracts. World Acad Sci Eng Technol 57:433–435
25. Al-Amiery AA, Musa AY, Kadhum AH, Mohamad A (2011) The use of umbelliferone in the synthesis of new heterocyclic compounds. Molecules 16:6833–6843. doi:10.3390/molecules16086833.

26. Kadhum AH, Al-Amiery AA, Musa AY, Mohamad A (2011) The antioxidant activity of new coumarin derivatives. Int J Mol Sci 12:5747–5761. doi:10.3390/ijms12095747.

27. Garratt DC (1964) The quantitative analysis of drugs. Chapman and Hall Ltd., Tokyo,3: pp 456–458

28. Duh PD, Tu YY, Yen GC (1999) Antioxidant activity of water extract of Harng Jyur (Chyrsanthemum morifolium Ramat). Lebn Wissen Technol 32:269

29. Roof I, Park S, Vogt T, Rassolov V, Smith M, Omar S, Nino J, Loye H (2008) Crystal growth of two new niobates, La_2KNbO_6 and Nd_2KNbO_6: structural, dielectric, photophysical, and photocatalytic properties. Chem Mater 20(10):3327–3335. doi:10.1021/cm703479k.

17

In silico identification of novel lead compounds with AT$_1$ receptor antagonist activity: successful application of chemical database screening protocol

Mahima Pal and Sarvesh Paliwal[*]

Abstract

Background: AT$_1$ receptor antagonists are clinically effective drugs for the treatment of hypertension, cardiovascular, and related disorders. In an attempt to identify new AT$_1$ receptor antagonists, a pharmacophore-based virtual screening protocol was applied. The pharmacophore models were generated from 30 training set compounds. The best model was chosen on the basis of squared correlation coefficient of training set and internal test set. The validity of the developed model was also ensured using catScramble validation method and external test set prediction.

Results: The final model highlighted the importance of hydrogen bond acceptor, hydrophobic aliphatic, hydrophobic, and ring aromatic features. The model satisfied all the statistical criteria such as cost function analysis and correlation coefficient. The result of estimated activity for internal and external test set compounds reveals that the generated model has high prediction capability. The validated pharmacophore model was further used for mining of 56000 compound database (MiniMaybridge). Total 141 hits were obtained and all the hits were checked for druggability, this led to the identification of two active druggable AT$_1$ receptor antagonists with diverse structure.

Conclusion: A highly validated pharmacophore model generated in this study identified two novel druggable AT$_1$ receptor antagonists. The developed model can also be further used for mining of other virtual database.

Keywords: angiotensin II receptor antagonists, N^2-aryl biphenyl triazolinone, pharmacophore mapping

1. Background

The renin-angiotensin system plays a fundamental role in blood pressure and fluid and electrolyte homeostasis [1]. Angiotensin II (AII), an octapeptide produced by the renin-angiotensin system, is a powerful endogenous vasopressor. Angiotensin converting enzyme inhibitors work by blocking the production of angiotensin II from angiotensin I. An alternative and possibly superior approach would be to block the action of AII at the level of its receptor. Two distinct subtypes of AII receptors [type 1 (AT$_1$) and type 2 (AT2)] have been identified, and both belong to the G protein-coupled receptors super family (GPCRs) [2,3]. Most of the biological actions of AII are mediated by the AII receptors of the AT$_1$ subtype. The AT$_1$ receptor subtype mediates virtually all the known physiological actions of AII in cardiovascular, neuronal, endocrine, and hepatic cells as well as in other ones. Since AT$_1$ receptor is GPCR the interaction of AII with the AT$_1$ receptor induces a conformational change, which promotes the coupling with the G protein(s) and leads to the signal transduction via several effector systems (phospholipases C, D, A2, adenyl cyclase, etc.). The AT$_1$ receptors play a major role in the pressor and trophic actions of the AII, and much effort has been spent in developing nonpeptide antagonists for this receptor for the treatment of hypertension and congestive heart failure [4].

---

* Correspondence: paliwalsarvesh@yahoo.com
Department of Pharmacy, Banasthali University, Banasthali, Tonk, Rajasthan, India

Like other GPCR families, AT_1 receptors are transmembrane proteins and such macromolecules are not easily crystallized for structural analysis by X-ray crystallography [5]. In the absence of three-dimensional (3D) structure for AT_1 receptor, a rational design of antagonists using a structure-based approach is not feasible [1]. For this reason, 3D pharmacophore models from the ligand-based approach are very useful for analyzing the ligand-receptor interactions. Moreover, a pharmacophore can also be used as a query in a 3D database search to identify new structural classes of potential lead compounds. In the recent years, the development of a 3D-pharmacophore and its use in the virtual screening of the chemical databases appear to be a more relevant and time-saving approach. Thus, the construction of an accurate pharmacophore is a key objective in many drug discovery efforts.

The pharmacophore generation methods of the Catalyst software have been successfully used in drug discovery research and toxicology [6-8] as evident from pharmacophore-based development of protein farnesyl transferase, human immunodeficiency virus (HIV) protease, and HIV reverse transcriptase inhibitors [9,10].

In this study, our approach of pharmacophoric exploration via set of diverse 3D structures has resulted in development of a highly validated and predictive pharmacophore model for AT_1 receptor antagonists. The developed phamacophore was subsequently used for virtual screening of chemical databases for identification of novel lead compounds with nanomolar activity range.

2. Results and discussion

2.1. HypoGen model
Pharmacophore models were generated using 30 training set compounds representing two series of structurally diverse compounds with AT_1 receptor antagonist activity. All the generated pharmacophore hypotheses were evaluated for their statistical fitness on the basis cost difference values, correlation coefficients (r), and rms deviations. The pharmacophoric features and statistical data for a set of ten chosen hypothesis are listed in Additional file 1.

Out of ten, hypothesis1 was identified as best pharmacophore model, since this hypothesis showed a cost difference of 20.17 between null cost 148.75 and total cost 128.58 satisfying the range recommended in the cost analysis of the catalyst procedure. Hypothesis1 had total cost close to fixed cost (124.52), lower error cost (103.409), lowest root-mean-square (RMS) divergence (0.408), best correlation ($r = 0.977$), and good internal test set prediction ($r_{test-set} = 0.93$). The configuration cost of the hypothesis exceeded the limit of 17 bits but can be accepted as the model achieves other validation criterion [11,12].

The chosen hypothesis comprised of one hydrogen-bond acceptor (HBA), hydrophobic aliphatic region, and hydrophobic (HY) and one ring aromatic (RA) sites in a specific 3D orientation. The results of tolerance and weight fit to the features of the training set compounds are given in Additional file 2. The pharmacophore model mapped well to the training and test set compounds. The values of actual and predicted activity for the training and internal test set compounds are given in Additional files 3 and 4. The model was found to be quite good in predicting the activity of external test set compounds [13] with correlation co-efficient value of 0.71 and the values of actual and predicted activity are given in Additional file 5.

2.2. Fisher's cross validation test
The Fisher's randomization test was used to validate the strong correlation between chemical structures and biological activity. The generated pharmacophore model was assessed for quality by Fischer randomization test method using Cat Scramble technique in Catalyst at 98% confidence. The results are shown in Figure 1 and the resultant data clearly shows that none of the outcome hypothesis had a lower cost score than the initial hypothesis. The results obtained clearly supported the validity of selected pharmacophore model.

2.3. Mapping of training set compounds
Hypothesis1 is presented in Figure 2, aligned with the most active compound (**6b**: 0.072 nM) of the training set molecules. For this compound, HBA feature mapped to the S = O group of sulfonamide moiety. The HY aliphatic group mapped to the butyl chain at the triazolinone ring and the other HY feature mapped to the chlorophenyl ring. Ring aromatic feature mapped to one of the phenyl ring of biphenyl ring.

Figures 3 and 4 depict one of the conformations of compounds **7a** and **16** in the training set mapped onto Hypothesis1. As seen from these figures, both the compound fit all features of the developed pharmacophore model very well similar to the most active compound.

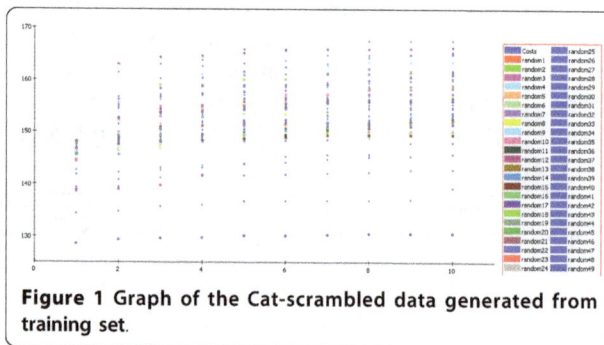

Figure 1 Graph of the Cat-scrambled data generated from training set.

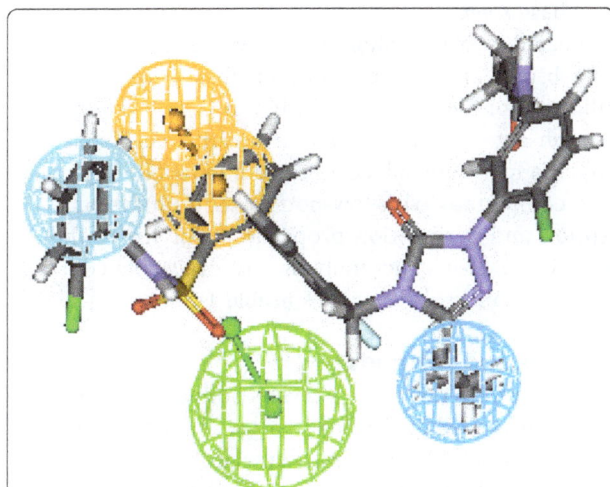

Figure 2 Best conformation of compound **6b** fit to the generated pharmacophore model of AT_1 receptor antagonists.

Moreover, compounds **7a** and **16** were reasonably well estimated with a fit value of 9.42 and 9.15, respectively (actual activity (**7a**) 0.14 nM; estimated 0.13 nM and actual activity (**16**) 0.26 nM; estimated 0.251 nM).

The most active compounds in the dataset assumed conformations that allowed proper mapping of all the feature of the generated hypotheses, whereas least active

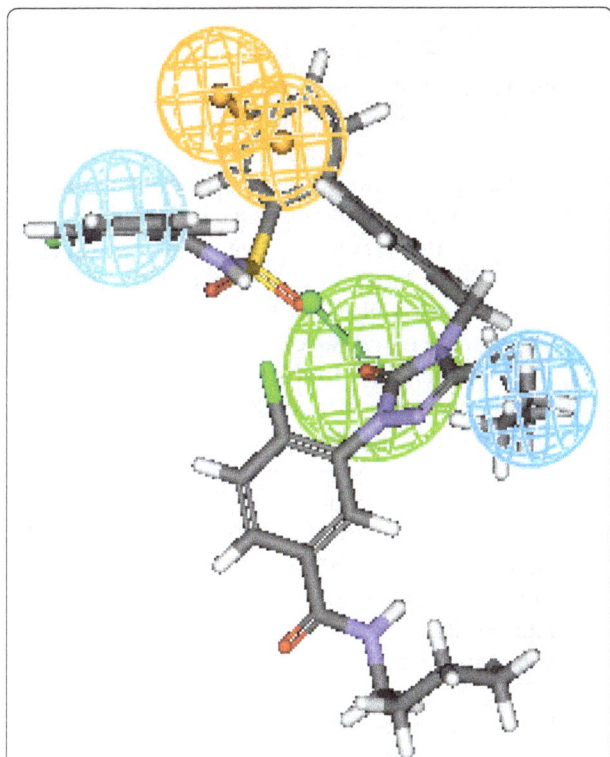

Figure 4 Best conformation of compound **16** fit to the generated pharmacophore model of AT_1 receptor antagonists.

compounds were unable to map HY aliphatic or ring aromatic. Pharmacophore mapping of the least active compound **33e** is shown in Figure 5.

2.4. Mapping of test set compounds

Hypothesis1 was further studied for its mapping pattern for the compounds of test set. The mapping analysis of the compounds, namely **5b** in the test set, revealed that none of the essential pharmacophoric features were missed and all features mapped with the least displacement from the centroid of all features (Figure 6). The

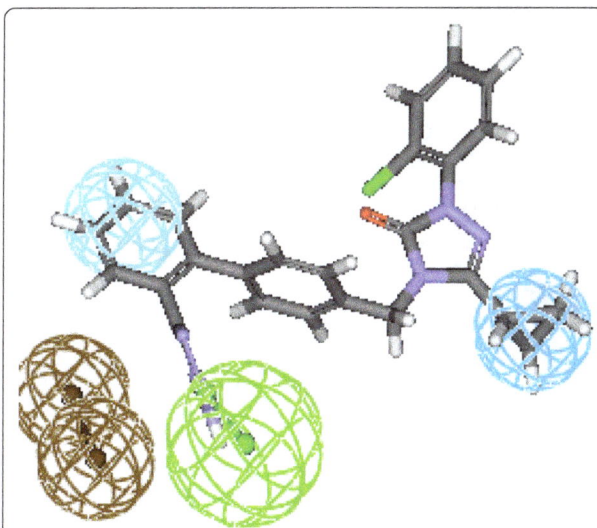

Figure 3 Best conformation of compound **7a** fit to the generated pharmacophore model of AT_1 receptor antagonists.

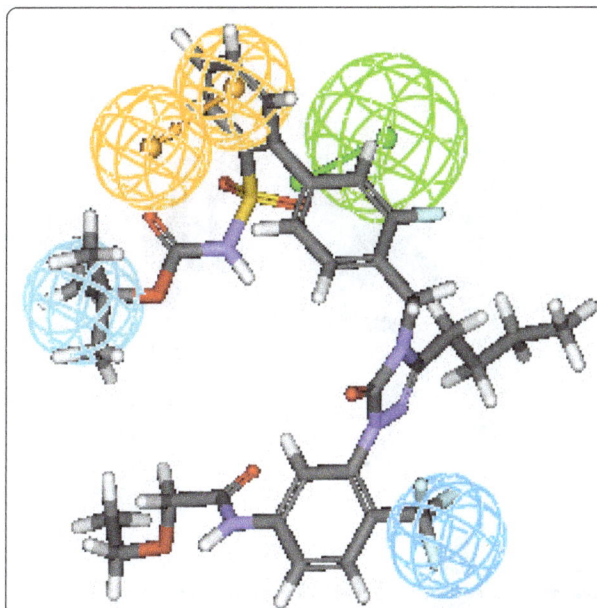

Figure 5 Best conformation of compound **33e** fit to the generated pharmacophore model of AT_1 receptor antagonists.

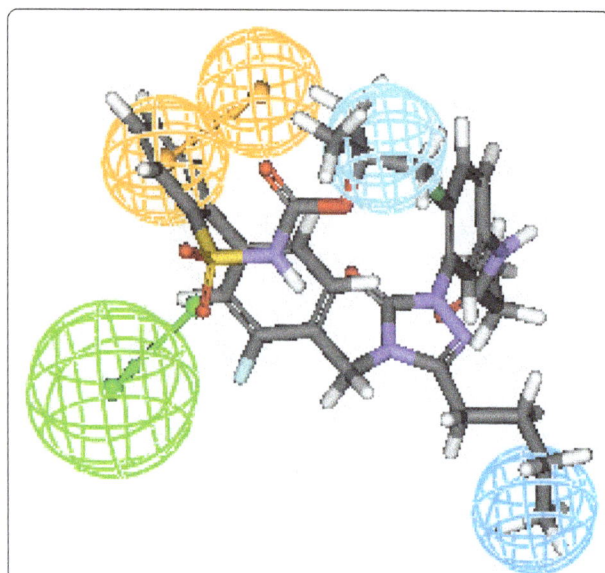

Figure 6 Best conformation of compound **5b** fit to the generated pharmacophore model of AT_1 receptor antagonists.

t-butyl group of **5b** mapped well with the HY feature of the pharmacophoric model, and the butyl group mapped with HY feature. The oxygen of the SO_2 mapped to the HBA feature, while the ring aromatic feature mapped to the phenyl ring of the biphenyl ring groups of compound **5b**. The moderate and lesser active compounds missed to map one pharmacophoric features and thereby justifying their corresponding categories. The moderately active compounds **35e** and **36e** missed the HY feature while the lesser active compound **38e** (Figure 7) missed the ring aromatic feature. These results revealed the importance of HY functionalities and ring aromatic feature in imparting good AT1 receptor antagonist activity.

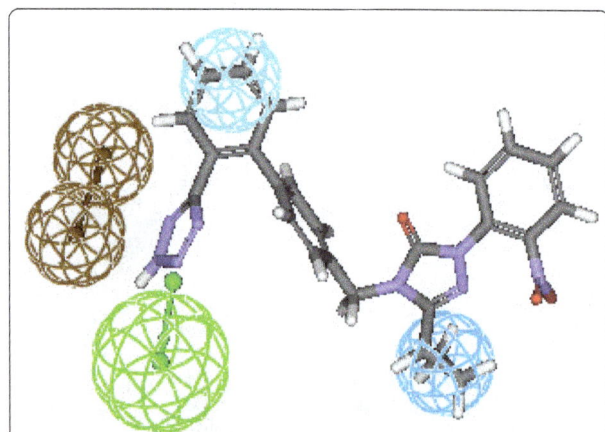

Figure 7 Best conformation of compound **38e** fit to the generated pharmacophore model of AT_1 receptor antagonists.

2.5. Database search

The validated pharmacophore model was used to search MiniMaybridge and NCI chemical databases [14,15] for identification of new AT_1 antagonists. By employing the fast search algorithm, 141 hits were retrieved. Subsequently, the hits were subjected to additional filtering to exclude compounds with low potency and unfavorable absorption and permeation properties. This led to the repossession of five structurally diverse druggable compounds with nanomolar activities (Table 1).

3. Materials and methods

Discovery studio, version 2.0, Accelrys Software Inc., San Diego, CA, was used to develop pharmacophore hypothesis for structurally diverse series of triazolinone derivatives reported in the literature [16,17] with activity range from 0.072 to 250 nM. Chemical structures of various N^2-aryltriazolinone biphenylsulfonamides with their experimental IC_{50} values for the AT_1 receptor subtype are listed in Additional file 6.

3.1. Selection of the training set and test set

The most important aspect of the hypothesis generation in HypoGen is the selection of the training set of molecules. The selection has to follow some basic requirements; such as a minimum of 16 structurally diverse compounds should be selected to avoid any chance correlation, most active compound should be included and the activity data should have a range of 3.5-5 orders of magnitude [18].

On the basis of above criteria, the dataset was divided into training set and test set. The training set comprised of 30 compounds, whereas internal test set was composed of 27 compounds. The most active compounds were included in the training set so that they would provide critical information for pharmacophore requirements. Several moderately active and inactive compounds were also included to spread the activity ranges as wide as possible. The important aspect of such selection scheme is that each active compound should teach something new to the HypoGen module to help it uncover as much critical information as possible for predicting biological activity.

3.2. Generation of pharmacophores

Details of the pharmacophore development procedures have been described in the literature [9,18]. In brief, conformational models of all training set molecules with AT_1 receptor antagonist activity were generated using the best quality conformational search option in Catalyst employing a constraint of a 20 kcal/mol energy threshold above the global energy minimum using CHARMm force field. A maximum of 250 conformations were generated to ensure maximum coverage in the conformational space [19]. Instead of using just the lowest energy conformation

Table 1 List of hits obtained from the MiniMaybridge and NCI database with their corresponding fit value and estimated activity

Number	Hits retrieved	Fit value	Estimated activity (nM)
1 (MiniMaybridge HITS)	SP 01066	9.239	0.205
2	KM 09509	8.524	1.062
3(NCI HITS)	NSC 122371	9.517	0.108
4	NSC 157629	9.515	0.108
5		9.356	0.156

of each compound, all conformational models for molecules in each training set were used in for pharmacophore hypothesis generation. The Catalyst software can generate pharmacophore hypotheses consisting of a maximum of five features. An initial analysis revealed that four chemical feature types such as HBA, HY, hydrophobic aliphatic (HY-ALI), and ring aromatic (RA) could effectively map all critical chemical features of all molecules in the training set. The minimum and maximum counts for HBA, HY, HY-ALI, and RA were set to 0 and 3, respectively. These four feature types were used to generate ten pharmacophore hypothesis from the training set. The uncertainty value was defaulted to 3 which is a ratio range of uncertainty in the activity value and MinPoints and MinSubsetPoints were 4 (default value). The MinPoints parameter controls the minimum number of location constraints required for any hypothesis. The MinSubsetPoint parameter defines the number of chemical features that a hypothesis must match in all the compounds set [20].

3.3. Evaluation of the HypoGen model

3.3.1. Cost function analysis

All the hypotheses generated were subjected to cost function analysis which is considered as stringent quality check tool. Two important theoretical cost calculations that determine the success of any pharmacophore hypothesis are "fixed cost" and "null cost". Fixed cost represents the simplest model that fits all data perfectly, and the second null cost represents the highest cost of a pharmacophore with no features and which estimates activity to be the average of the activity data of the training set molecules. The null cost value is equal to the maximum occurring error cost. The greater the difference between null cost and total cost and closer the total cost of the generated hypothesis to the fixed cost, the more statistically significant is the generated hypothesis. Another important cost is the overall cost of HypoGen model which consist of three cost components, the weight cost, the error cost, and the configuration cost. The quality of each hypothesis can be judged on the basis of total cost which is sum of error cost, weight cost, and configuration cost. The configuration cost, which is also known as the entropy cost, depends on the complexity of the pharmacophore hypothesis space. The error cost is dependent on the RMS differences between the estimated and the actual activities of the training set molecules. In standard HypoGen model, the configuration should not be greater than 17.0. The RMS deviations represent the quality of the correlation between the estimated and the actual activity data. The error cost is the most important part of the total cost and increases as the RMS difference between the estimated and the actual affinity for the training set increases. The RMS value is related to the quality of prediction of the hypothesis. Error cost provides the highest contribution to total cost and it is directly related to the capacity of the particular pharmacophore as 3D QSAR model, i.e., in correlating the molecular structures to the corresponding biological responses. The weight cost is a value that increases in a gaussian form as the difference between the actual and ideal weights of the features deviates. According to the

documentation, the ideal value of the weight is 2 because higher weight values tend to force unrealistic conformations of the compounds to fit such features [20].

3.3.2. Test set prediction

The ability of the models to predict the biological activity of compounds outside the model development procedure is a common method of validation [21]. Internal test set of 27 and external test set of 46 compounds were employed to assess statistical significance of the developed model. All test set molecules were built and minimized as well as used in conformational analysis like the training set molecules. Predictions were made to evaluate the level of similarity between actual and predicted activity.

3.3.3. Statistical validation

Statistical cross-validation study was performed to assess the significance of the best hypotheses using the cat-Scramble program available in Catalyst. The statistical significance is given by the equation.

$$\text{Significance} = [1 - (1 + x)/y] \times 10$$

where x is the total number of hypotheses having a total cost lower than best significant hypothesis and y the number (HypoGen runs initial + random runs). To obtain a 95% confidence level, 19 random spreadsheets are generated ($y = 20$) and every generated spreadsheet is submitted to HypoGen using the same experimental conditions (functions and parameters) as the initial run.

4. Database mining

The generated validated pharmacophore was used as query to search the virtual chemical compound database (NCI and MiniMaybridge) to identify new lead compounds with AT_1 receptor antagonist activity.

5. Conclusion

The quantitative pharmacophore models were developed using the training set of molecules with the help of HypoGen module implemented in the Catalyst. The best pharmacophore model provided a statistically significant correlation and well-estimated AT_1 activities for the test set compounds. Pharmacophore models generated for AT_1 antagonists in this study highlight the structural requirements for antagonistic activity. This study also helped in the identification of five structurally diverse AT_1 receptor antagonists.

Additional material

Additional file 1: Pharmacophoric hypotheses generated with training set of molecules using the HypoGen algorithm. The file contains the details of the generated pharmacophore models using two series of structurally diverse compounds with AT_1 receptor antagonist activity alongwith their statistical fitness on the basis of cost difference values, correlation coefficients (r), and rms deviations.

Additional file 2: Pharmacophoric features and corresponding weights, tolerances, and 3D coordinates of best model. The file contains the details of the features retrieved (hydrogen-bond acceptor, hydrophobic aliphatic, hydrophobic, and ring aromatic) and the tolerance and weight fit to the features of the training set compounds.

Additional file 3: Actual versus estimated activity and the selected chemical features of the final pharmacophoric model for training set of compounds. The file contains the comparison of the estimated and actual activity along with feature mapping status for training set of compounds.

Additional file 4: Actual versus estimated activity and the selected chemical features of the final pharmacophoric model for internal test set of compounds. The file contains the comparison of the estimated and actual activity along with feature mapping status for internal test set of compounds.

Additional file 5: Actual versus estimated activity and the selected chemical features of the final pharmacophoric model for external test set of compounds. The file contains the comparison of the estimated and actual activity along with feature mapping status for external test set of compounds.

Additional file 6: Chemical structures of various N^2-aryltriazolinone biphenylsulfonamides with their experimental IC_{50} values for the AT_1 receptor subtype. The file contains the structural and activity details of the series of the compound used in present study.

Acknowledgements
This study was supported by grants from the Council of Scientific and Industrial Research, New Delhi. The authors also thank the Vice Chancellor, Banasthali University, for extending all the necessary facilities.

Competing interests
The authors declare that they have no competing interests.

References
1. Tuccinardi T, Calderone V, Rapposelli S, Martinelli A (2006) Proposal of a new binding orientation for non-peptide AT_1 antagonists. J Med Chem 49:4305–4316. doi:10.1021/jm060338p.
2. Ellis ML, Patterson JH (1996) A new class of antihypertensive therapy: angiotensin II receptor antagonists. Pharmacotherapy 16:849–860
3. Israili ZH, Hall WD (1992) Cough and angioneurotic edema associated with angiotensin-converting enzyme inhibitor therapy. A review of the literature andpathophysiology. Ann Intern Med 117:234–242
4. Bondensgaard K, Ankersen M, Thogersen H, Hansen BS, Wulff BS, Bywater RP (2004) Recognition of privileged structures by G-protein coupled receptors. J Med Chem 47:888–899. doi:10.1021/jm0309452.
5. Sprague PW (1995) Automated chemical hypothesis generation and database searching with catalyst. Perspect Drug Discov Des 3:1. doi:10.1007/BF02174464.
6. Langer T, Krovat EM (2003) Chemical feature based pharmacophores and virtual library screening for discovery of new-leads. Curr Opin Drug Discovery Dev 6:370–376
7. Clark DE, Westhead DR, Sykes RA, Murray CW (1996) Active site-directed 3D database searching: pharmacophore extraction and validation of hits. J Comput Aided Mol Des 10:397–416. doi:10.1007/BF00124472.
8. Al-Sha'er MA, Taha MO (2010) Elaborate ligand-based modeling reveals new nanomolar heat shock Protein 90α Inhibitors. J Chem Inf Model 50:1706–1723. doi:10.1021/ci100222k.
9. Mukherjee S, S Mullick S, Mukherjee A, Saha A (2007) Pharmacophore mapping of selective binding affinity of estrogen modulators through classical and space modeling approaches: exploration of bridged-cyclic

compounds with diarylethylene linkage. J Chem Inf Model 47:475–487. doi:10.1021/ci600419s.
10. Chang LL, Ashton WT, Flanagan KL, Chen TB, O'Malley SS, Zingaro GJ, Siegl PKS, Kivlighn SD, Lotti VJ, Chang RSL, Greenlee WJ (1994) Triazolinone biphenylsulfonamides as angiotensin II receptor antagonists with high affinity for both the AT_1 and AT_2 subtypes. J Med Chem 37:4464–4478. doi:10.1021/jm00052a006.
11. Ashton WT, Chang LL, Flanagan KL, Hutchins SM, Naylor EM, Chakravarty PK, Patchett AA, Greenlee WJ, Chen TB, Faust KA, Chang RSL, Lotti VJ, Zingaro GJ, Schorn TW, Siegl PKS, Kivlighn SD (1994) Triazolinone biphenylsulfonamide derivatives as orally active Angiotensin II antagonists with potent AT_1 receptor affinity and enhanced AT2 affinity. J Med Chem 37:2808–2824. doi:10.1021/jm00043a020.
12. Fischer R (1966) The principle of experimentation illustrated by a psychophysical experiment. Hafner Publishing Co., New York, 8
13. Manallack DT (1996) Getting that hit: 3D database searching in drug discovery. Drug Discover Today 1:231–238. doi:10.1016/1359-6446(96)88990-2.
14. Chang LL, Ashton WT, Flanagan KL, Chen TB, O'Malley SS, Zingaro GJ, Kivlighn SD, Siegl PKS, Lotti VJ, RSL Greenlee WJ (1995) Potent and orally active angiotensin II receptor antagonists with equal affinity for human AT_1 and AT_2 subtype. J Med Chem 38:3741–3758. doi:10.1021/jm00019a004.
15. Chang LL, Ashton WT, Flanagan KL, Strelitz RA, MacCoss M, Greenlee WJ, Chang RSL, Lotti VJ, Faust KA, Chen TB, Bunting P, Zingaro GJ, Kivlighn SD, Siegl PKS (1993) Triazolinones as nonpeptide angiotensin II antagonists. 1. Synthesis and evaluation of potent 2,4,5-trisubstituted triazolinones. J Med Chem 36:2558–2568. doi:10.1021/jm00069a015.
16. Smellie A, Teig S, Towbin P (1995) Poling: promoting conformational variation. J Comput Chem 16:171–187. doi:10.1002/jcc.540160205.
17. Mason JS, Good AC, Martin EJ (2001) 3-D pharmacophores in drug discovery. Curr Pharm Des 7:567–597. doi:10.2174/1381612013397843.
18. Greenidge PA, Weiser J (2001) A comparison of methods for pharmacophore generation with the Catalyst software and their use for 3DQSAR: application to a set of 4-aminopyridine thrombin inhibitors. Mini Rev Med Chem 1:79–87. doi:10.2174/1389557013407223.
19. Brooks BR, Bruccoleri RE, Olafson BD, States DJ, Swaminathan S, Karplus M (1983) CHARMM: a program for macromolecular energy minimization, and dynamics calculations. J Comput Chem 4:187–217. doi:10.1002/jcc.540040211.
20. Paliwal S, Pal M, Yadav D, Singh S, Yadav R (2011) Ligand-based drug design studies using predictive pharmacophore model generation on 4H-1,2,4-triazoles as AT1 receptor antagonists. Med Chem Res. DOI 10.1007/s00044-011-9756-4
21. Toba S, Srinivasan J, Maynard AJ, Sutter J (2006) Using pharmacophore models to gain insight into structural binding and virtual screening: An application study with CDK2 and human DHFR. J Chem Inf Model 46:728–35. doi:10.1021/ci050410c.

18

Plant polyphenols as electron donors for erythrocyte plasma membrane redox system: validation through *in silico* approach

Rajesh Kumar Kesharwani[1], Durg Vijay Singh[2], Krishna Misra[1] and Syed Ibrahim Rizvi[3*]

Abstract

Background: The plasma membrane redox system (PMRS) has extensively been studied in erythrocytes. The PMRS plays an important role in maintaining plasma redox balance and provides a protective mechanism against oxidative stress. Earlier it was proposed that only NADH or NADPH provided reducing equivalents to PMRS; however, now it is acknowledged that some polyphenols also have the ability to donate reducing equivalents to PMRS.

Methods: Two different docking simulation softwares, Molegro Virtual Docker and Glide were used to study the interaction of certain plant polyphenols viz. quercetin, epigallocatechin gallate, catechin epicatechin and resveratrol with human erythroyte NADH-cytochrome b5 reductase, which is a component of PMRS and together with the identification of minimum pharmacophoric feature using Pharmagist.

Results: The derived common minimum pharmacophoric features show the presence of minimum bioactive component in all the selected polyphenols. Our results confirm wet lab findings which show that these polyphenols have the ability to interact and donate protons to the Human NADH-cytochrome b5 reductase.

Conclusion: With the help of these comparative results of docking simulation and pharmacophoric features, novel potent molecules can be designed with higher efficacy for activation of the PMRS system.

Keywords: *In Silico*, QSAR, Polyphenols, Pharmacophoric, Docking simulation, Glide, Molegro Virtual Docker

Background

The property of erythrocytes to reduce membrane impermeant anions was first reported by Orringer and Roer [1]. Later researches established the existence of trans-membranous NADH dehydrogenases in several other cell types [2,3]. Evidence is now clear for the presence of a trans-plasma membrane electron transport or plasma membrane redox system (PMRS) in all organisms including bacteria, yeast, animals and plants [4,5]. It is accepted that PMRS is involved in transferring reducing equivalents from intracellular donors to extracellular acceptors mainly oxidized ascorbate. In this way the PMRS helps the cells to respond to changes in redox potential thereby regulating a variety of physiological functions including cell metabolism, ion channels, growth and death [6,7].

The PMRS has extensively been studied in erythrocytes basically due to the fact that erythrocytes lack mitochondria and PMRS is the only mechanism for trans-plasma membrane electron transport. Importantly, erythrocytes encounter a variety of oxidants in the blood during their life span. Recent reports show that erythrocyte PMRS plays an important role in providing protection against oxidative stress during human aging [8,9] and in type 2 diabetes mellitus [10]. The basic structure of PMRS includes three major entities: the intracellular electron donor species, electron carrier proteins and oxidoreductases and extracellular electron acceptors. An important enzyme of PMRS in erythrocyte is the cytochrome b_5 reductase (EC 1.6.2.2).

Cytochrome b_5 reductase is encoded by the CYB5R3 locus located on chromosome 22q 13-qter (287). The

* Correspondence: sirizvi@gmail.com
[3]Department of Biochemistry, University of Allahabad, Allahabad 211002, India
Full list of author information is available at the end of the article

tertiary folding structure of human cyt b$_5$ red, revealed by X-ray crystallography shows similarity with other flavin-linked oxido reductases such as ferredoxin: NADP +reductase and phthalate dioxygenase reductase [11]. Cyt b$_5$ reductase contains two functional lobes: a flavin adenine dinuceotide FAD-binding amino terminal domain (residues 33-147) and NADH-binding carboxyl end domain (residues 148-170). The two domains are linked by a hinge region (residues 148-170), which is critical for the protein conformation and enzymatic activity. Cyt b$_5$ red. catalyses one-electron reduction reactions in association with FAD and cytochrome b$_5$.

In erythrocytes, cytochrome b5 reductase primarily helps in maintaining hemoglobin in its reduced state

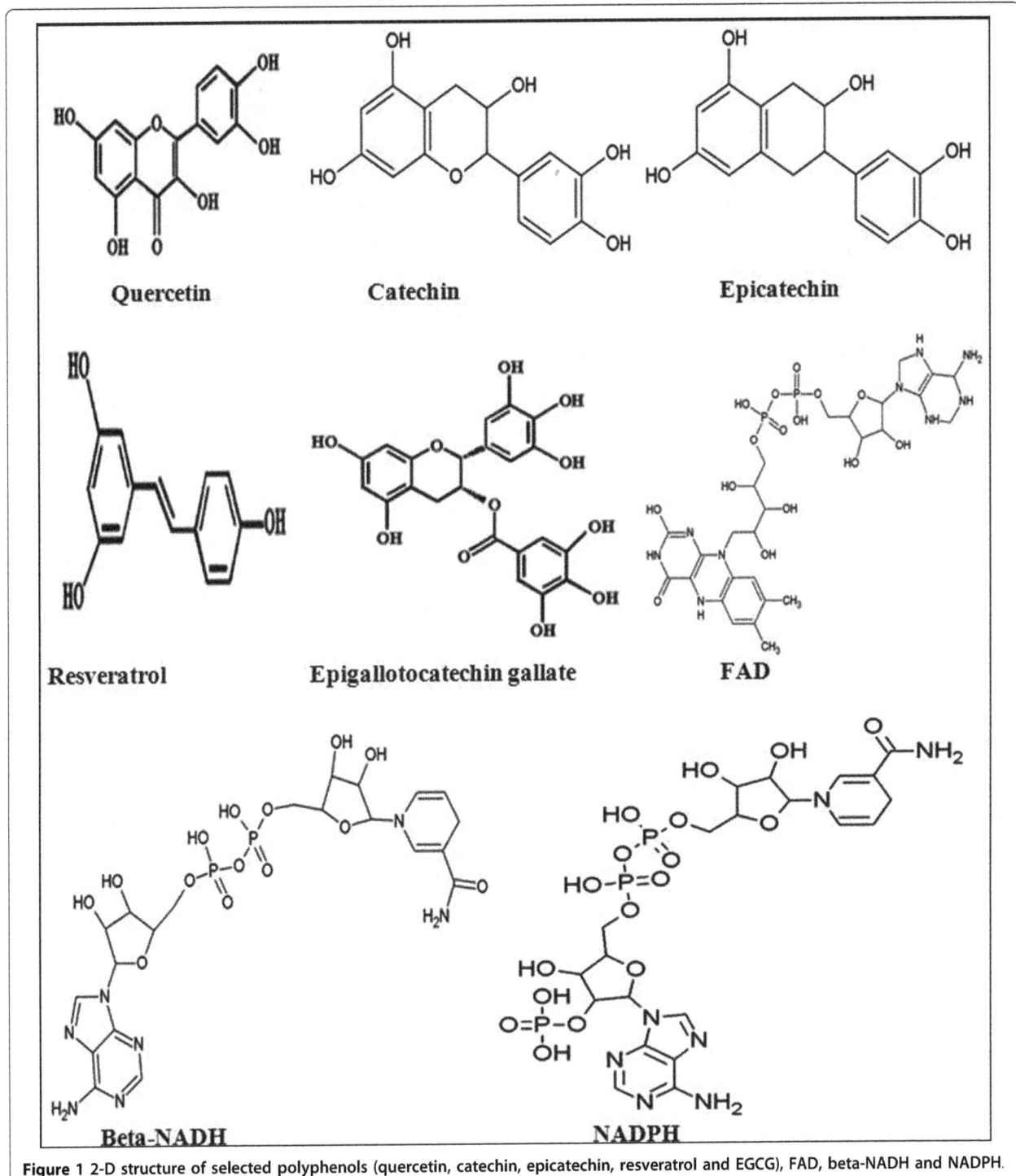

Figure 1 2-D structure of selected polyphenols (quercetin, catechin, epicatechin, resveratrol and EGCG), FAD, beta-NADH and NADPH.

Table 1 Comparative docking simulation result of selected polyphenols, NADPH and beta-NADH with Human NADH-cytochrome b5 reductase together with FAD, ligand from X-ray Crystallized data of protein data bank (1umk.pdb) using MVD

Serial Number	Ligands	MoleDockScore	H-bonding energy
1.	FAD	-232.638	-20.532
2.	NADPH	-209.954	-13.985
3.	beta-NADH	-208.235	-13.506
4.	EGCG	-131.595	-9.012
5.	Quercetin	-113.611	-10.033
6.	Catechin	-110.472	-9.063
7.	Epicatechin	-102.952	-14.638
8.	Resveratrol	-102.074	-10.272

Table 2 Comparative docking simulation result of selected polyphenols, FAD, NADPH and beta-NADH with Human NADH-cytochrome b5 reductase using Glide docking simulation software

Serial number	Ligands	GScore	Lipophilic EvdW	HBond	Electro
1	FAD	-12.18	-5.07	-2.14	-0.71
2	NADPH	-10.86	-4.45	-2.13	-0.68
3	beta-NADH	-10.48	-4.43	-1.72	-0.79
4	EGCG	-9.10	-4.13	-1.33	-0.51
5	Catechin	-7.83	-4.41	-1.75	-0.95
6	Quercetin	-7.82	-4.19	-1.58	-0.94
7	Epicatechin	-7.57	-3.12	-1.33	-1.07
8	Resveratrol	-4.29	-3.8	-1.5	-0.54

Where *GScore*: It is GlideScore called as Docking Score

LipophilicEvdW: It is term derived from hydrophobic grid potential and fraction of the total protein-ligand Van der Waals energy; *HBond*: Hydrogen-bonding term.

Electro: This term represents Electrostatic rewards

and also plays a crucial role in reducing extracellular ascorbate-free radical to ascorbate. Earlier it was proposed that only NADH or NADPH provided reducing equivalents to PMRS, however, now it is acknowledged that some polyphenols and ascorbate also have the ability to donate reducing equivalents to PMRS. It is now known that resveratrol, quercetin, myricetin, and epigallocatechin gallate (EGCG) may be taken up by erythrocytes from the plasma and actively promote PMRS activity [12,13]. In view of the important role of PMRS during aging and the emerging opinion that activation of erythrocyte PMRS may be an effective anti-aging strategy [14], this study was undertaken to determine the comparative molecular binding indices of some polyphenols (quercetin, catechin, epicatechin, resveratrol and EGCG together with FAD, NADPH and NADH (Figure 1) with an important component of erythrocyte PMRS, the cytochrome b5 reductase, through computational docking simulation using Molegro Virtual Docker (MVD) [15], Glide module (supplied by Schrödinger suite) [16] and ligand-based pharmacophoric feature derivation using PharmaGist server [17].

Methods
Protein structure and preparation
Three-dimensional X-ray crystallized structure of Human NADH-cytochrome b5 reductase (PDB: 1UMK, resolution = 1.75 Å) was downloaded from the Protein Data Bank [18,19]. The downloaded protein has single chain A with 275 residues together with FAD-binding region and contains bound FAD as a ligand molecule. It also contains 753 water molecules of crystallization. The protein structure was prepared using the protein preparation module of Schrödinger software [20]. The co-crystallized ligands and water molecules were removed. Some residues and side chain atom are missing in crystallized structure of protein that was modeled using Prime 2.2.108 followed by

refinement of the protein structure. The final modeled protein was taken as receptor protein and found the most suitable-binding site using sitemap script of Schrödinger. On the basis of priority of site, FAD-binding site has been selected for docking with the FAD, NADPH, beta-NADH, catechin, quercetin, epicatechin, EGCG and resveratrol.

Ligands structure preparation
All the selected ligands were assigned an appropriate bond order using the LigPrep 2.4.107 script and converted to .mae format (Maestro, Schrödinger, Inc.) followed by optimization by means of the OPLS_2005 force field [21].

Experimental
Docking study with MVD
It is an automated docking software with fast processing. The preparation of selected polyphenols and protein were done using default parameters, which automatically adds the missing hydrogen atoms. The software has module to create surface over receptor molecule and to give possible binding site for its activity. The active site region of receptor Human NADH-cytochrome b5 reductase protein was chosen for docking, which is already known from literature with the selected polyphenols. It gives ten conformations for each ligand and returns five outputs with MoleDockScore and other thermodynamically calculated values. The MoleDockScore is an anonymous value on which we have to suggest the best docked ligand with its conformation. It also shows hydrogen bond information together with other thermodynamic values, which suggest the formation of stable complex between ligand and receptor molecule [15].

Table 3 Human NADH-cytochrome b5 reductase protein residues interact with selected polyphenols, NADPH and beta-NADH using MVD (highlighted residues are involved in H-bonding interaction with ligands) and FAD from X-ray Crystallized data of protein data bank

Serial Number.	ligands	Interacting residues of receptor Human NADH-cytochrome b5 reductase	No. of H-bond interaction
1.	FAD	Arg91, Pro92, Tyr93, Val108, Ile109, Lys110, Tyr112, Phe113, Phe120, Gly123, Gly124, Lys125, Ser127, Thr181, Thr184	13
2.	NADPH	His77, Arg91, Pro92, Tyr93, Thr94, Val108, Ile109, Try112, His117, Phe120, Gly123, Ser127, Thr181, Thr184, Pro185	12
3.	beta-NADH	Arg91, Pro92, Tyr93, Thr94, Val108, Ile109, Lys110, Phe113, His117, Gly123, Gly124, Lys125, Thr181, Thr184	10
4.	EGCG	Arg91, Tyr93, Tyr112, Phe113, His17, Phe120, Gly123, Gly124, Lys125	5
5.	Catechin	His77, Pro92, Tyr93, Thr94, Val108, Ile109, Thr184, Pro185, Phe300	6
6.	Quercetin	His77, Pro92, Tyr93, Thr94, Val108, Ile109, Thr181, Thr184, Cys273, Phe300	7
7.	Epicatechin	Pro92, Tyr93, Thr94, Val108, Ile109, Lys110, Thr181, Thr184, Pro185, Phe300	8
8.	Resveratrol	His77, Pro92, Tyr93, Thr94, Val108, Ile109, Lys110, Thr181, Thr184, Pro185, Phe300	5

Where MoleDock Score is molegro docking scoring function or Energy Score (E_{Score})

Docking study with glide

The Protein ligand docking studies were performed using Maestro 9.1.107. Default parameters were selected with Glide Extra Precision (XP Glide), version 4.5.19. After the complete preparation of ligands and protein for docking, receptor-grid files were generated. For running the grid generation module we have scaled van der Waal radii of receptor atoms by 1.00 Å with a partial atomic charge of 0.25. A grid box of size 25 × 25 × 25 Å with coordinates X = 37.955433, Y = -6.749032 and Z = 39.920372 was generated at the centroid of the FAD-binding site predicted by sitemap script of Schrödinger suite 10.0. After the formation of receptor-grid file, flexible ligands with rigid receptor docking were performed. Glide generates conformations internally and passes these through a series of filters. The final energy evaluation is done with GlideScore and a single best pose is generated as the output for a particular ligand [16].

Pharmacophoric study

It is highly efficient method for the derivation of a minimum pharmacophoric features which is spatial arrangement of physico-chemical properties in a set of ligand,

essential for the interaction with a specific receptor. It takes three dimensional structure of set of ligands as an input to multiply align flexible ligands in a deterministic manner and to focus on the input ligands. It searches shared large common substructure for the detection of both outer molecules and alternative binding modes and finally derived pharmacophoric features shared by a large number of ligand molecules as an output [17].

Results and discussion

The binding site cavity detection and docking simulation was performed by using two different docking softwares, namely MVD and Glide simulation module (supplied by Schrödinger suite) for the selected polyphenols together with FAD NADPH and beta-NADH at Human NADH-cytochrome b5 reductase.

The results obtained using MVD and Glide, shown in terms of MoleDockScore; H-bonding energy and Glide score; LipophilicEvdW enrgy; HBond energy; Electro energy respectively are given in Table 1 and 2.

The comparative result of docking simulation given in Tables 3 and 4, shows active site residues and proves

Table 4 Human NADH-cytochrome b5 reductase protein residues interact with selected polyphenols, NADPH, beta-NADH using Glide docking simulation software (highlighted residues are H-bonding interacting residues) and FAD from X-ray Crystallized data of protein data bank

S. No.	ligands	Interacting residues of receptor Human NADH-cytochrome b5 reductase	No. of H-bond interaction
1.	FAD	Arg91, Pro92, Tyr93, Thr94, Val108, Ile109, Lys110, Phe113, Phe120, Gly123, Gly124, Lys125, Met126, Ser127, Gly179, Gly180, Thr181, Thr184	17
2.	NADPH	Thr94, Lys110, Try112, His117, Gly179, Gly180, Thr181, Thr184, Gln210, Cys273, Pro275	8
3.	beta-NADH	Tyr93, Lys110, Tyr112, Gly179, Gly180, Thr181, Gln210, Asp239, Phe251, Val252, Pro275	8
4.	EGCG	His117, Asn209, Gln210, Asp239, Phe251, Met278	4
5.	Catechin	Lys110, Tyr112, Gly180, Ala208, Asn209, Gln210, Phe251, Val252, Pro275	6
6.	Quarcetin	Lys110, Tyr112, Ala208, Asn209, Asp239, Phe251	4
7.	Epicatechin	Lys110, Tyr112, Gly180, Ala208, Gln210, Asp239, Phe251, Val252, Pro275	7
8.	Reserveratrol	Lys110, Tyr112, Ala208, Gln210, Phe251, Val252	3

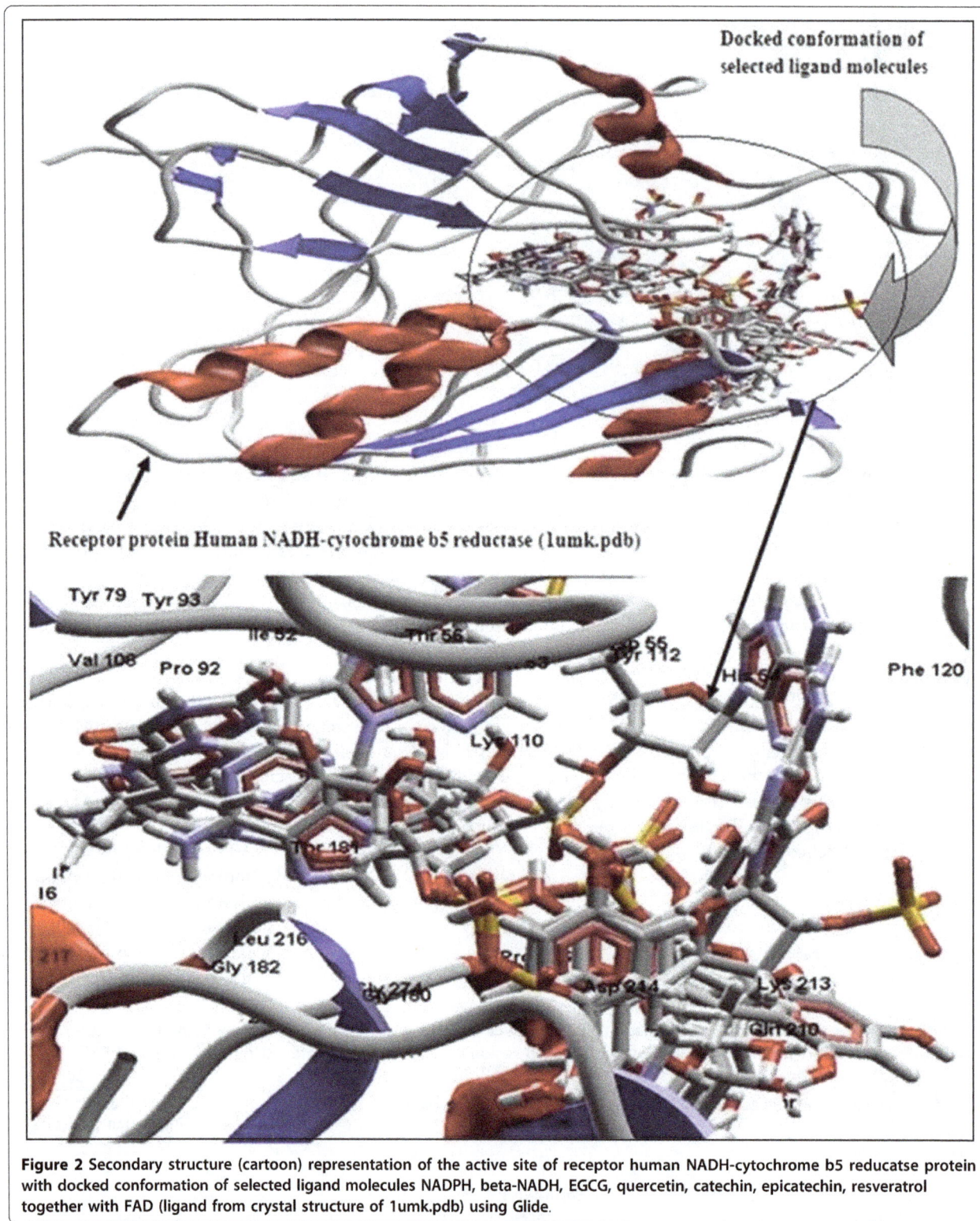

Figure 2 Secondary structure (cartoon) representation of the active site of receptor human NADH-cytochrome b5 reducatse protein with docked conformation of selected ligand molecules NADPH, beta-NADH, EGCG, quercetin, catechin, epicatechin, resveratrol together with FAD (ligand from crystal structure of 1umk.pdb) using Glide.

that a number of hydrogen bonds are involved in interaction between selected polyphenols, FAD, NADPH and beta-NADH with the receptor Human NADH-cytochrome b5 reductase.

The binding affinity of selected polyphenols, NADPH, beta-NADH and FAD at the active site of Human NADH-cytochrome b5 reductase using MVD and Glide in decreasing order is: FAD>NADPH>beta-

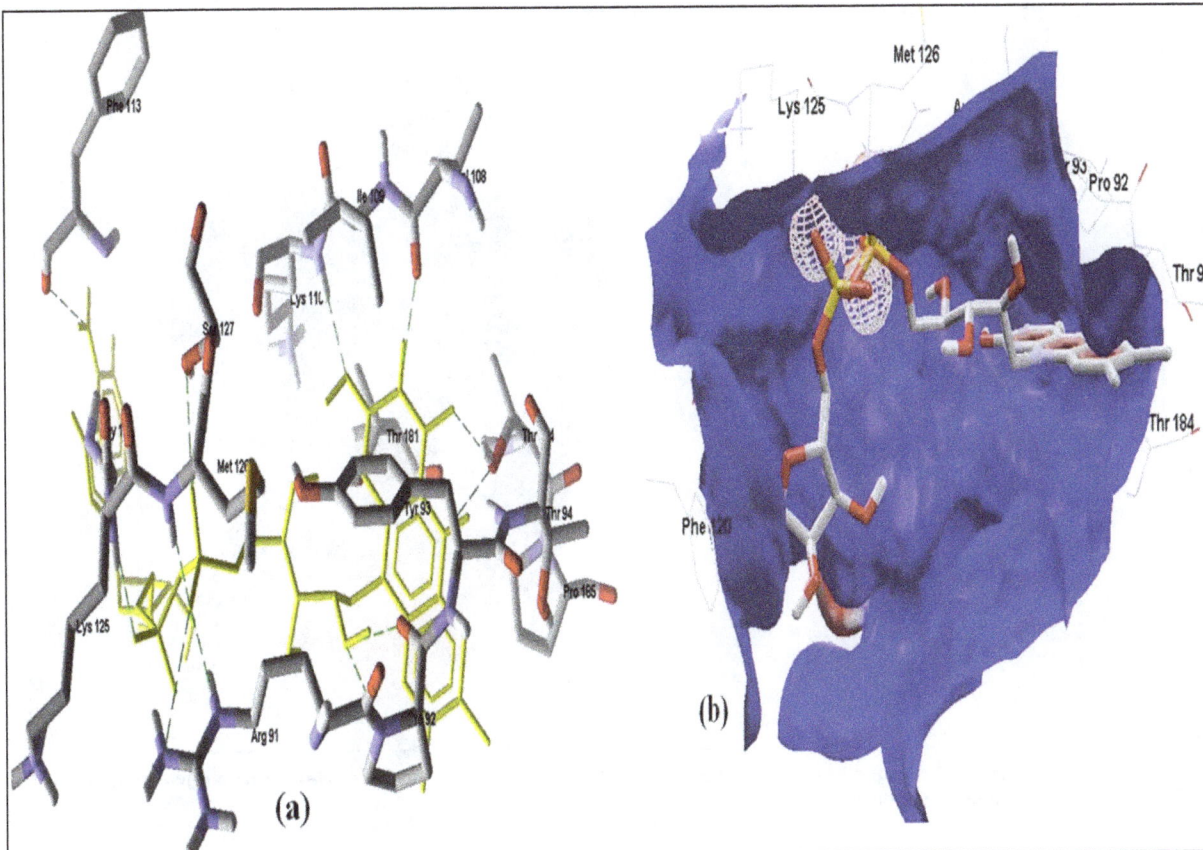

Figure 3 Docked conformation of hydrogen bonding view and 3.b with Electrostatic interaction of FAD with interacting amino acids of human NADH-cytochrome b5 reducatse protein at the active site cavity.

NADH>EGCG>quercetin>catechin>epicatechin>resveratrol and FAD>NADPH>beta-NADH>FAD>NADPH>-beta-NADH>EGCG>catechin>quercetin>epicatechin>-resveratrol respectively.

The Figure 2 of Glide docking simulation results shows low energy bound conformation of selected polyphenols, NADPH, beta-NADH and together with FAD (ligand from crystal structure of PDB:1UMK) at the active site of Human NADH-cytochrome b5 reductase. The low energy bound conformation of selected ligands shows hydrogen bonding and electrostatic interactions as shown in Figure 3 (a, b), 4 (a, b), 5 (a, b), 6(a, b), 7 (a, b), 8(a, b), 9 (a, b) and 10(a, b) for FAD, NADPH, beta-NADH, epigallocatechin gallate, catechin, quarcetin, epicatechin and resveratrol respectively.

Figure 2 of Glide docking simulation results shows low energy bound conformation of selected polyphenols, NADPH, beta-NADH, and together with FAD (ligand from crystal structure of PDB:1UMK) at the active site of Human NADH-cytochrome b_5 reductase. The low energy bound conformation of selected ligands shows hydrogen bonding and electrostatic interactions as shown in Figures 3a, b, 4a, b, 5a, b, 6a, b, 7a, b, 8a, b,

9a, b, and 10a, b for FAD, NADPH, beta-NADH, EGCG, catechin, quarcetin, epicatechin, and resveratrol, respectively

Computational methods provide aids for not only designing and interpretation of hypothesis-driven experiments in the field of drug discovery research but may also be used to compare in vitro results for rapid generation of new hypotheses. The binding affinity was higher for FAD because it is a natural ligand of the receptor protein having highest number of hydrogen bonds. The formation of hydrogen bonds provides additional force to stabilize the ligand-protein complex required for the activity of the Human NADH-cytochrome b5 reductase. The results obtained using two different docking simulation softwares were compared and their findings were common, which also strongly supports our *in silico* findings. An analysis of pharmacophoric features of the docked conformation for all the selected polyphenols, NADPH, beta-NADH and FAD, in the study provided the minimum common phormacophoric features shown in Figure 11, which include one aromatic ring, two donor atoms and one acceptor atom derived from PhrmaGist server [17]. The presence of

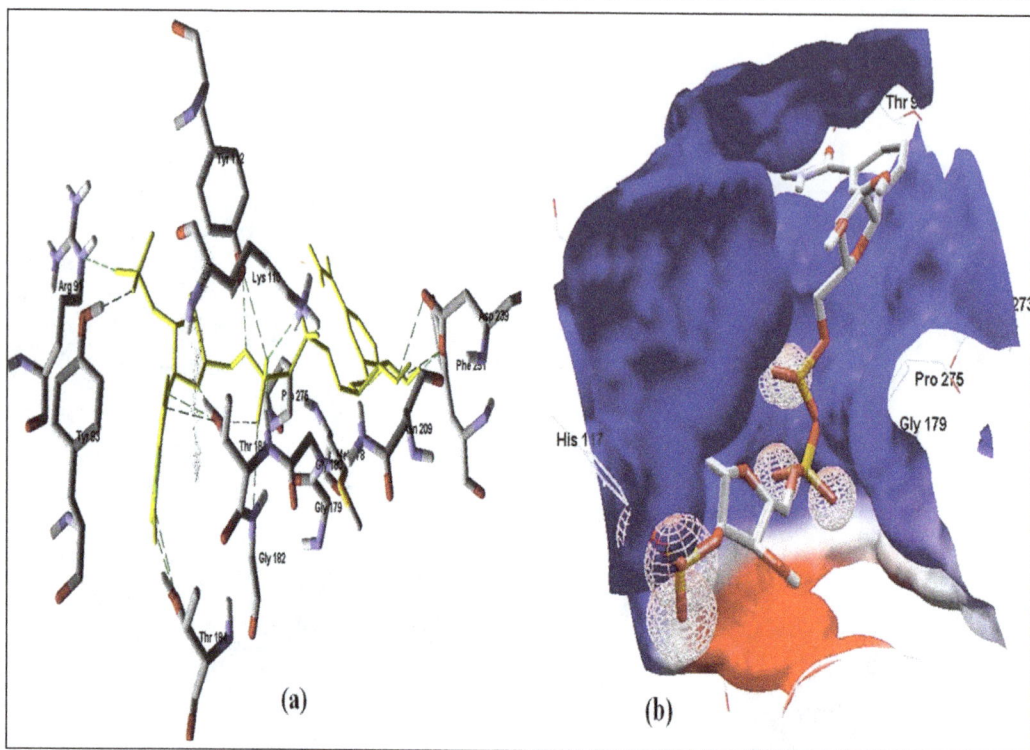

Figure 4 Docked conformation of hydrogen bonding view and 4.b with Electrostatic interaction of NADPH with interacting amino acids of human NADH-cytochrome b5 reducatse protein at the active site cavity.

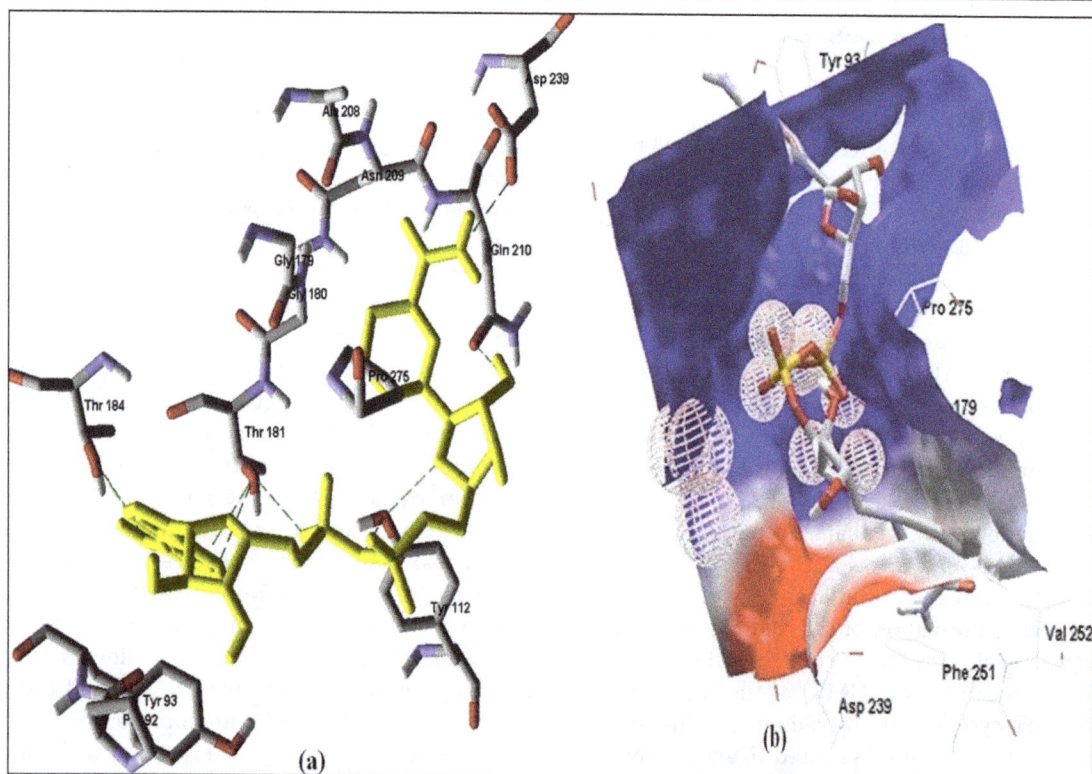

Figure 5 Docked conformation of hydrogen bonding view and 5.b with Electrostatic interaction of beta-NADH with interacting amino acids of human NADH-cytochrome b5 reducatse protein at the active site cavity.

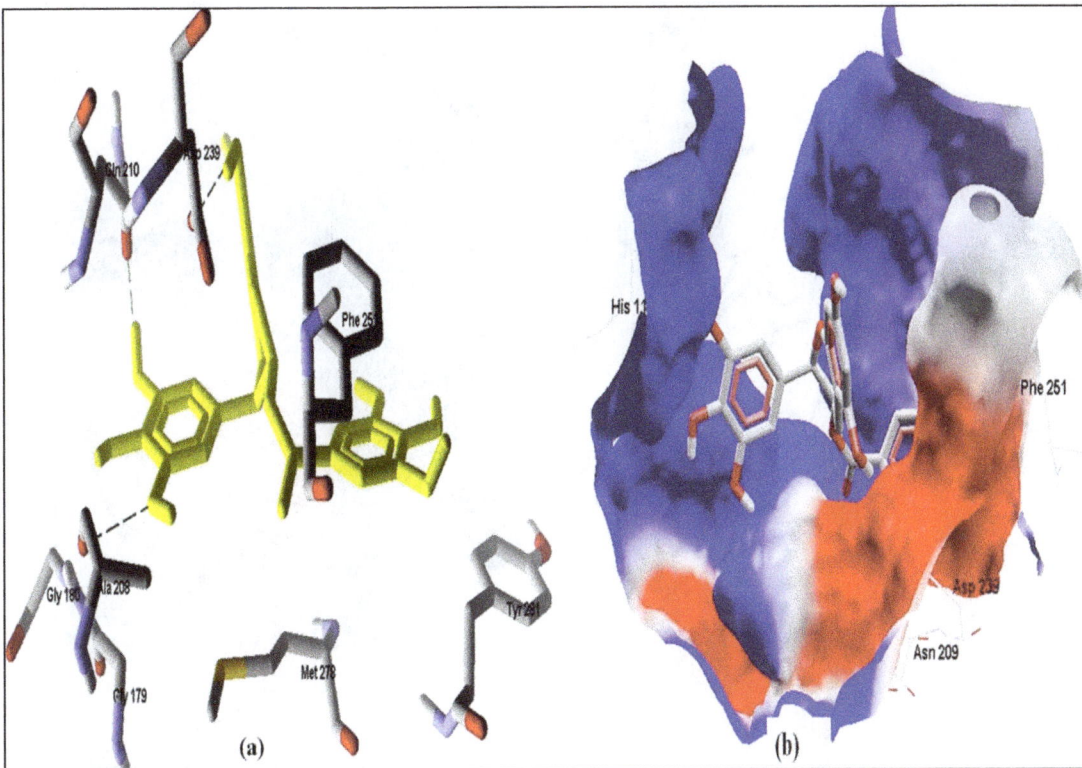

Figure 6 Docked conformation of hydrogen bonding view and 6.b, Electrostatic interaction of EGCG with interacting amino acids of human NADH-cytochrome b5 reducatse protein at the active site cavity.

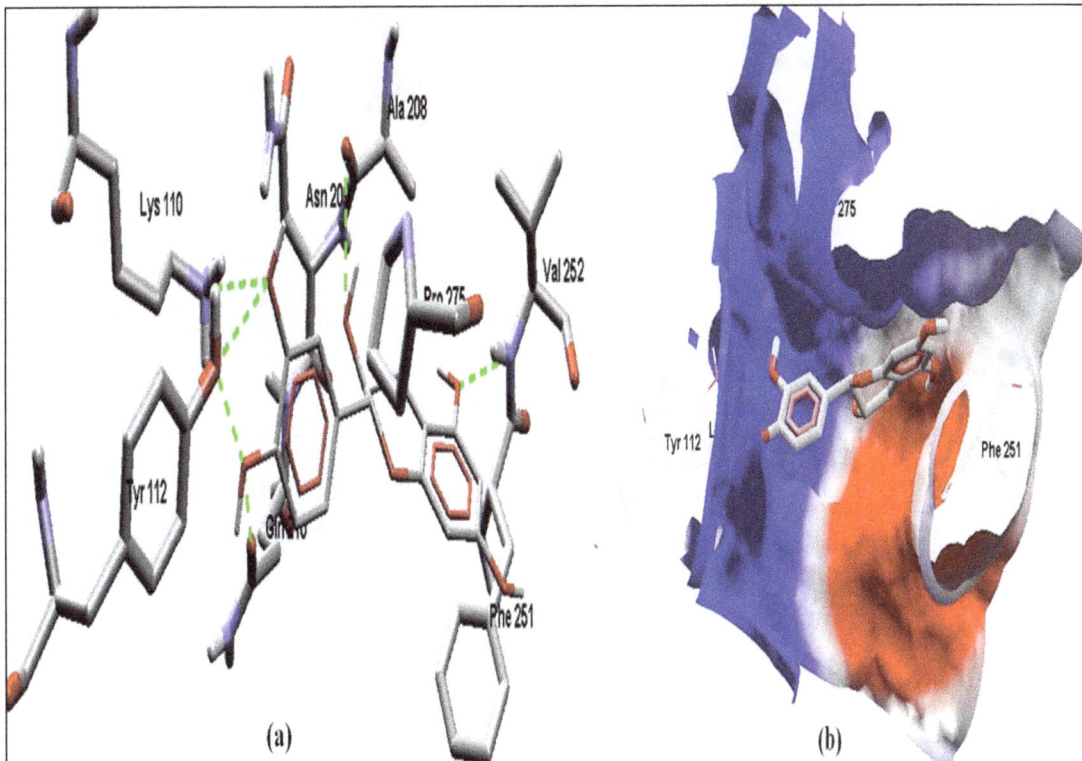

Figure 7 Docked conformation of hydrogen bonding view and 7.b with Electrostatic vnteraction of Catechin with interacting amino acids of human NADH-cytochrome b5 reducatse protein at the active site cavity.

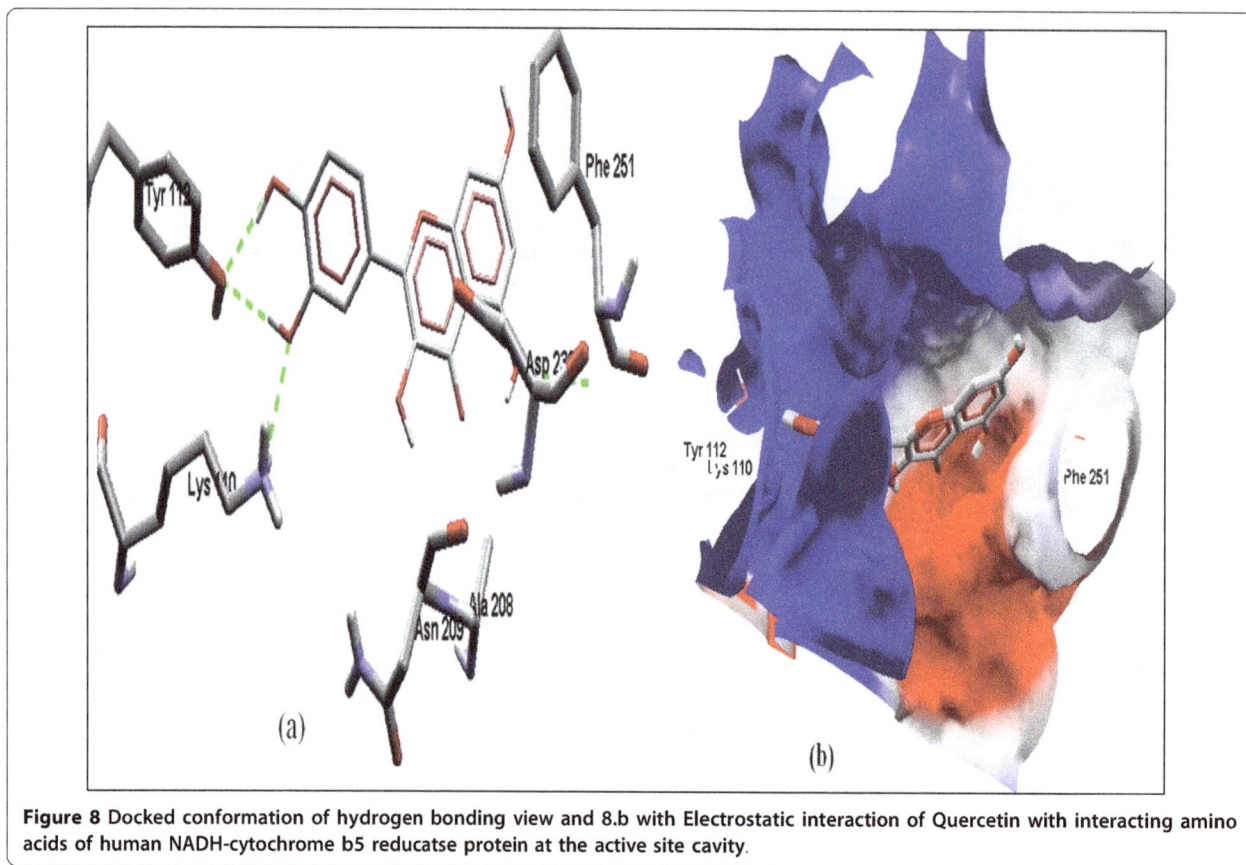

Figure 8 Docked conformation of hydrogen bonding view and 8.b with Electrostatic interaction of Quercetin with interacting amino acids of human NADH-cytochrome b5 reducatse protein at the active site cavity.

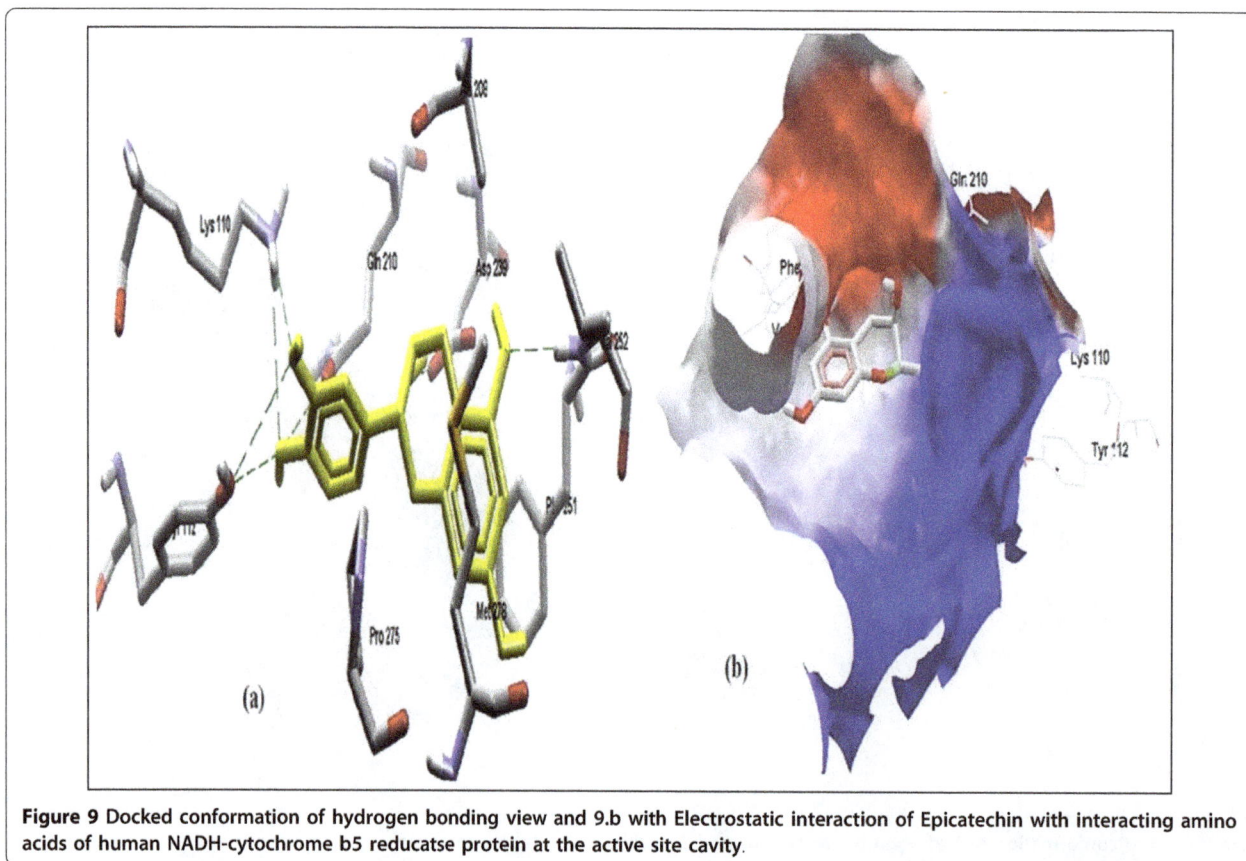

Figure 9 Docked conformation of hydrogen bonding view and 9.b with Electrostatic interaction of Epicatechin with interacting amino acids of human NADH-cytochrome b5 reducatse protein at the active site cavity.

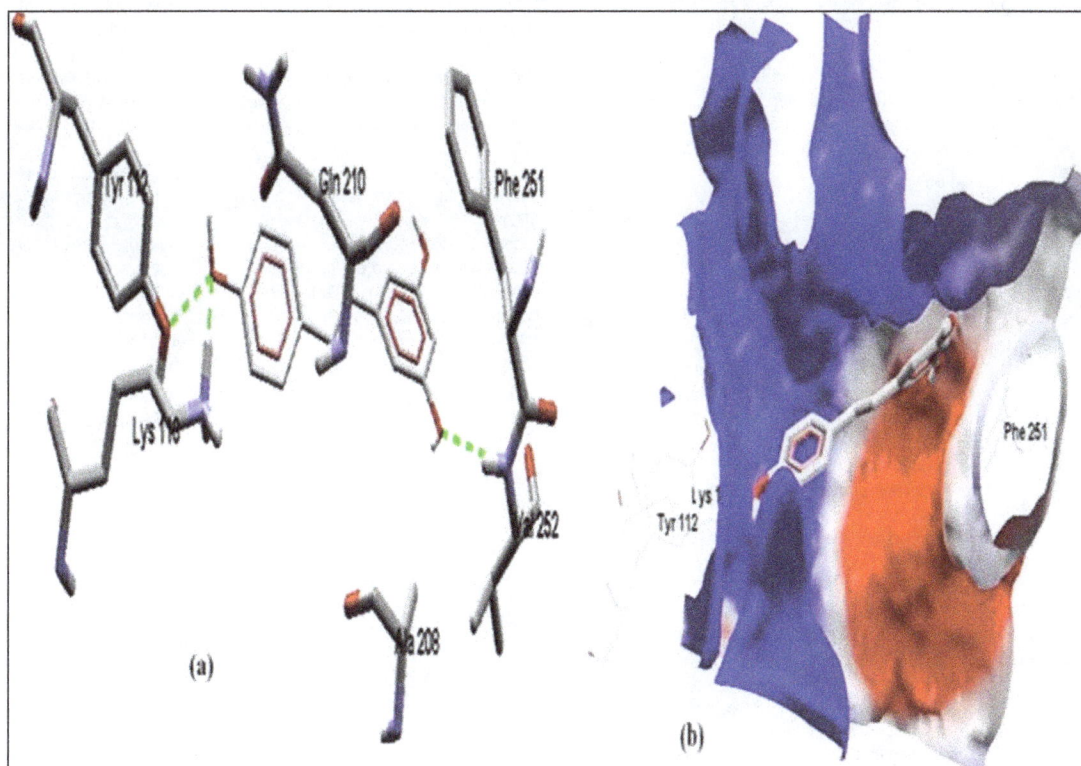

Figure 10 Docked conformation of hydrogen bonding view and 10.b with Electrostatic interaction of Resveratrol with interacting amino acids of human NADH-cytochrome b5 reducatse protein at the active site cavity.

minimum common pharmacophoric features in all the selected polyphenols proves the wet lab findings [12,13] which show that these polyphenols have the ability to interact and donate protons to the Human NADH-cytochrome b5 reductase.

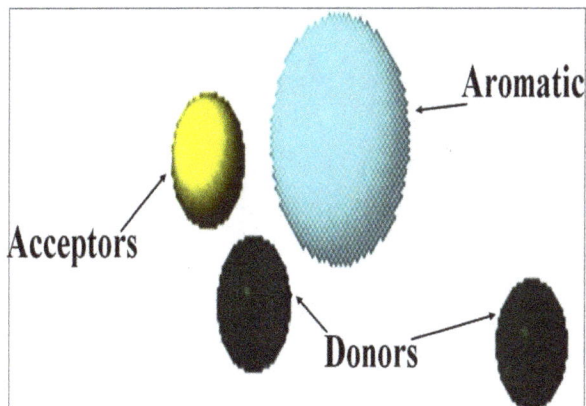

Figure 11 Derived Common pharmacophoric features for all the selected polyphenols (NADPH, beta-NADH, EGCG, Quercetin, Catechin, Epicatechin, Resveratrol and FAD) using PharmaGist sever.

Conclusion

Given the importance of human PMRS system during human aging and life span determination [8,9,22], our findings provide important insight into the docking and binding characteristics of the selected polyphenols on the Human NADH-cytochrome b5 reductase. With the help of these comparative results for docking simulation and pharmacophoric features, molecules having higher electron donor/acceptor efficacy for activation of the PMRS system can be designed. It is significant that activation of PMRS is being viewed as a putative mechanism for designing anti-aging agents [14]. Our in silico study may also lead to important information regarding the use of polyphenols as immunomodulating agents.

Abbreviations
EGCG: Epigallocatechin gallate; PMRS: Plasma membrane redox system.

Acknowledgements
One of the authors (RKK) gratefully acknowledges the Director, IIIT, Allahabad for providing necessary facilities for carrying out the computational work.

Author details
[1]Division of Applied Science & Indo-Russian Center For Biotechnology [IRCB], Indian Institute of Information Technology, Allahabad 211012, India
[2]Department of Bioinformatics, UIET, CSJM University, Kanpur 208024, India

[3]Department of Biochemistry, University of Allahabad, Allahabad 211002, India

Authors' contributions

RKK carried out docking simulation study, DVS performed pharmacophoric study, KM supervised docking and pharmacophoric studies, and SIR conceived the study, drafted the manuscript. All authors read and approved the final manuscript.

Competing interests

The authors declare that they have no competing interests.

References

1. Orringer EP, Roer ME (1979) An ascorbate mediated transmembrane reducing system of the human erythrocytes. J Clin Invest 63:53–58. doi:10.1172/JCI109277.
2. Greibing C, Crane FL, Low H, Hall K (1984) A transmembranous NADH dehydrohgenase in human erythrocyte membranes. J Bioenerg Biomembr 16:517–533. doi:10.1007/BF00743243.
3. Kilberg MS, Christensen HN (1979) Electron transferring enzymes in the plasma membrane of the Ehrlich ascites tumor cell. Biochemistry 18:1525–1530. doi:10.1021/bi00575a021.
4. Crane FL, Sun IL, Clark MG, Grebing C, Low H (1985) Transplasma membrane redox systems in growth and development. Biochim Biophys Acta 811:233–264
5. Rubinstein B, Luster DG (1993) Plasma membrane redox activity: components and role in plant processes. Ann Rev Plant Physiol Plant Mol Biol 44:131–155. doi:10.1146/annurev.pp.44.060193.001023.
6. Herst PM, Berridge MV (2006) Plasma membrane electron transport: a new target for cancer drug development. Curr Mol Med 6:895–904. doi:10.2174/156652406779010777.
7. Ly JD, Lawen A (2003) Transplasma membrane electron transport: enzymes involved and biological function. Redox Rep 8:3–21. doi:10.1179/135100003125001198.
8. Rizvi SI, Jha R, Maurya PK (2006) Erythrocyte plasma membrane redox system in human aging. Rejuvenation Res 9:470–474. doi:10.1089/rej.2006.9.470.
9. Rizvi SI, Pandey KB, Jha R, Maurya PK (2009) Ascorbate recycling by erythrocytes during aging in humans. Rejuvenation Res 12(1):3–6. doi:10.1089/rej.2008.0787.
10. Rizvi SI, Srivastava N (2010) Erythrocyte plasma membrane redox system in first degree relatives of type 2 diabetic patients. Int J Diab Mellitus 2:119–121. doi:10.1016/j.ijdm.2010.05.005.
11. Correll CC, Batie CJ, Ballou DP, Ludwig ML (1992) Pthalate dioxygenase reductase: a modular structure for electron transfer from pytidine nucleotides to [2Fe-2S]. Science 258:1604–1610. doi:10.1126/science.1280857.
12. Rizvi SI, Pandey KB (2011) Activation of the erythrocyte plasma membrane redox system by resveratrol: a possible mechanism for antioxidant properties. Pharmacol Rep 62(4):726–732
13. Rizvi SI, Jha R, Pandey KB (2010) Activation of erythrocyte plasma membrane redox system provides a useful method to evaluate antioxidant potential of plant polyphenols Methods Mol Biol 594:341–348
14. Rizvi SI, Jha R (2011) Strategies for the discovery of anti-aging compounds. Expert Opin Drug Dis 2011, 8(1):89–102
15. Thomsen R, Christensen MH (2006) MolDock: a new technique for high-accuracy molecular docking. J Med Chem 49(11):3315–3321. doi:10.1021/jm051197e.
16. Friesner RA, Murphy RB, Repasky MP, Frye LL, Greenwood JR, Halgren TA, Sanschagrin PC, Mainz DT (2006) Extra precision glide: docking and scoring incorporating a model of hydrophobic enclosure for protein-ligand complexes. J Med Chem 149(21):6177–6196
17. Schneidman-Duhovny D, Dror O, Inbar Y, Nussinov R, Wolfson HJ (2008) Deterministic pharmacophore detection via multiple flexible alignment of drug-like molecules. J Comput Biol 15(7):737–754. doi:10.1089/cmb.2007.0130.
18. Bando S, Takano T, Yubisui T, Shirabe K, Takeshita M, Nakagawa A (2004) Structure of human erythrocyte NADH-cytochrome 5 reductase. Acta Cryst 60(11):1929–1934
19. Dutta S, Burkhardt K, Swaminathan GJ, Kosada T, Henrick K, Nakamura H, Berman HM (2009) Data Deposition and Annotation at the Worldwide Protein Data Bank. Mol Biotechnol 42(1):1–13. doi:10.1007/s12033-008-9127-7.
20. Jacobson MP, Pincus DL, Rapp CS, Day TJ, Honig B, Shaw DE, Friesner RA (2004) A hierarchical approach to all-atom protein loop prediction. Proteins 55(2):351–367. doi:10.1002/prot.10613.
21. Albers HMHG, Hendrickx LJD, van Tol RJP, Hausmann J, Perrakis A, Ovaa H (2011) Structure-based design of novel boronic acid-based inhibitors of autotoxin. J Med Chem 54(13):4619–4626. doi:10.1021/jm200310q.
22. Rizvi SI, Kumar D, Chakravarti S, Singh P (2011) Erythrocyte plasma membrane redox system may determine maximum life span. Medical Hyp 76(4):547–549. doi:10.1016/j.mehy.2010.12.014.

19

Cytotoxic and potent CYP1 inhibitors from the marine algae *Cymopolia barbata*

Simone Badal[1], Winklet Gallimore[2], George Huang[3], Tzuen-Rong Jeremy Tzeng[3] and Rupika Delgoda[1*]

Abstract

Background: Extracts from the marine algae *Cymopolia barbata* have previously shown promising pharmacological activity including antifungal, antitumor, antimicrobial, and antimutagenic properties. Even though extracts have demonstrated such bioactivity, isolated ingredients responsible for such bioactivity remain unspecified. In this study, we describe chemical characterization and evaluations of biological activity of prenylated bromohydroquinones (PBQ) isolated from the marine algae *C. barbata* for their cytotoxic and chemopreventive potential.

Methods: The impact of PBQs on the viability of cell lines (MCF-7, HT29, HepG, and CCD18 Co) was evaluated using the MTS assay. In addition, their inhibitory impact on the activities of heterologously expressed cytochrome P450 (CYP) enzymes (CYP1A1, CYP1A2, CYP1B1, CYP2C19, CYP2D6, and CYP3A4) was evaluated using a fluorescent assay.

Results: 7-Hydroxycymopochromanone (PBQ1) and 7-hydroxycymopolone (PBQ2) were isolated using liquid and column chromatography, identified using ^{1}H and ^{13}C NMR spectra and compared with the spectra of previously isolated PBQs. PBQ2 selectively impacted the viability of HT29, colon cancer cells with similar potency to the known chemotherapeutic drug, fluorouracil (IC_{50}, 19.82 ± 0.46 μM compared to 23.50 ± 1.12 μM, respectively) with impact toward normal colon cells also being comparable (55.65 ± 3.28 compared to 55.51 ± 3.71 μM, respectively), while PBQ1 had no impact on these cells. Both PBQs had potent inhibition against the activities of CYP1A1 and CYP1B1, the latter which is known to be a universal marker for cancer and a target for drug discovery. Inhibitors of CYP1 enzymes by virtue of the prevention of activation of carcinogens such as benzo-a-pyrene have drawn attention as potential chemopreventors. PBQ2 potently inhibited the activity of CYP1B1 (IC_{50} 0.14 ± 0.04 μM), while both PBQ1 and PBQ2 potently inhibited the activity of CYP1A1 (IC_{50}s of 0.39 ± 0.05 μM and 0.93 ± 0.26 μM, respectively). Further characterizations showed partial noncompetitive enzyme kinetics for PBQ2 with CYP1B1 with a K_i of 4.7 × 10^{-3} ± 5.1 × 10^{-4} μM and uncompetitive kinetics with CYP1A1 (K_i = 0.84 ± 0.07 μM); while PBQ1 displayed partial non competitive enzyme kinetics with CYP1A1 (K_i of 3.07 ± 0.69 μM), noncompetitive kinetics with CYP1A2 (K_i = 9.16 ± 4.68 μM) and uncompetitive kinetics with CYP1B1 (K_i = 0.26 ± 0.03 μM) .

Conclusions: We report for the first time, two isolated ingredients from *C. barbata*, PBQ1 and PBQ2, that show potential as valuable chemotherapeutic compounds. A hydroxyl moiety resident in PBQ2 appears to be critical for selectivity and potency against the cancer colon cells, HT29, in comparison to the three other malignant cell lines studied. PBQs also show potency against the activities of CYP1 enzyme which may be a lead in chemoprevention. This study, the first on isolates from these marine algae, exemplifies the value of searching within nature for unique structural motifs that can display multiple biological activities.

Keywords: *Cymopolia barbata*, Dasycladaceae, Anticancer, CYP450, Chemoprevention, Chemoprotection.

* Correspondence: thejani.delgoda@uwimona.edu.jm
[1]Natural Products Institute, Faculty of Pure and Applied Sciences, University of the West Indies, Mona, West Indies, Jamaica
Full list of author information is available at the end of the article

Background

Cymopolia barbata (Linnaeus) V.Lamouroux (Dasycladaceae) is widespread in shallow waters and is seen covering rocks by the shorelines in tropical marine habitats. Known to grow to about 10-cm high, these green algae (Chlorophyta) have tufts at the end of their stems that are lightly calcified. Extracts from this plant have previously shown significant pharmacological properties such as antifungal, antitumor, antimicrobial, and antimutagenic activities [1-8]. Although the cymopols are known halogenated natural products which have been isolated from *C. barbata*, active ingredients responsible for the displayed biological activities remain unspecified. In this study, we investigated bioactivities of prenylated bromohydroquinones (PBQ), cymopol-related metabolites which are known to accumulate in *C. barbata*, and report, for the first time, biological activities from single ingredients isolated from this marine algae. Two of these compounds namely, 7-Hydroxycymopochromanone (PBQ1) and 7-hydroxycymopolone (PBQ2), shown in Figure 1 were investigated for cytotoxicity against three cancerous cell lines, one normal cell line, in addition to their potential for chemoprevention via inhibition of cytochrome P450 (CYP) 1 enzymes.

The CYP1 family of enzymes and in particular CYP1B1 appears to be a universal molecular cancer marker and a target for drug discovery. Findings of the overexpression of CYP1B1 in many tumor tissues compared with normal surrounding cells have led to the search for prodrugs reliant on CYP1B1 metabolism for the conversion into cytotoxic therapeutics [9]. The modification in the expression levels of CYP1B1 has been shown to modulate tumor progression [10] and thus specific inhibitors are expected to be of therapeutic/preventive benefit. Further, the involvement of CYP1 enzymes in the bioactivation of procarcinogens such as polycyclic aromatic hydrocarbons (PAHs), heterocyclic amines, aromatic amines, and nitro polycyclic hydrocarbons [11], in addition to the biotransformation of anticancer drugs, has stimulated research into inhibitors of CYP1 enzyme activity [12,13]. Such inhibitors are thought to be potential anti-carcinogens if they could inhibit the activities of

CYP1B1 and CYP1A1 to metabolize PAHs to toxic intermediates and/or decrease their ability to detoxify cancer drugs. A number of natural products have been found to be direct inhibitors of CYP1 enzymes, as well as generate metabolites that are CYP inhibitors with cytotoxic properties. In the study described in this article, PBQ2 demonstrated potent inhibition against CYP1B1 activity, together with promising and specific activity against the colon cancer cell line HT29. The examination of a close structural relative, PBQ1, also allows identification of structural motifs critical for biological activity.

Methods

Chemicals

All chemicals for the MTS and CYP inhibition assays were purchased from Sigma-Aldrich (St. Louis, MO, USA). All CYP substrates and metabolites were purchased from Gentest Corporation (Worburn, MA, USA).

Cell lines and CYP microsomes

All cell lines along with their respective media and supplements were purchased from ATCC (Manassas, VA, USA). *Escherichia coli* membranes expressing human CYP1A1, CYP1A2, CYP1B1, CYP2D6, CYP3A4, and CYP2C19 co-expressed with CYP reductase were purchased from Cypex Ltd. (Dundee, UK).

Cell culture and cytotoxicity assays

Cell lines (CCD18 Co, HepG2 and MCF-7) were maintained in ATCC-formulated Eagle's Minimum Essential Medium and HT29 was maintained in McCoy's 5a Modified Medium supplemented with 10% fotal bovine serum (Atlas; Fort Collins, CO, USA), 10 mM HEPES solution, 100 mM L-glutamine penicillin streptomycin solution, 3 g/L glucose, and 1.5 g/L of sodium bicarbonate. Cells were maintained at 37°C with 5% CO_2 in Corning 75 cm^2 culture flasks. Cells were exposed to a given isolate or known anticancer agent for 24 h. Following the appropriate treatments, cell viability was evaluated using an MTS assay according to the manufacturer's instructions [14]. All assays were performed at least three times and were monitored spectrophotometrically at 590 nm [15]. Cell viability was recorded as percentage relative to vehicle solvent-treated control.

CYP inhibition assays

The test compounds were evaluated for their ability to inhibit the catalytic activity of human CYP1 enzymes by means of high throughput fluorometric detection assays conducted in 96-well microtitre plates as described elsewhere [16,17]. 7-Ethoxyresorufin (ERes) was used as a substrate for detecting activity of CYP1B1 and 7-ethoxy-3-cyanocoumarin (CEC) was used as a substrate for both

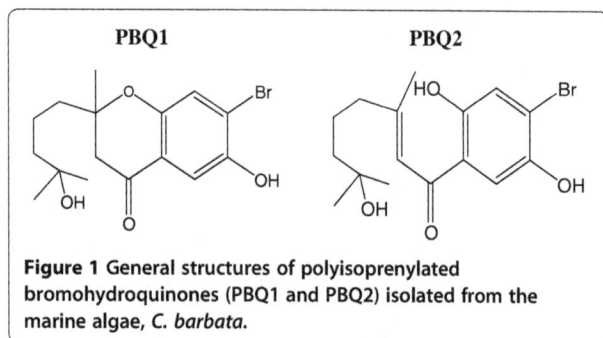

Figure 1 General structures of polyisoprenylated bromohydroquinones (PBQ1 and PBQ2) isolated from the marine algae, *C. barbata*.

CYP1A1 and CYP1A2. Further, the substrates, 3-[2-(N, N-diethyl-N-methylamino)ethyl]-7-methoxy-4methyl-coumarin (AMMC), 7-benzyloxy-4-trifluoromethylcoumarin (BFC), and CEC were used as substrates for CYP2D6, CYP3A4, and CYP2C19, respectively. The reactions were monitored fluorometrically at 37°C, using a Varian Cary Eclipse fluorescence spectrophotometer. All inhibitors were dissolved in a solvent of 20% acetonitrile in water and less than 0.3% of acetonitrile was used in the final assay.

Data analysis

IC_{50} and K_i values were determined by fitting the data in Sigma Plot (version 10.0) and enzyme kinetics module, using nonlinear regression analysis. The apparent K_i values were determined on the basis of visual inspection of Eadie-Hofstee and various statistics to evaluate goodness of fit, such as the size of the sum of squares of residuals, Akaike information criterion, and standard error (Enzyme kinetics module, version 1.3). The data listed represent the average values from three different determinations.

Results and discussion

Two PBQs (Figure 1) were isolated from the marine alga *C. barbata* and investigated for biological activity. The ability of these compounds to interfere with the reduction of the tetrazolium salt in the MTS assay was examined as a measure of impact on cell viability (Figure 2) using normal and cancer colon cells (CCD18 Co and HT29, respectively) along with liver and breast cancer cells (HepG2 and MCF-7, respectively). IC_{50} values were

calculated for test compounds and positive control known drug entities, doxorubicin, fluorouracil, and tamoxifen (Table 1). PBQ2 selectively impacted the viability of colon cells, HT29 with comparable potency to fluorouracil (for HT29 cancer cells: IC_{50}, 19.82 ± 0.46 μM compared to 23.50 ± 1.12 μM and normal colon cells, CCD18 Co IC_{50}, 55.65 ± 3.28 compared to 55.51 ± 3.71 μM, respectively). PBQ1 had no significant impact (<10% at 60 μM) on any of the cell lines tested.

To verify the accuracy of experimental techniques employed to detect CYP inhibition, assays with known inhibitors were carried out with furafylline (against CYP1A2 activity), ketoconazole (against activities of CYP1A1, CYP1B1, and CYP3A4), (−)-N-3-Benzyl-phenobarbital (against 2 C19) and quinidine (against CYP2D6 activity) and the obtained IC_{50} values (0.8 ± 0.2, 0.04 ± 0.01, 6.3 ± 1.7, 0.06 ± 0.01, 0.3 ± 0.01, 0.03 ± 0.01 μM, respectively) compared well with published values (0.99, <10, <10, 0.06, 0.25, and 0.04 μM, respectively; [17-20]). Michaelis constant, K_M, was determined for each marker substrate under the specified experimental conditions, in order to determine suitable substrate concentrations for assessing inhibitory potential of test compounds [21].

Both PBQs 1 and 2 potently ($IC_{50} < 1$ μM) inhibited the activity of CYP1A1 (IC_{50}s of 0.39 ± 0.05 and 0.93 ± 0.26 μM, respectively). PBQ2 also potently inhibited the activity of CYP1B1 (IC_{50}, 0.14 ± 0.04 μM) as shown in Figure 3. For those interactions yielding an $IC_{50} < 10$ μM against the activities of CYP1 family, further kinetic characterization was carried out to determine the nature of the inhibition, and Eadie-Hofstee plots are illustrated

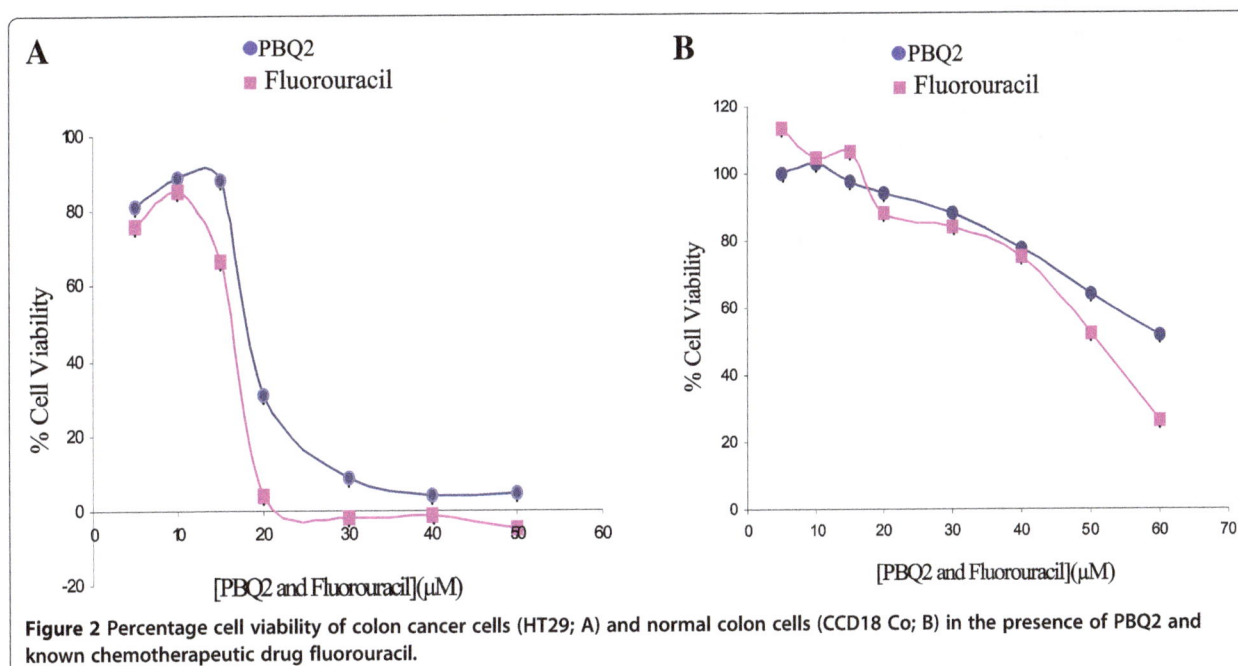

Figure 2 Percentage cell viability of colon cancer cells (HT29; A) and normal colon cells (CCD18 Co; B) in the presence of PBQ2 and known chemotherapeutic drug fluorouracil.

Table 1 IC$_{50}$ values (µM) obtained from the interaction of isomers of PBQs with colon cancer cell line (HT29) and the normal colon cell line (CCD18Co) along with positive controls

Compound	Cell lines			
	CCD18 Co	HT29	HepG	MCF-7
PBQ1	NI	NI	NI	NI
PBQ2	55.65 ± 3.28	19.82 ± 0.46	NI	NI
Tamoxifen	NA	NA	NA	17.28 ± 0.06
Fluorouracil	55.51 ± 3.71	23.50 ± 1.12	ND	ND
Doxorubicin	NA	NA	18.61 ± 0.58	NA

Key NI, no impact (<10% inhibition at 60 µM); NA, not applicable; ND, not determined.

in Figure 4. Reversible enzyme kinetics was observed for PBQ1 with partial noncompetitive inhibition of CYP1A1 activity, noncompetitive inhibition of CYP1A2 activity (K_is of 3.07 ± 0.69 and 9.16 ± 4.68 µM, respectively) and uncompetitive inhibition of CYP1B1 activity (K_i of 0.26 ± 0.03 µM). PBQ2 displayed uncompetitive inhibition of the activity of CYP1A1 (K_i of 0.84 ± 0.07 µM) and partial noncompetitive inhibition of the activity of CYP1B1 (K_i of 4.7 × 10^{-3} ± 5.1 × 10^{-4} µM).

Further characterization of the isolated test compounds against other major drug metabolizing P450 enzymes (CYP2C19, CYP2D6, and CYP3A4) was carried out. A summary table with all IC$_{50}$ data is presented in Table 2. As seen therein, while both PBQs 1 and 2 moderately (IC$_{50}$ > 1 µM) inhibited the activities of CYP2D6

(IC$_{50}$s, 1.03 ± 0.40 and 2.75 ± 0.96 µM, respectively) and CYP3A4 (IC$_{50}$s, of 5.07 ± 3.54 and 8.31 ± 4.67 µM, respectively). PBQ1 and PBQ2 potently inhibited the activity of CYP2C19 (0.08 ± 0.03 and 0.12 ± 0.06 µM, respectively).

From the panel of cell lines tested, the impact on the viability of malignant colon (HT29) and normal colon (CCD18 Co) cells by PBQ2 was similar to that imparted by the chemotherapeutic drug, fluorouracil, with comparable IC$_{50}$ values. PBQ2 also displayed selective cytotoxicity toward HT29 cells with no impact on cancerous liver (HepG2) and breast (MCF-7) cells. PBQ1, its structural isomer on the other hand, had no impact on any of the cell lines investigated and thus the presence of a tertiary hydroxyl group on PBQ2 appears to be critical for the observed bioactivity. Be it the formation of hydrogen bonds with key residues within the cell or during receptor-mediated cell permeability, the conjugated, open ring, and hydroxyl group presence in PBQ2 plays a crucial role in impacting cell viability compared with epoxy moiety of PBQ1.

Inhibitors of CYPs1A1 and 1B1 enzymes have received particular interest due to their role in reducing the activation of carcinogens and thus as chemoprotectors and chemotherapeutics. Several classes of natural compounds [22], including flavonoids [23,24] and organosulfur compounds [13,25,26], have demonstrated great potential in chemoprevention and thus provide the impetus for the search for others. Both PBQs potently (IC$_{50}$ < 1 µM) inhibited the activity of CYP1A1while PBQ2 also

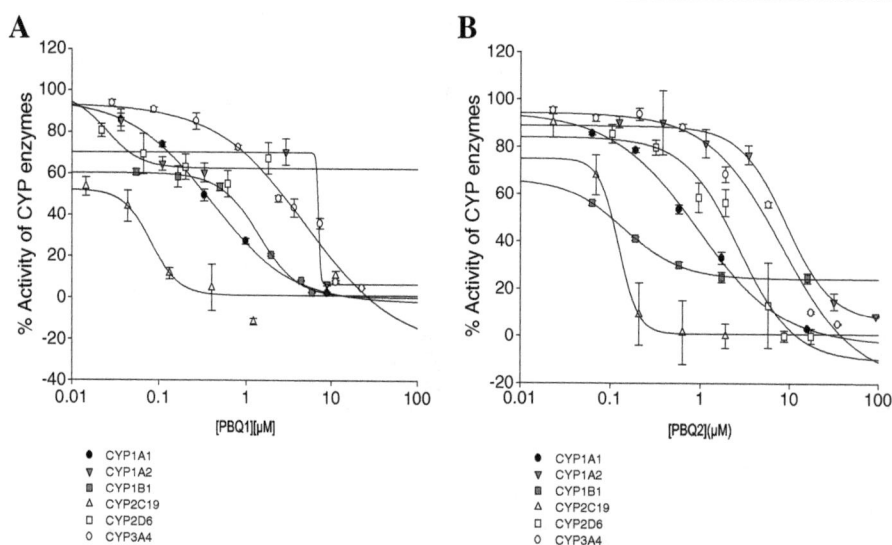

Figure 3 Inhibition of activities of CYP isoforms by PBQs 1 (A) and PBQ2 (B). Human recombinant CYP1B1-catalyzed dealkylation of ERes (0.37 µM), CYP1A1, CYP1A2, and CYP2C19-catalyzed dealkylation of CEC (0.5, 5, and 25 µM, respectively) CYP2D6-catalyzed dealkylation of AMMC (1.5 µM) and CYP3A4-catalyzed debenzylation of BFC (50 µM) were determined in the presence of varying concentrations of PBQs ranging between 0 and 900 µM, as described in the section "methods". Control enzyme activity (mean ± SEM) for CYP1B1, CYP1A2, CYP1A1, CYP2C19, CYP2D6, and CYP3A4 was 0.34 ± 0.08, 0.23 ± 0.04, 0.86 ± 0.01, 0.25 ± 0.02, 0.10 ± 0.003, and 1.28 ± 0.07 µM/min/pmol of CYP, respectively. Data are expressed as mean percentage of control enzyme activity for three independent experiments.

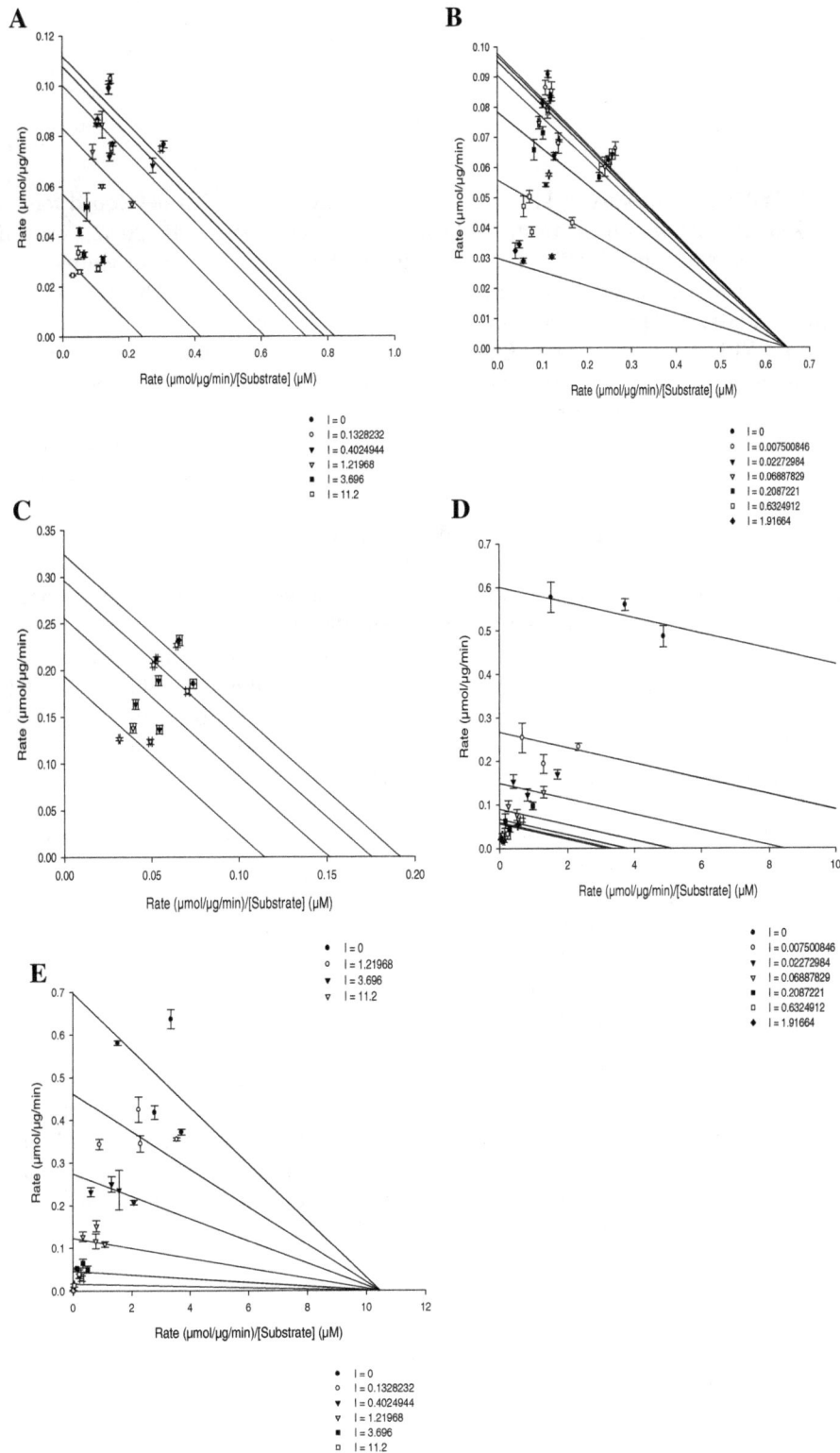

Figure 4 Eadie-Hofstee plots for inhibition of activities of CYP1A1 (A), CYP1A2(B), and CYP1B1(C) by PBQ1 along with inhibition of activities of CYP1A1 (D) and CYP1B1 (E) by PBQ2. CEC dealkylation catalyzed by recombinant CYP1A1 and CYP1A2 was determined in the absence and presence of six different concentrations of PBQs along with ERes dealkylation catalyzed by recombinant CYP1B1. Each point represents the mean ± SEM of three independent experiments.

Table 2 IC$_{50}$ values (µM) obtained from the interaction of isomers of PBQs with CYP enzymes

Compounds	CYP I isoforms					
	1A1	1A2	1B1	2 C19	2D6	3A4
PBQ1	0.39 ± 0.05	9.75 ± 0.0365	1.42 ± 0.14	0.08 ± 0.03	1.03 ± 0.40	5.07 ± 3.54
PBQ2	0.93 ± 0.26	10.55 ± 6.75	0.14 ± 0.04	0.12 ± 0.06	2.75 ± 0.96	8.31 ± 4.67

displayed potency toward CYP1B1. Studies using knock-out mice models have linked CYP1B1 with the activation of several carcinogens, such as B[*a*]P and DMBA [11] and have also been shown to play an important role in modulating tumor progression [10,27]. Thus, the potency toward both CYP1B1 and CYP1A1 activities by PBQ2 suggests potential chemopreventive bioactivity in vivo. Conversely, PBQ1 with demonstrated CYP1A1 inhibition, devoid of cytotoxicity on all cells examined in this study, also highlights it as an attractive candidate with potential for development as a chemoprotector.

The development of novel classes of therapeutics that can target both drug metabolizing enzymes and disease pathways is a multi-targeted approach that may well suit the multi-factorial origins of a disease such as cancer. Examples of such compounds include isothiocyanate which impact both Nrf-2 transcription factors, and inhibit the nuclear factor κß pathway to exhibit potent anti-inflammatory properties [28]. Such attractive dual qualities are displayed by PBQ2 in this study, with potent and selective targeting of HT29 colon cancer cells, as well as the inhibition of CYP1A1 and CYP1B1enzyme activities.

The potency of PBQ2 can be put into perspective with the reported inhibitory effect of eight flavonoids tested against recombinant human CYP1B1 and CYP1A1 enzyme activities which showed a range in IC$_{50}$s between 0.3 and 27 µM [29]. They made ideal chemoprotectants against prostate cancer [30]. PBQ2 had an IC$_{50}$ of 0.14 µM, which appears to be more potent at inhibiting CYP1B1 activity than all the eight flavonoids tested by Chaudhary and Willet [29], making this isolate an ideal candidate for further research.

PBQs examined in this study displayed reversible, non or uncompetitive (partial or full) kinetics on CYP1 enzyme activities. In noncompetitive inhibition, typically the IC$_{50}$ value is equal to the K_i, while in uncompetitive inhibition IC$_{50}$ will equal twice the value of the K_i for experiments where the substrate concentration is close to the K_m value [31], as designed in our experiments. Such approximations are observed in the kinetics of PBQ1 with CYPs1A2, 1B1 and of PBQ2 with CYP1A1, although deviations from these approximations were seen for interactions of PBQ1 with CYP1A1 and PBQ2 with CYP1B1 where the partial noncompetitive kinetics were observed and such mixed type binding may complicate relations between IC$_{50}$ and K_is. Due to the non and uncompetitive nature of PBQ binding with CYP1A1,

previous active site models developed for CYP1A1 using natural product quassinoids [20,32], were therefore not useful in shedding light on structure–activity relationships within the active site. The dietary flavonoid, galangin, shown to display inhibition of DMBA-induced CYP1A1 in MCF-7 breast cancer cells, was of a non-competitive, dose-dependent manner [33] similar to that of PBQ1.

Investigating the impact of these PBQs against the other major drug metabolising enzymes (CYP2C19, CYP2D6, and CYP3A4) allowed for the predictions of drug interaction potential. The impacts on CYP3A4 and CYP2D6, the enzymes responsible for metabolism of over 90% of drugs on the market, were only moderate by the two PBQs, suggesting unlikely metabolism-based drug interactions via these important enzymes. However, both compounds potently inhibited CYP2C19 activity. CYP2C19 is also involved in the process of carcinogenesis *albeit* with lower impact than the CYP1 family, and the CYP2C19 inhibition by the PBQs may prove useful in chemopreventive value, although drug interactions possibility via this enzyme that metabolises important therapeutics such as omeprazole and theophylline will remain a concern compounded by likely variations in inhibition reliant on the expression levels of this polymorphic enzyme.

Experimental

Plant material

Cymopolia barbata was collected from the shoreline of the north eastern coast of Jamaica at Fairy Hill Beach in the parish of Portland at a depth of 0.5 m in June 2004. A voucher specimen (#UWI-Mona 35, 438) was deposited in the Herbarium at the University of the West Indies, Mona, Jamaica.

Extraction and isolation

The air-dried sample (962.15 g) was extracted with methanol:dichloromethane (1:1) to yield a dark green gum (30.91 g), a portion of which (12.8 g) was subjected to vacuum liquid chromatography on silica gel in a 2-L sintered funnel with a gradient elution system consisting of increasing proportions of CH_2Cl_2 in hexanes, 100% CH_2Cl_2 with final elution in 20% methanol:CH_2Cl_2. Of the 56 fractions obtained, fraction 22–24 (2.35 g), which eluted in 20% methanol:CH_2Cl_2, underwent further gravity column chromatography to afford 172 sub fractions.

From this column, sub fraction 20–22 was found to contain 7-hydroxycymopochromanone (PBQ1). Another portion of the crude extract (2.0130 g) was subjected to column chromatography on a Sephadex LH-20 column in methanol resulting in 11 main combined fractions. The fifth combined fraction from this column was subjected to silica gel chromatography in 30% acetone:hexane to afford 37 fractions. Fraction 23–28 was found to contain 7-hydroxycymopolone (PBQ2). Both PBQs were identified by comparison of their ^{1}H and ^{13}C NMR data with the literature [1,34].

NMR data for 7-hydroxycymopochromanone (PBQ1)
^{1}H NMR(CDCl$_3$, ppm): 1.05, 3 H, s (H-8), 1.20, 3 H, s (H-9), 1.30, 2 H, m (H-6), 1.35, 3 H, s (H-10), 1.61, 2 H, m (H-4), 1.61, 2 H, m (H-5), 2.99, 1 H, s (H-2), 3.00, 1 H, s (H-2), 5.35, 1 H, br s (OH-6'), 7.13, 1 H, s (H-4'), 7.66, 1 H, s (H-1'), 12.00, 1 H, s (OH-7).

^{13}C NMR (CDCl$_3$, ppm): 16.3 (C-5), 27.1 (C-10), 28.2 (C-8), 32.2 (C-9), 34.5 (C-4), 36.3 (C-6), 52.7 (C-2), 72.2 (C-7), 73.9 (C-3), 118.3 (C-1'), 118.8 (C-5'), 120.8 (C-4'), 121.1 (C-2'), 144.2 (C-6'), 156.1 (C-3'), 205.4 (C-1).

NMR data for 7-hydroxycymopolone (PBQ2)
^{1}H NMR (CDCl$_3$, ppm):1.28, 6 H, s (H-8, 9), 1.55, 2 H, m (H-6), 1.67, 2 H, m (H-5), 2.20, 3 H, s (H-10), 2.30 2 H, t, J = 7.5 Hz (H-4), 6.69, 1 H, s (H-2), 7.18, 1 H, s (H-4'), 7.43, s (H-1'), 12.32, 1 H, s (OH-7).

^{13}C NMR (CDCl$_3$, ppm): 20.5 (C-10), 22.6 (C-5), 29.7 (C-8), 29.7 (C-9), 42.3 (C-4), 43.5 (C-6), 71.5 (C-7), 115.6 (C-1'), 119.0 (C-5'), 119.8 (C-2), 120.9 (C-2'), 121.9 (C-4'), 145.0 (C-6'), 157.2 (C-3'), 162.6 (C-3), 195.9 (C-1).

Conclusions

The polyisoprenylated bromohydroquinone, PBQ2, was found to affect cell viability of colon cells (HT29) comparable to the chemotherapeutic drug fluorouracil, with selectivity, making this compound an ideal lead candidate suitable for further experimentation in chemotherapy of colon cancer cells. In addition, it showed potent inhibition against CYP1B1 enzyme activities, a marker for cancer and target for drug discovery. Compounds such as PBQ2 that can target both drug metabolizing enzymes and disease state cells are of high value. Such chemotherapeutic and chemopreventive potential implied by the displayed bioactivity validate the on-going search for treatment leads among natural products from endemic tropical biodiversity including marine habitats.

Competing interests
The authors declare that they have no competing interests.

Authors' contribution
SB carried out all CYP inhibition and cell culture assays, WG carried out extraction and purification of natural products, GH designed and assisted all cytotoxicity assays, TJT participated in coordination of cytotoxicity assays, RD conceived of the study and participated in its design and coordination. All authors read and approved final manuscript.

Acknowledgments
We are grateful to the International Foundation for Science (IFS), Sweden, the University of the West Indies post graduate fund, the Forestry Conservation fund, and the Luther Speare Scholarship (for SB) for financial support.

Author details
[1]Natural Products Institute, Faculty of Pure and Applied Sciences, University of the West Indies, Mona, West Indies, Jamaica. [2]Department of Chemistry, Faculty of Pure and Applied Sciences, University of the West Indies, Mona, West Indies, Jamaica. [3]Department of Biological Sciences, Clemson University, Clemson SC 29634, USA.

References
1. Dorta E, Darias J, Martin AS, Cueto M (2002) New Prenylated bromoquinols from the green alga Cymopolia barbata. J Nat Prod 65:329–333
2. Högberg HE, Thomson RH, King TJ (1976) The cymopols, a group of prenylated bromohydroquinones from the green calcareous alga Cympolia barbata. J Chem Soc 1:1696–1701
3. Martínez-Nadal NG, Rodríguez LV, Casillas S (1964) Isolation and characterization of sarganin complex, a new broad spectrum antibiotic isolated from marine algae. Antimicrob Agents Chemother 10:131
4. Estrada DM, Martín JD, Pérez CA (1987) New Brominated monoterpenoid quinol from Cymopolia barbata. J Nat Prod 50:735–737
5. Wall EM, Wani MC, Manikumar G, Taylor H, Hughes TJ, Gerwick WH, McPhail AT, McPhail DR (1989) Plant antimutagenic agents 7. Structure and antimutagenic properties of cymobarbatol and 4-isocymbarbatol, new cymopols from green alga (Cymopolia barbata). J Nat Prod 52:1092–1099
6. McConnell OJ, Hughes PA, Targett NM, Daley J (1982) Effects of secondary metabolites from marine algae on feeding by the sea urchin. Lytechinus variegatus. J Chem Ecol 8:1427
7. Park M, Fenical W, Hay M (1992) Debromoisocymobarbatol, a new chromanol feeding deterrent from the marine alga Cymopolia barbata. Phytochemistry 31:4115–4118
8. Targett NM, McConnell OJ (1989) Detection of secondary metabolites in marine macroalgae using the marsh periwinkle, Littorina irrorata say, as an indicator organism. J Chem Ecol 8:115
9. Swanson HI, Njar VCO, Yu Z, Castro DJ, Gonzalez FJ, Williams DE, Huang Y, Kong AT, Doloff JC, Ma J, Waxman DJ, Scott EE (2010) Targeting drug-metabolizing enzymes for effective chemoprevention and chemotherapy. Drug Metab Dispos 38:539–544
10. Castro DJ, Baird WM, Pereira CB, Giovanni J, Löhr C, Fischer K, Yu Z, Gonzalez FJ, Krueger SK, Williams DE (2008) Fetal mouse cyp1b1 and transplacental carcinogenesis from maternal exposure to Dibenzo[a, l] pyrene. Cancer Prev Res 1:128–134
11. Shimada T, Fujii-Kuriyama Y (2004) Metabolic activation of polycyclic aromatic hydrocarbons to carcinogens by cytochrome P50 1A1 and 1B1. Cancer Sci 95:1–6
12. Shimada T, Oda Y, Gillam EMJ, Guengerich FP, Inoue K (2001) Metabolic activation of polycyclic aromatic hydrocarbons and their dihydrdiol derivation and other procarcinogens by cytochrome P450 1A1 and 1B1 allelic variants and other human cytochrome P450 enzymes in Salmonella typhimurium NM2009. Drug Metab Dispos 29:1179–1182
13. Skupinska K, Misiewicz-Krzeminska I, Stypulkowski R, Lubelska K, Kasprzycka-Guttman T (2009) Sulforaphane and its analogues inhibit CYP1A1 and CYP1A2 activity induced by benzo[a]pyrene. J Biochem Mol Toxicol 23 (1):18–28
14. Palmari J, Dussert C, Berthois Y, Penel C, Martin PM (1996) Distribution of estrogen receptor heterogeneity in growing MCF-7 cells measured by quantitative microscopy. Cytometry 27:26–35
15. Heusch WL, Maneckjee R (1999) Effects of bombesin on methadone-induced apoptosis of human lung cancer cells. Cancer Lett 136:177–185
16. Crespi CL, Miller VP, Penman BW (1997) Microtitre plate assays for inhibition of human, drug metabolising cytochromes P450. Anal Biochem 48:188–190

17. Powrie RH (2007) High-throughput inhibition screening of five major human cytochrome P450 enzymes using an *in vitro* substrate cocktail., CXR Biosci, Available at http://www.cxrbiosciences.com/cmsimages/media/pdfs/Microsoft%20PowerPoint%20-%20P450%20inhibition%20poster.pdf. Accessed 20 Apr 2010

18. Stresser DM, Broudy MI, Ho T, Cargil CE, Blnachard AP, Sharma R, Dandeneau AA, Goodwin JJ, Turner SD, Erve JCL, Patten CJ, Dehal SS, Crespi CL (2004) Highly selective inhibition of human CYP3A in vitro by azmulin and evidence that inhibition is irreversible. Drug Metab Dispos 32:105–112

19. Cali J (2003) Screen for CYP450 inhibitors using P450-GLOTM luminescent cytochrome P450 assays. Cell Notes Issue, Available at www.promega.com

20. Cai X, Wang RW, Edom RW, Evans DC, Shou M, Rodrigues D, Liu W, Dean DC, Baillie TA (2004) Validation of (−)-*N*-3-benzyl-phenobarbital as a selective inhibitor of CYP2C19 in human liver microsomes. Drug Metab Dispos 32:584–586

21. Badal S, Williams SA, Huang G, Francis S, Vendantam P, Dunbar O, Jacobs H, Tzeng TJ, Gangemi J, Delgoda R (2011) Cytochrome P450 1 enzyme inhibition and anticancer potential of chromene amides from *Amyris plumieri*. Fitoterapia 82:230–236

22. Gerhauser C, Klimo K, Heiss E, Neumann I, Gamal-Eldeen A, Knauft J, Liu GY, Sitthimunchai S, Frank N (2003) Mechanism-based in vitro screening of potential cancer chemopreventive agents. Mutat Res 523–524:163–172

23. Leung H, Wang Y, Chan H, Leung L (2007) Developing a high throughput system for the screening of cytochrome P450 1A1—inhibitory polyphenols. Toxicol In Vitro 21:996–1002

24. Ren W, Qiao Z, Wang H, Zhu L, Zhang L (2003) Flavonoids: promising anticancer agents. Med Res Rev 3:519–534

25. Xiao D, Pinto JT, Gundersen GG, Weinstein IB (2005) Effects of a series of organosulfur compounds on mitotic arrest and induction of apoptosis in colon cancer cells. Mol Cancer Ther 4:1388–1398

26. Gusman J, Malonne H, Atassi G (2001) A reappraisal of the potential chemopreventive and chemotherapeutic properties of resveratrol. Carcinogenesis 22:1111–1117

27. Carnell DM, Smith RE, Daley FM, Barber PR, Hoskin PJ, Wilson GD, Murraly GI, Everett SA (2004) Target validation of cytochrome P450 CYP1B1 in prostate carcinoma with protein expression in associated hyperplastic and premalignant tissue. Int J Radiat Oncol Biol Phys 58:500–509

28. Prawan A, Buranrat B, Kukongviriyapan U, Sripa B, Kukongviriyapan V (2009) Inflammatory cytokines suppress NAD(P)H:quinone oxidoreductase-1 and induce oxidative stress in cholangiocarcinoma cells. J Cancer Res Clin Oncol 135:515–522

29. Chaudhary A, Willet KL (2006) Inhibition of human cytochrome CYP1 enzymes by flavonoids of St John's wort. Toxicology 217:194–205

30. Marchand LL (2002) Cancer preventive effects of flavonoids—a review. Biomed Pharmacother 58:296–301

31. Zhang ZY, Wong YN (2005) Enzyme kinetics for clinically relevant CYP inhibition. Curr Drug Metab 6:241–257

32. Shields M, Niazi U, Badal S, Yee T, Sutcliffe M, Delgoda R (2009) Inhibition of CYP1A1 by quassinoids found in *Picrasma excelsa*. Planta Medica 75:137–141

33. Ciolino H, Yeh G (1999) The flavonoid galangin is an inhibitor of CYP1A1 activity and an agonist/antagonist of the aryl hydrocarbon receptor. Br J Cancer 79(9–10):1340–1346

34. Gallimore WW, Sambo T, Campbell T (2009) Debromocymopolone from the green alga, *Cymopolia barbata*. J Chem Res 3:160–161

20

Four butyrolactones and diverse bioactive secondary metabolites from terrestrial *Aspergillus flavipes* MM2: isolation and structure determination

Mohamed MS Nagia[1,3], Mohammad Magdy El-Metwally[2], Mohamed Shaaban[1,3*], Soheir M El-Zalabani[4] and Atef G Hanna[1]

Abstract

The chemical constituents and biological activities of the terrestrial *Aspergillus flavipes* MM2 isolated from Egyptian rice hulls are reported. Seven bioactive compounds were obtained, of which one sterol: ergosterol (**1**), four butyrolactones: butyrolactone I (**2**), aspulvinone H (**3**), butyrolactone-V (**6**) and 4,4'-diydroxypulvinone (**7**), along with 6-methylsalicylic acid (**4**) and the cyclopentenone analogue; terrien (**5**). Structures of the isolated compounds were deduced by intensive studies of their 1D & 2D NMR, MS data and comparison with related structures. The strain extract and the isolated compounds (**1-7**) were biologically studied against number of microbial strains, and brine shrimp for cytotoxicity. In this article, the taxonomical characterization of *A. flavipes* MM2 along with its upscale fermentation, isolation and structural assignment of the obtained bioactive metabolites, and evaluate their antimicrobial and cytotoxic activities were described.

Keywords: *Aspergillus flavipes* MM2, butyrolactones, biological studies

1. Background

In recent years, numerous metabolites possessing uncommon structures and potent bioactivity have been isolated from strains of bacteria and fungi collected from diverse environments, such as soils, animals, plants and sediments [1,2]. It was noted until Alexander Fleming discovered penicillin G from *Penicillium notatum* almost 83 years ago (1928) that fungal microorganisms suddenly became a hunting ground for novel drug leads [3,4]. Therefore, many pharmaceutical companies and research groups were motivated to start sampling and screening large collections of fungal strains for antibiotics [3,5,6]. Antimycotics [7,8], antivirals [9], anticancers [10] and pharmacologically active agents [11]. The Aspergilli represents a large diverse genus, containing ca. 180 filamentous fungal species, of substantial

pharmaceutical and commercial values [12]. In the research program to explore promising bioactive secondary metabolites from fungi, the terrestrial fungi, *Aspergillus flavipes* sp. isolate MM2 obtained from rice hulls, was investigated. The strain extract revealed the presence of promising antimicrobial activity against some pathogenic test organisms. Chemical screening (TLC investigation) of the strain extract showed numerous characteristic bands. Therefore, the strain was applied to large-scale fermentation by using Czapeck-Dox medium [13]. Working up of the strain cells produced ergosterol (**1**), while the filtrate extract afforded six diverse metabolic compounds: butyrolactone-I (**2**), aspulvinone H (**3**), 6-methylsalicylic acid (**4**), terrien (**5**), butyrolactone-V (**6**) and 4,4'-diydroxypulvinone (**7**). The chemical structures of the isolated compounds (**1-7**) were identified with the help of NMR (1D & 2D) and mass spectrometry (ESI, EI, HRESIMS) (Figure 1). The antimicrobial activity was tested against some microorganisms and cytotoxicity was examined by using brine shrimp.

* Correspondence: mshaaba_99@yahoo.com
[1]Division of Pharmaceutical Industries, Chemistry of Natural Compounds Department, National Research Centre, El-Behoos st. 33, Dokki, Cairo 12622, Egypt
Full list of author information is available at the end of the article

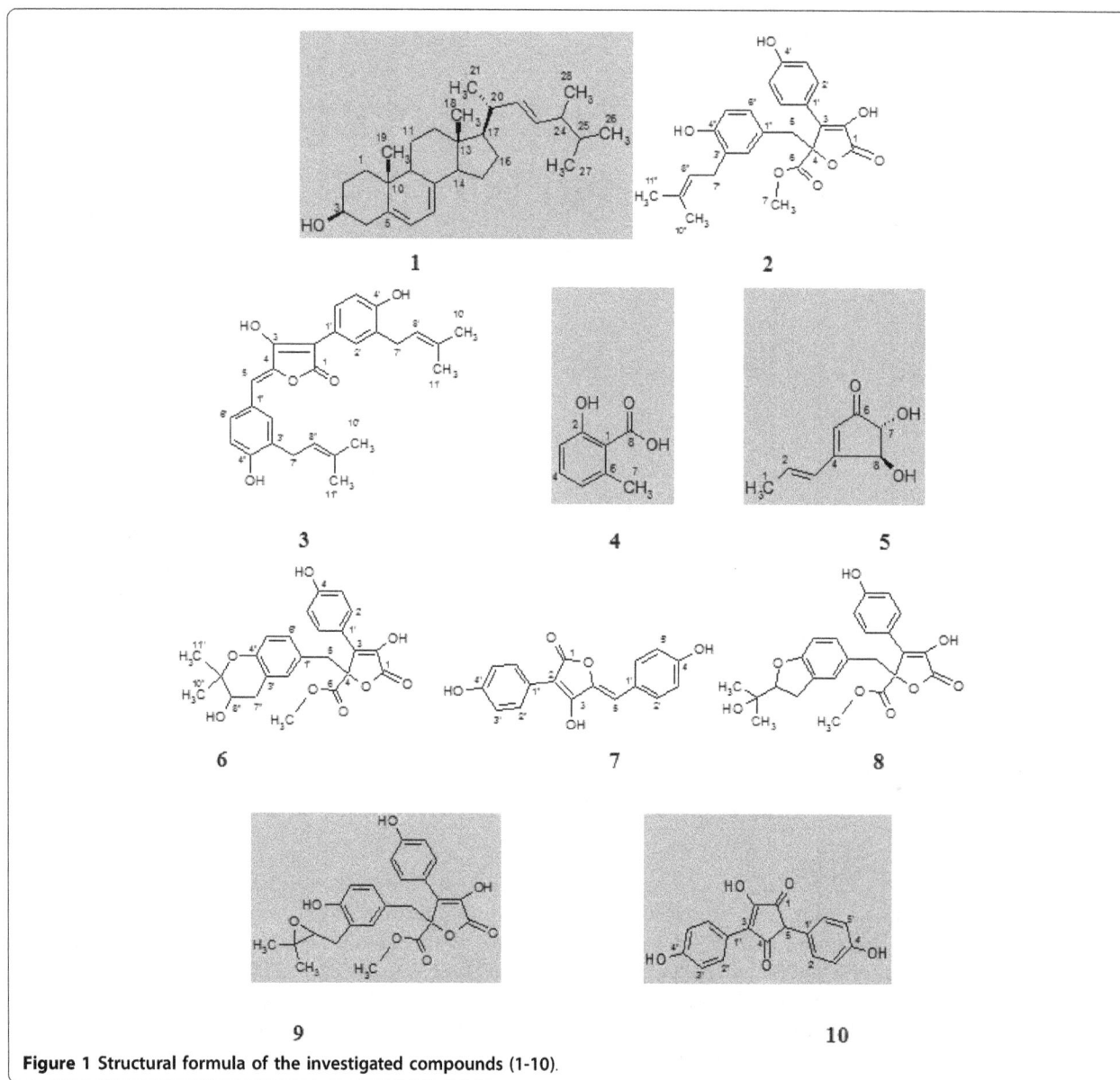

Figure 1 Structural formula of the investigated compounds (1-10).

2. Results and discussion

2.1. Taxonomical characterization of the fungal strain

The grown colonies of the fungal strain on Czapek-Dox medium showed bright whit-faint yellow colonies on the agar plate with a brown staining background [13]. The colonies are growing rather slowly, showing whitish from conidial masses, with brownish conidiophores shining through, reverse yellow-brown to red brown conidial heads spas, loosely columnar, conidiophores smooth-walled, pale yellow to light brown 2.4-3.2 μm in diameter. According to its morphological and microscopic characteristics and comparison with the taxonomical keys of Raper and Fennel [14], the strain was assigned as A. flavipes MM2.

2.2. Fermentation, working up and isolation

Based on the pre-screening study, the fungal strain A. flavipes MM2, cultivated on Czapeks-Dox for 10 days at 28°C, was shown to exhibit biological and chemical interest results. Therefore, the fungal strain was scaled up as 10 L culture using the same cultivating conditions applied for screening studies. After harvesting, both supernatant and mycelial cake phases were individually worked up. Purification of the mycelial extract using silica gel column, followed by washing the afforded major fraction by methanol and purification with Sephadex LH-20, yielded ergosterol (1). An application of the culture filtrate extract of A. flavipes MM2 to silica gel column chromatography, followed by diverse chromatographic techniques, resulted in the isolation of six compounds: butyrolactone-I (2), aspulvinone H (3), methylsalicylic acid (4), terrine (5), butyrolactone-V (6) and 4,4'-diydroxypulvinone (7).

2.3. Chemical characterization

2.3.1. Ergosterol (1)

Ergosterol (1) was obtained as colourless solid, showing UV activity during TLC, which turned violet on spraying with anisaldehyde/sulphuric acid and changed latter to blue. Structure of 1 was confirmed by different spectroscopic means (EI MS, ^{1}H, ^{13}C/APT NMR), chromatographic and comparison with literature [15,16]. Ergosterol plays an important role as inhibitor of lipid per-oxidation and showed strong DPPH radical scavenging activity as well [17,18], along with its cytotoxicity against HL-60 cells [19], MCF-7 cell line [20].

2.3.2. Butyrolactone-I (2)

The molecular weight of 2 was established as 424 Dalton by ESI MS, having the corresponding molecular formula $C_{24}H_{24}O_7$ and 13 unsaturation bonds. ^{1}H/H,H COSY NMR spectra of 2 showed two o-doublets ($J \sim$ 8.8 Hz) each of 2H at δ 7.57 and 6.86, being for 1,4-disubstituted aromatic residue, along with three signals at δ 6.50, 6.48 and 6.40 representing 1,3,4-trisubstituted aromatic ring. A triplet signal of 1H was at δ 5.05, representing an olefinic methine linked to a doublet methylene signal appeared at δ 3.06. A 3H methoxy group (3.76); doublet of an AB methylene group (δ 3.42) attached to sp^2 system; and further two singlet methyls were visible at δ 1.65 and 1.56, representing a prenyl system.

According to the ^{13}C NMR/HMQC spectra of compound 2, 22 carbon signals representing 24 carbons were displayed, including 2 carbonyls (δ 171.6 and 170.3), 2 sp^2 oxygenated carbons (δ 159.3, 155.0) of phenolic systems, along with 5 quaternary carbons (δ 139.6-123.1). Two 2CH sp^2 methine signals (130.4 and 116.6) for 1,4-disubstituted benzene ring beside to four sp^2 methines (δ 132.4-115.0). In the aliphatic region, signals for quaternary oxygenated methine (δ 86.8), methoxy (53.8), two methylenes (δ 39.6, 28.7) and two methyls (δ 25.9, 17.8) were assigned. Finally, structure of 2 was further deduced on the basis of HMBC experimental data, and comparison with literature as Butyrolactone-I [21,22]. Butyrolactone-I (2) was reported as a lipid lowering agent of Lovastatin × [19,23,24], showing antiproliferative activity against colon, pancreatic carcinoma, human lung cancer and prostatic cancer [25-30] (Figure 2).

2.3.3. Aspulvinone H (3)

Based on the ESI MS, the molecular weight of 3 was deduced as 432 Dalton, and the corresponding

molecular formula as $C_{27}H_{28}O_5$, containing 14 unsaturation bonds, as closely related to butyrolactone-I (2). ^{1}H NMR spectrum of 3 showed six confused doublets each of 1H between δ 7.81 and 6.73, being of two unsymmetrical tri-substituted aromatic residues, and singlet methine at δ 6.22. A multiplet of 2H (δ 5.36), 4H of two attached sp^2-bounded methylenes (δ 3.40-3.00) and multiplet signal (δ 1.75, 12H) of four sp^2-linked methyls, assigning two prenyl systems. Based on the revealed NMR data and molecular formula, and search in Anti-Base [2], structure of 3 was fixed as aspulvinone H [31].

2.3.4. 6-Methylsalicylic acid (4)

According to the ESI mass spectra, the molecular weight of 4 was deduced as 152 Dalton. The ^{1}H NMR spectrum displayed three 1H resonating signals in the aromatic region (7.07, 6.63, 6.59), being of 1,2,3-trisubstiuted aromatic ring ($J \sim$ 7.5-8.2 Hz) together with a singlet 3H of an aromatic bounded methyl (δ 2.56). Based on the ^{13}C NMR spectrum, compound 4 displayed eight carbon signals, including one quaternary (δ 176). Two further deep field quaternaries were visible (δ 162.7 and 142.7) for a-peri-hydroxy and methyl-sp^2 attached carbons, respectively. Three sp^2 methines (δ 132.2, 122.9, 115.1), one quaternary (δ 119.5) and a methyl signal (δ 23.3). In accordance, 2-Hydroxy-6-methyl-benzoic acid (4) was recognized [32,33] as antifungal substance [34], in addition to its analgesic [35], herbicidal [36] and antiacne activities [37].

2.3.5. Terrein (5)

The molecular weight of 5 was deduced as 154 Dalton ($C_8H_{10}O_3$), bearing four double bond equivalents. The ^{1}H NMR/H,H COSY spectrum of 5 showed two signals at δ 6.82 and 6.42 ($J \sim$ 15 Hz), representing a trans-olefinic double bond, attached to a doublet methyl (δ 1.97), constructing a terminal propene system. A further singlet (δ 5.99) being of an olefinic methine and two doublets each of 1H (δ 4.67, 4.07, $J \sim$ 2.8 Hz) corresponding to adjacent oxy-methines. According to ^{13}C NMR/HMQC spectra, eight carbon signals were displayed, including an acetophenone carbonyl (δ 205.6) and a deep field sp^2 quaternary carbon (δ 170.8); three sp^2 methines (δ 141.8, 126.4 and 125.9), two sp^3 oxymethines (δ 82.4, 78.1) and one sp^2-bounded methyl group (19.5).

A final interpretation of 5 was carried out by HMBC experiment (Figure 3), fixing the structure as 4,5-dihydroxy-3-propenyl-cyclopent-2-enone; terrein [38,39]. Terrein (5) has a hypopigmentary effect in Mel-Ab cells, and it is a strongly down-regulator of melanin synthesis by reducing tyrosinase production [40], and inhibit human platelet aggregation [41]. Terrein showed a strong antiproliferative effect on skin equivalents [42] and as proteasome inhibitor and anti-tumoral drug [43].

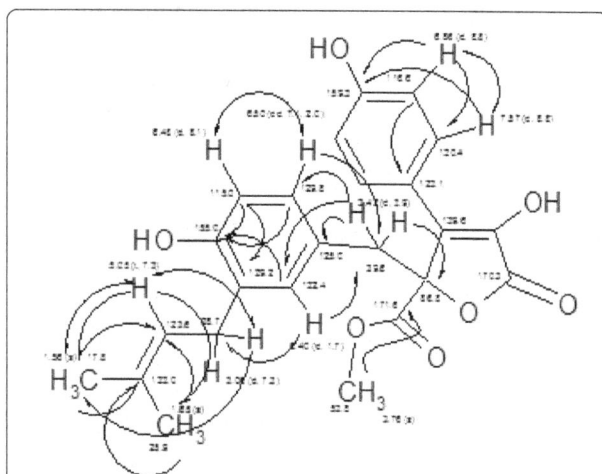

Figure 2 H,H COSY (↔) and HMBC (→) correlations of butyrolactone-I (2).

2.3.6. Butyrolactone-V (6)

The molecular weight of **6** was established as 440 Dalton ($C_{24}H_{24}O_8$), containing 13 double bond unsaturations. The ^1H NMR/H,HCOSY spectrum of compound **6** revealed the presence 1,4-disubstituted (δ 7.54 and 6.85, $J \sim 8.8$ Hz), and unsymmetrical tri-substituted (m, δ 6.48) aromatic systems. A 1H dd signal (δ 5.02) of an oxygenated methine attached to a dd signal (δ 2.80) of a methylene group, confirming their ABX property. A singlet of methoxy group (δ 3.77), 2H methylene singlet (δ 3.40) flanked by two sp^2 systems, and two methyl singlets (δ 1.25 and 1.16), being of gem dimethyl groups were deduced.

Based on the ^{13}C NMR/HMQC spectra of compound **6**, two carbonyls (δ 171.5 and 170.3), two phenolic carbons (δ 159.4 and 153.3), β-quaternary carbon (δ 139.6) of an ester or lactone system were deduced. Two 2CH sp^2 signals (δ 130.4, 116.6), and 3CH sp^2 signals (δ 132.9, 130.4, 117.2), being of 1,4-disubstitued and

unsymmetric tri-substituted phenolic residues were shown. Two sp^3 quaternary oxy-carbons (δ 86.8 and 78.0), one oxy-methine (δ 70.4), one carbomethoxy (δ 53.9) and two methylenes (δ 39.0, 2.80) were visible. Two gem dimethyl signals attached to an oxygenated quaternary carbon were displayed (δ 25.9, 20.9).

Based on the above spectroscopic data and molecular formula, compound **6** exhibited a strong close structural similarity to butyrolactone-I (**2**). In accordance, three structural formulas were proposed according to search in AntiBase: butyrolactone-V (**6**) [44,45], 4-hydroxy-2-[2-(1-hydroxy-1-methyl-ethyl)-2,3-dihydro-benzofuran-5-ylmethyl]-3-(4-hydroxy-phenyl)-5-oxo-2,5-dihydro-furan-2-carboxylic acid methyl ester (**8**) [21] and butyrolactone-III (**9**) [19].

The structure was confirmed by detailed 2D experiments; H,H COSY and HMBC (Figure 4) and comparison with literature as butyrolactone-V (**6**) [25,42,43]. Butyrolactone-V was reported to exhibit a moderate antimalarial activity against the malarial parasite *Plasmodium falciparum* K1 (IC50 7.9 µg/mL) [45].

2.3.7. 4,4'-Diydroxypulvinone (Aspulvinone E) (7)

Compound **7** was obtained with a molecular weight of 296 Dalton ($C_{17}H_{12}O_5$) by HRESI MS, bearing 12 double bond equivalents. The ^1H NMR spectrum of **7** showed five signals in the aromatic region for 9H (δ 8.06-5.88), representing two 1,4-disubstitued phenolic residues ($J \sim 8.6$ Hz). The fifth signal (1H) was shown as singlet at δ 5.88. Based on the revealed spectroscopic data and molecular formula and search in AntiBase, two alternatives, 4,4'-diydroxypulvinone (**7**) and Gyrocyanin (**10**) were displayed. However, the chemical shift of the singlet methine in compound **10** has high field shifting (δ 4.96), which was not matching with our revealed spectral data, establishing the structure as 4,4'-diydroxypulvinone (**7**) [46].

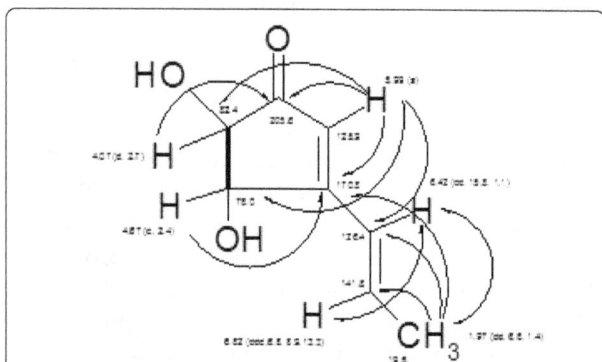

Figure 3 H, H COSY (−) and HMBC (→) correlations of Terrein (5).

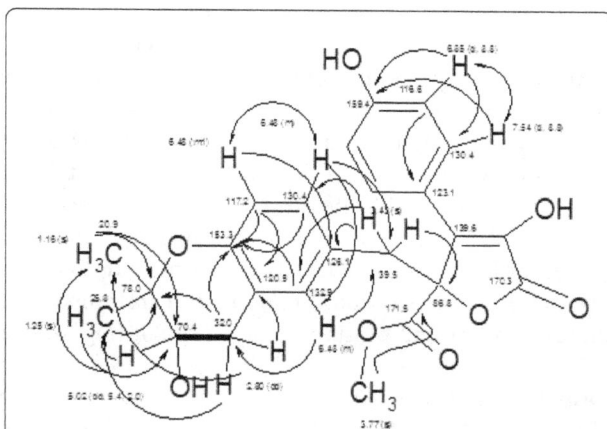

Figure 4 Full H,H COSY (↔, −) and HMBC (→) correlations of Butyrolactone-V (6).

2.4. Biological activities

Activity patterns of the mycelial and supernatant extracts produced by fungal strain A. *flavipes* MM2 against set of microorganisms namely, *Staphylococcus aureus*, *Pseudomonas aeruginosa*, *Candida albicans* and *Aspergillus niger* were carried out using agar disc method (25 µg/disc, Ø 5 mm). In accordance, both extracts showed high antibacterial (16-14 mm) and moderate anti-yeast and antifungal (10-14 mm) activities (Table 1).

Alternatively, the isolated compounds **1-7** were tested against *Bacillus subtilis*, *S. aureus*, *Streptomyces viridochromogenes* (Tü 57), *Escherichia coli*, *C. albicans*, *Mucor miehi*, *Chlorella vulgaris*, *Chlorella sorokiniana*, *Scenedesmus subspicatus*, *Rhizoctonia solani* and *Pythium ultimum* (40 µg/disc, Ø 9 mm). According to this study, only four compounds (**1, 2, 4, 7**) were active. Ergosterol (**1**) was highly and moderately active against *S. aureus* and *B. subtilis*. Compounds **7**, **4** and **3** showed high and moderate activity against *S. aureus*,. Finally, the whole studied compounds were tested against brine shrimp (10 µg/mL) for cytotoxic activities, exhibiting no cytotoxicity except ergosterol (**1**), which showed 100% cytotoxicity after 15 h (Table 2).

3. Experimental

NMR spectra were measured on Varian Unity 300 and Varian Inova 600 spectrometers. Electron spray ionization mass spectrometry (ESI HRMS): Finnigan LCQ ion trap mass spectrometer coupled with a Flux Instruments (Basel, Switzerland) quaternary pump Rheos 4000 and a HP 1100 HPLC (nucleosil column EC 125/2, 100-5, C 18) with autosampler (Jasco 851-AS, Jasco Inc., Easton, MD, USA) and a Diode Array Detector (Finnigan Surveyor LC System). High-resolution mass spectra (HRMS) were recorded by ESI MS on an Apex IV 7 Tesla Fourier-Transform Ion Cyclotron Resonance Mass Spectrometer (Bruker Daltonics, Billerica, MA, USA). EI MS at 70 eV with Varian MAT 731, Varian 311A, AMD-402, high-resolution with perflurokerosine as standard. R_f values were measured on Polygram SIL F/UV$_{254}$ (Merck, pre-coated sheets). Size exclusion chromatography was done on Sephadex LH-20 (Pharmacia).

3.1. Isolation and taxonomy of the producing strain

The terrestrial A. *flavipes* MM2, which was identified according to the Raper and Fennel [14], has been isolated from rice hulls sample by placing the rice hulls over water agar medium (g/L): Agar-agar (20) and water (100%) with incubation at 28°C for 7 days the developing colony was transferred to Czapeks agar with incubation at 28°C for 10 days. Bright whit-faint yellow colonies with a brown straining background of the fungal strain were grown. The colonies are growing rather slowly, showing whitish from conidial masses, with brownish conidiophores shining through, reverse yellow-brown to red brown Conidial heads spas, loosely columnar, conidiophores smooth-walled, pale yellow to light brown 2.4-3.2 µm diameter. According to its morphological and microscopic characteristics and comparison with literature, the fungal strain was assigned as A. *flavipes* MM2 [14]. The strain is deposited in Dr Mohammad Magdy El Metwally collection in Microbiology Department, Soil & Water and Environment Research Institute, ARC, Giza, Egypt.

3.2. Fermentation, extraction and isolation

Small pieces (1 cm^2) of well grown sub-cultures of A. *flavipes* MM2 were inoculated into thirty 1-L Erlenmeyer flasks, each containing 300 mL of sterilized Czapeck-Dox medium (g/L): Sucrose (30), NaNO$_3$ (3), K$_2$HPO$_4$ (1), KCl (0.5), MgSO$_4$ (0.5), FeSO$_4$ (0.01) and distilled water (1 L) at pH = (7.3). The inoculated flasks were incubated for 10 days at 28°C and 100 rpm. After harvesting, the fungal mate and supernatant were separated by filtration. The fungal mat was then applied to maceration in methanol (3 × 0.5 L). The methanol extract was concentrated in vacuum and the remaining aqueous solution was re-extracted by ethyl acetate followed by concentration to yield 845 mg as brown crude extract. The supernatant was passed through XAD-16 column (4 × 120 cm). After washing with water, the absorbed organic extract was eluted by methanol, followed by concentration under vacuum, and the aqueous residue was re-extracted by ethyl acetate, followed by concentration in vacuo to afford 818 mg as brown crude extract.

The mycelial extract (845 mg) was subjected to fractionation using silica gel column chromatography (cyclohexane-CH$_2$Cl$_2$-MeOH) to afford 200 mg as major fraction, which was then washed by MeOH to deliver a colourless precipitate. The last precipitate was purified on Sephadex LH-20 (CH$_2$Cl$_2$/40% MeOH) to afford Ergosterol (**1**, 12 mg) as colourless solid.

Table 1 Pre-antimicrobial assays of A. *flavipes* MM2 (φ mm)

Medium no.	Inhibition zone (mm)							
	Culture filtrate extract				Cells extract			
	St. aureus	Ps. aeruginosa,	C. albicans	A. niger	St. Aureus	Ps. aeruginosa,	C. albicans	A. niger
Czapeck-Dox	15	16	14	12	14	14	10	10

Table 2 Antimicrobial assays of *A. flavipes* MM2 compounds (φ mm)

Compound (No.)	Inhibition zone (mm) of tested microorganisms											
	B. sub.	St. aur	St. Virid	E. coli	C. alb	M. miehi	Ch. vulg	Ch. Sorok	Sce. sub	R. solani	P. ultim	Brine shrimp
Ergosterol (**1**)	11	19	ND	ND	ND	ND	ND	ND	ND	ND	ND	100%
Butyrolactone I (**2**)	ND	ND	ND	ND	ND	ND	ND	ND	ND	ND	ND	ND
Aspulvinone H (**3**)	ND	11	ND	ND	ND	ND	ND	ND	ND	ND	ND	ND
6-methylsalicylic acid (**4**)	ND	15	ND	ND	ND	ND	ND	ND	ND	ND	ND	ND
Terrien (**5**)	ND	ND	ND	ND	ND	ND	ND	ND	ND	ND	ND	ND
Butyrolactone-V (**6**)	ND	ND	ND	ND	ND	ND	ND	ND	ND	ND	ND	ND
4,4'-diydroxypulvinone (**7**)	ND	18	ND	ND	ND	ND	ND	ND	ND	ND	ND	ND

The filtrate crude extract (818 mg) was fractionated on silica gel column and eluted by cyclohexane-CH_2Cl_2-MeOH gradient to give five fractions (I-V). Fraction FIII was further fractionated using Sephadex LH-20 column (MeOH) to afford two sub-fractions, FIIIa (44 mg) and FIIIb (73 mg). Purification of FIIIa by Sephadex LH-20 (MeOH) afforded a colourless solid of butyrolactone-I (**2**, 4 mg). PTLC purification (CH_2Cl_2/5%MeOH) of FIIIb followed by Sephadex LH-20 (MeOH) afforded Aspulvinone H (**3**) as colourless solid (3 mg). A further fractionation of FIV on Sephadex LH-20 (MeOH) led to sub-fractions FIVa (35 mg) and FIVb (120 mg). Purification of sub-fraction FIVa using Sephadex LH-20 (MeOH), PTLC (CH_2Cl_2/5% MeOH), and then Sephadex LH-20 (MeOH) resulted in 6-methylsalicylic acid (**4**, 10 mg) as colourless solid. Sub-fraction FIVb was purified on Sephadex LH-20 (MeOH) to afford Terrien (**5**, 10 mg) and butyrolactone-V (**6**, 2 mg) as two colourless solids. Finally, fraction FV was purified using two subsequent Sephadex LH-20 columns (MeOH) to give a yellow solid of 4,4'-diydroxypulvinone (**7**, 4 mg).

3.2.1. Ergosterol; ergosta-5,7,22-triene-3β-ol (1)

$C_{28}H_{44}O$ (396), colourless solid, UV-absorbing, turned violet with anisaldehyde/sulphuric acid, R_f = 0.46 (CH_2Cl_2/5%MeOH); ^{1}H NMR ($CDCl_3$, 300 MHz): δ = 5.57 (dm, 1H, H-6), 5.38 (dm, 1H, H-7), 5.17 (m, 2H, H-22,23), 3.62 (m, 1H, H-3), 2.46 (dm, 1H, H-5), 2.35 (m, 2H, H-20, 24), 2.09-1.93 (m, 3H), 1.92-1.89 (m, 4H), 1.88-1.55 (m, 4H), 1.50-1.40 (m, 3H), 1.38-1.16 (m, 3H), 1.02 (d, J = 7.2, 3H, CH_3-21), 0.93 (s, 3H, CH_3-19), 0.91 (d, J = 7.2, 3H, CH_3-28), 0.82 (d, J = 6.8, 3H, CH_3-27), 0.80 (d, J = 6.8, 3H, CH_3-26), 0.61 (s, 3H, CH_3-18); ^{13}C NMR ($CDCl_3$, 75 MHz): δ = 141.3 (C_q-8), 139.8 (C_q-5), 135.5 (CH-22), 131.9 (CH-23), 119.6 (CH-7), 116.3 (CH-6), 70.4 (CH-3), 55.7 (CH-17), 54.5 (CH-14), 46.2 (CH-9), 42.8 (C_q-13), 42.8 (CH-24), 40.7 (CH_2-4), 40.4 (CH-20), 39.1 (CH_2-12), 38.4 (CH_2-1), 37.0 (C_q-10), 33.1 (CH-25), 32.0 (CH_2-2), 28.3 (CH_2-16), 23.0 (CH_2-11), 21.1 (CH_2-15), 21.1 (CH_3-21), 19.9 (CH_3-27), 19.6 (CH_3-26), 17.6 (CH_3-28), 16.2 (CH_3-19), 12.0 (CH_3-18); **EI-MS (70 EV):** m/z (%) = 396 ([M]$^+$, 87), 378 ([M-H_2O]$^+$,

12), 363 ([M-(H_2O+CH_3)]$^+$, 100), 271 (25), 253 (52), 211 (33).

3.2.2. Butyrolactone-I (2)

$C_{24}H_{24}O_7$ (424), colourless solid, UV-absorbing, turned violet with anisaldehyde/sulphuric acid, R_f = 0.39 (CH_2Cl_2/5% MeOH); ^{1}H NMR (CD_3OD, 300 MHz): δ = 7.57 (d, J = 8.8 Hz, 2H, H-2',6'), 6,86 (d, J = 8.8 Hz, 2H, H-3',5'), 6.50 (dd, J = 7.1, 2.0 Hz, 1H, H-6"), 6.48 (d, J = 8.1 Hz, 1H, H-5"), 6.40 (d, J = 1.7, 1H, H-2"), 5.05 (t, J = 3.7 Hz, 1H, H-8"), 3.76 (s, 3H, 7-OCH_3), 3.42 (d, J = 3.9, 2H, CH_2-5), 3.06 (d, J = 7.3 Hz, 2H, CH_2-7"), 1.65 (s, 3H, CH_3-10"), 1.56 (s, 3H, CH_3-11"); ^{13}C NMR (CD_3OD, 75 MHz): δ = 171.6 (C_q-6), 170.3 (C_q-1), 159.3 (C_q-4'), 155.0 (C_q-4"), 139.6 (C_q-3), 133.0 (C_q-9"), 132.4 (CH-2"), 130.4 (CH-2',6'), 129.8 (CH-6"), 129.2 (C_q-3"), 125.0 (C_q-1"), 123.1 (C_q-1'), 123.6 (CH-8"), 116.6 (CH-3',5'), 115.0 (CH-5"), 86.8 (C_q-4), 53.8 (OCH_3-7), 39.6 (CH_2-5), 28.7 (CH_2-7"), 25.9 (CH_3-10"), 17.8 (CH_3-11"); -(+)ESI MS: m/z (%) = 447 ([M+Na]$^+$, 81), 871 ([2M+Na]$^+$, 100); -(-)ESI MS: m/z (%) = 423 ([M-H]$^-$, 13), 847 ([2M-H]$^-$, 4); (+)-HRESI: m/z = 447.1414 [M+Na]$^+$ (calc. 447.1414 for $C_{24}H_{24}NaO_7$); (-)-HRESI: m/z 423.1435 [M-H]$^-$ (calc. 423.1449 for $C_{24}H_{23}O_7$).

3.2.3. Aspulvinone H (3)

$C_{27}H_{28}O_5$ (432), colourless solid, UV-blue fluorescent, turned yellow with anisaldehyde/sulphuric acid, R_f = 0.62 (CH_2Cl_2/10% MeOH), ^{1}H NMR (CD_3OD, 300 MHz): δ = 7.81 (d, J = 1.8 Hz, 1H, H-2'), 7.68 (m, 1H, H-6'), 7.59 (m, 1H, H-6"), 7.44 (d, J = 1.6 Hz, H-2"), 6.73 (m, 2H, H-5',5"), 6.22 (s, H-5), 5.36 (m, 2H, H-8',8"), 3.40-3.00 (m, 4H, $H_{2a, b}$-7', $H_{2a, b}$-7"), 1.75 (m, 12H, H_3-10',11',10",11"); -(+)ESI MS: m/z (%) = 455 ([M+Na]$^+$, 56), 477 ([M+2Na-H]$^+$, 100), 887 ([2M+Na]$^+$, 5); -(-)ESI MS: m/z (%) = 431 ([M-H]$^-$, 100), 863 ([2M-H]$^-$, 4), (+)-HRESI: m/z 455.1808 [M+Na]$^+$ (calc. 455.1829 for $C_{27}H_{28}NaO_5$); (-)-HRESI: m/z 431.1860 [M-H]$^-$ (calc. 431.1864 for $C_{27}H_{27}O_5$).

3.2.4. 6-Methylsalicylic acid (4)

$C_8H_8O_3$ (152), colourless solid, UV-absorbing, R_f = 0.24 (CH_2Cl_2/5%MeOH); ^{1}H NMR (CD_3OD, 300 MHz): δ = 7.07 (t, J = 7.7 Hz, 1H, 4-H), 6.63 (d, J = 8.2 Hz, 1H, 3-

H), 6.59 (d, J = 7.5 Hz, 1H, 5-H), 2.56 (s, 3H, CH_3-7); ^{13}C NMR (CD_3OD, 75 MHz): δ = 176 (C_q-8), 162.7 (C_q-2), 142.7 (C_q-6), 132.1 (CH-4), 122.9 (CH-3), 119.5 (C_q-1), 115.1 (CH-5), 23.3 (CH_3-7); -(+)ESI MS: m/z (%) = 175 ([M+Na]$^+$, 25), 371 ([2M+3Na-2H]$^+$, 55); -(-)ESI MS: m/z (%) = 151 ([M-H]$^-$, 100), 303 ([2M-H]$^-$, 4).

3.2.5. Terrine (5)

$C_8H_{10}O_3$ (154), colourless solid, UV-absorbing, turned dark green on spraying with anisaldehyde/sulphuric acid, R_f = 0.51 (CH_2Cl_2/10%MeOH); ^{1}H NMR (CD_3OD, 300 MHz): δ = 6.82 (ddd, J = 13.7, 8.9, 6.8 Hz, 1H, H-2), 6.42 (dd, J = 15.8, 1.1 Hz, 1H, H-3), 5.99 (s, 1H, H-5), 4.67 (d, J = 2.4 Hz, 1H, H-8), 4.07 (d, J = 2.7 Hz, 1H, H-7), 1.97 (dd, J = 6.8, 1.4 Hz, 3H, 1-CH_3); ^{13}C NMR (CD_3OD, 75 MHz): δ = 205.6 (C_q-6), 170.8 (C_q-4), 141.8 (CH-2), 126.4 (CH-3), 125.9 (CH-5), 82.4 (CH-7), 78.1 (CH-8), 19.5 (CH_3-1); -(+)ESI MS: m/z (%) = 177 ([M+Na]$^+$, 62), 331 ([2M+Na]$^+$, 100); -(-)ESI MS: m/z (%) = 153 ([M-H]$^-$, 34), 307 ([2M-H]$^-$, 4); (+)-HRESI MS: m/z 177.0528 [M+Na]$^+$ (calc. 177.0522 for $C_8H_{10}NaO_3$); (-)-HRESI MS: m/z 153.0553 [M-H]$^-$ (calc. 153.0557 for $C_8H_9O_3$).

3.2.6. Butyrolactone-V (6)

$C_{24}H_{24}O_8$ (440), colourless solid, UV-absorbing, turned pink with anisaldehyde/sulphuric acid, R_f = 0.12 (CH_2Cl_2/5% MeOH), ^{1}H NMR (CD_3OD, 300 MHz): δ = 7.54 (d, J = 8.8 Hz, 2H, H-2',6'), 6.85 (d, J = 8.8 Hz, 2H, H-3',5'), 6.48 (m, 3H, H-2",5",6"), 5.02 (dd, J = 5.2, 2.0 Hz, 1H, H-8"), 3.77 (s, 3H, OCH_3-7), 3.40 (s, 2H, CH_2-5), 2.80 (dd, J = 5.2, 16.9 Hz, 2H, CH_2-7"), 1.25 (s, 3H, CH_3-10"), 1.16 (s, 3H, CH_3-11"); ^{13}C NMR (CD_3OD, 75 MHz): δ = 171.5 (C_q-6), 170.3 (C_q-1), 159.4 (C_q-4'), 153.3 (C_q-4"), 139.6 (C_q-3), 132.9 (CH-2"), 130.4 (CH-2',6'), 130.4 (CH-6"), 120.5 (C_q-3"), 126.0 (C_q-1"), 123.1 (C_q-1'), 116.6 (CH-3',5'), 117.2 (CH-5"), 86.8 (C_q-4), 78.0 (C_q-9"), 70.4 (CH-8"), 53.9 (OCH_3-7), 39.5 (CH_2-5), 32.0 (CH_2-7"), 25.8 (CH_3-10"), 20.9 (CH_3-11"); -(+)ESI MS: m/z (%) = 441 ([M+H]$^+$, 30), 463 ([M+Na]$^+$, 57.5), 881 ([2M+H]$^+$, 25), 903 ([2M+Na]$^+$, 50); -(-)ESI MS: m/z (%) 439 ([M-H]$^-$, 3); (+)-HRESI: m/z 463.1370 [M+Na]$^+$ (calc. 463.1363 for $C_{24}H_{24}NaO_8$); (-)-HRESI: m/z 439.1399 [M-H]$^-$ (calc. 439.1389 for $C_{24}H_{23}O_8$).

3.2.7. 4,4'-Diydroxypulvinone (7)

$C_{17}H_{12}O_5$ (296), colourless solid, UV yellow fluorescence, R_f = 0.15 (CH_2Cl_2/5% MeOH); ^{1}H NMR (DMSO-d_6, 300 MHz): δ = 9.42 (brs, 1H, 4'-OH), 8.70 (brs, 1H, 4"-OH), 8.06 (d, J = 8.6 Hz, 2H, H-2',6'), 7.51 (d, J = 8.7 Hz, 2H, H-2",6"), 6.75 (d, J = 8.7 Hz, 2H, H-3', 5'), 6.16 (d, J = 8.7 Hz, 2H, H-3", 5"), 5.88 (s, 1H, H-5); ^{13}C NMR (DMSO-d_6, 300 MHz): δ = 156.1 (C_q-4',4"), 152.4 (C_q-4), 130.4 (CH-2',2",6',6"), 126.1 (C_q-1', 1"), 124.6 (CH-5), 115.3 (CH-3',5'), 114.1 (CH-3",5"); -(+)-ESI MS: m/z (%) = 319 ([M+Na]$^+$, 20), 314 ([M+2Na-H]$^+$, 30); -(-)ESI MS: m/z (%) = 295 ([M-H]$^-$,

100); (+)-HRESI MS: m/z 319.0587 [M+Na]$^+$ (calc. 319.0577 for $C_{17}H_{12}NaO_5$). (-)-HRESI: m/z 295.0616 [M-H]$^-$ (calc. 295.0612 for $C_{17}H_{11}O_5$).

3.3. Biological activities

3.3.1. Antimicrobial activity

Antimicrobial assays were conducted utilizing the disc-agar method [47]. This has been carried out gainst diverse sets of microorganisms. A. flavipes MM2 extract was dissolved in CH_2Cl_2/10% MeOH at a concentration of 1 mg/mL. Aliquots of 40 µL were soaked on filter paper discs (9 mm Ø, no. 2668, Schleicher & Schüll, Germany) and dried for 1 h at room temperature under sterilized conditions. The paper discs were placed on inoculated agar plats and incubated for 24 h at 38°C for bacterial and 48 h (30°C) for the fungal isolates, while the algal test strains were incubated at approximately 22°C in day light for 8-10 days. The pure compounds were examined against the test microorganisms: B. subtilis, S. aureus, S. viridochromogenes (Tü 57), E. coli, C. albicans, M. miehi, C. vulgaris, C. sorokiniana, S. subspicatus, R. solani and P. ultimum.

3.3.2. Brine shrimp microwell cytotoxicity assay

The cytotoxic assay was performed according to Sajid et al.'s screening [48].

Acknowledgements

The authors are deeply thankful to Prof. H. Laatsch for his Lab facilities and unlimited support. We thank Dr. H. Frauendorf and Mr. R. Machinek for the spectral measurements. We appreciate to Miss F. Lissy for testing biological activity and Mr. A. Kohl for his technical assistance. This research work is financed by German Egyptian Scientific Projects (GESP) No. 7.

Author details

^{1}Division of Pharmaceutical Industries, Chemistry of Natural Compounds Department, National Research Centre, El-Behoos st. 33, Dokki, Cairo 12622, Egypt ^{2}Microbial Activity Unit, Microbiology Department, Soil & Water and Environment Research Institute, ARC, Giza, Egypt ^{3}Institute of Organic and Biomolecular Chemistry, University of Göttingen, Tammannstrasse 2, D-37077 Göttingen, Germany ^{4}Pharmacognosy Department, Faculty of Pharmacy, Cairo University, Cairo, Egypt

Competing interests

The authors declare that they have no competing interests.

References

1. Faulkner DJ (2006) Marine bacterial metabolites. In: Proksch P, Muller WEG (eds) Frontiers in marine biotechnology. Horizon Bioscience pp 225–288
2. Laatsch H (2010) A data base for rapid structural determination of microbial natural products and annual updates. Chemical Concepts, Weinheim, Germany
3. Larsen TO, Smedsgaard J, Nielsen KF, Hansen ME, Frisvad JC (2005) Phenotypic taxonomy and metabolite profiling in microbial drug discovery. Nat Prod Rep 22:672–695. doi:10.1039/b404943h.
4. Hassan AEHA (2007) Novel natural products from endophytic fungi of Egyptian medicinal plants–chemical and biological characterization. Dissertation, Düsseldorf, Germany
5. Butler MS (2004) The role of natural product chemistry in drug discovery. J Nat Prod 67:2141–2153. doi:10.1021/np040106y.

6. Rasmussen TB, Skinderso ME, Bjarnsholt T, Phipps RK, Christensen KB, Andersen JB, Koch B, Larsen TO, Hentzer M, Hoiby N, Givskov M (2005) Identity and effects of quorum-sensing inhibitors produced by Penicillium species. Microbiology 151:1325–1340. doi:10.1099/mic.0.27715-0.

7. Li JY, Strobel GA (2001) Jesterone and hydroxyjesterone antioomycete cyclohexenenone epoxides from the endophytic fungus: Pestalotiopsis jesteri. Phytochemistry 57:261–265. doi:10.1016/S0031-9422(01)00021-8.

8. Brady SF, Clardy J (2000) CR377, a new pentaketide antifungal agent isolated from an endophytic fungus. J Nat Prod 63:1447–1448. doi:10.1021/np990568p.

9. Singh SB, Zink DL, Guan Z, Collado J, Pelaez F, Felock PJ, Hazuda DJ (2003) Isolation, structure and HIV-1 integrase inhibitory activity of xanthoviridicatin E and F two novel fungal metabolites produced by Penicillium chrysogenum. Helv Chim Acta 86:3380–3385. doi:10.1002/hlca.200390281.

10. Zhang HW, Song YC, Tan RX (2006) Biology and chemistry of endophytes. Nat Prod Rep 23:753–771. doi:10.1039/b609472b.

11. Song YC, Li H, Ye YH, Shan CY, Yang YM, Tan RX (2004) Endophytic naphthopyrone metabolites are co-inhibitors of xanthine oxidase, SW1116 cell and some microbial growths. FEMS Microbiol Lett 241:67–72. doi:10.1016/j.femsle.2004.10.005.

12. Lubertozzi D, Keasling JD (2009) Developing Aspergillus as a host for heterologous expression. Biotechnol Adv 27:53–75. doi:10.1016/j.biotechadv.2008.09.001.

13. Zhang Z (2009) A new species of Aspergillus. Int J Biol 1:78–80

14. Raper KB, Fennel DI (1965) The genus Aspergillus. Williams and Wilkins Baltimore. USA

15. Liebermann C (1885) Ueber das oxychinoterpen, Berichte. 18:1803–1807

16. Mourao F, Umeo SH, Takemura OS, Linde GA, Colauto NB (2011) Antioxidant activity of Agaricus brasiliensis basidiocarps on different maturation phases. Braz J Microbiol 42:197–202. doi:10.1590/S1517-83822011000100024.

17. Dissanayake DP, Abeytunga DTU, Vasudewa NS, Ratnasooriya WD (2009) Inhibition of lipid peroxidation by extracts of Pleurotus ostreatus. Pharmacogn Mag 5:266–271

18. Chen A, Chen H, Shao Y, Fan M (2009) Active components and free radical scavenging activity of fermented mycelia and broth of Paecilomyces tenuipes. Shipin Kexue 30:25–28

19. Han X, Lin Z, Tao H, Liu P, Wang Y, Zhu W (2009) Cytotoxic metabolites from symbiotic fungus Penicillium sp. HK13-8 with Rhizophora stylosa. Zhongguo Haiyang Yaowu 28:11–16

20. Yan D, Bao HY, Bau T, Li Y, Kim YH (2009) Antitumor components from Naematoloma fasciculare. J Microbiol Biotechnol 19:1135–1138

21. Nitta K, Fujita N, Yoshimura T, Arai K, Yamamoto U (1983) Metabolic products of Aspergillus terreus. IX: biosynthesis of butyrolactone derivatives isolated from strain IFO 8835 and 4100. Chem Pharm Bull 31:1528–1533. doi:10.1248/cpb.31.1528.

22. Zain ME, Awaad AS, Al-Jaber NA, Maitland DJ (2008) New phenolic compounds with antifungal activity from Aspergillus terreus isolated from desert soil. J Saudi Chem Soc 12:107–113

23. Nuclear P, Sommit D, Boonyuen N, Pudhom K (2010) Butenolide and furandione from an endophytic Aspergillus terreus. Chem Pharm Bull 58:1221–1223. doi:10.1248/cpb.58.1221.

24. Rao KV, Sadhukhan AK, Veerender M, Ravikumar V, Mohan EVS (2000) Butyrolactones from Aspergillus terreus. Chem Pharm Bull 48:559–562. doi:10.1248/cpb.48.559.

25. Parvatkar RR, Souza CD, Tripathi A, Naik CG (2009) Aspernolides Α and Β, butenolides from a marine-derived fungus. Aspergillus terreus. Phytochemistry 70:128–132

26. Kitagawa M, Okabe T, Ogino H, Matsumoto H, Suzuki-Takahashi I (1993) Butyrolactone I, a selective inhibitor of cdk2 and cdc2 kinase. Oncogene 8:2425–2432

27. Someya A, Tanaka N, Okuyama A (1994) Inhibition of cell cycle oscillation of DNA replication by a selective inhibitor of the cdc2 kinase family, butyrolactone I, in Xenopus egg extracts. Biochem Biophys Res Commun 198:536–545. doi:10.1006/bbrc.1994.1079.

28. Kitagawa M, Higashi H, Takahashi IS, Okabe T, Ogino H (1994) A cyclin-dependent kinase inhibitor, butyrolactone I, inhibits phosphorylation of RB protein and cell cycle progression. Oncogene 9:2549–2457

29. Nishio K, Ishida T, Arioka H, Kurokawa H, Fukuoka K (1996) Antitumor effects of butyrolactone I, a selective cdc2 kinase inhibitor, on human lung cancer cell lines. Anticancer Res 16(6B):3387–3395

30. Suzuki M, Hosaka Y, Matsushima H, Goto T, Kitamura T, Kawabe K (1999) Butyrolactone I induces cyclin B1 and causes G2/M arrest and skipping of mitosis in human prostate cell lines. Cancer Lett 138:121–130. doi:10.1016/S0304-3835(98)00381-4.

31. Ojima N, Takahashi I, Ogura K, Shuichi SS (1976) New metabolites from Aspergillus terreus related to the biosynthesis of aspulvinones. Tetrahedron Lett 13:1013–1014

32. Venkatasubbaiah P, Van Dyke CG, Chilton WS (1992) Phytotoxic metabolites of phoma sorghina, a new foliar pathogen of pokeweed. Mycologia 84:715–723. doi:10.2307/3760381.

33. Shao C, Guo Z, Peng H, Peng G, Huang Z (2007) A new isoprenyl phenyl ether compound from mangrove fungus. Chem Nat Comp 43:377–380. doi:10.1007/s10600-007-0142-x.

34. Yamasaki S, Nobusada M, Sasaki T, Shimada A (1999) 6-Methylsalicylic acid, an antifungal substance, produced by an unidentified fungus, No 3. Kyushu Kyoritsu Daigaku Kogakubu Kenkyu Hokoku 23:67–71

35. Sievertsson H, Nilsson JLG (1970) Analgesic properties of methylsalicylic acids. Acta Pharm Suecica 7:289–292

36. Thomas GJ (1984) Herbicidal activity of 6-methylanthranilic acid and analogs. J Agric Food Chem 32:747–749. doi:10.1021/jf00124a011.

37. Kubo I, Muroi H, Kubo A (1994) Naturally occurring antiacne agents. J Nat Prod 57:9–17. doi:10.1021/np50103a002.

38. Nielsen KF, Smedsgaard J (2003) Fungal metabolite screening: database of 474 mycotoxins and fungal metabolites for dereplication by standardised liquid chromatography-UV-mass spectrometry methodology. J Chromatog A 1002:111–136. doi:10.1016/S0021-9673(03)00490-4.

39. Harper JK, Mulgrew AE, Li JY, Barich DH, Strobel GA, Grant DM (2001) Characterization of stereochemistry and molecular conformation using solid-state NMR tensors. J Am Chem Soc 123:9837–9842. doi:10.1021/ja010997l.

40. Park SH, Kim DS, Kim WG, Ryoo IJ, Lee DH, Huh CH, Youn SW, Yoo ID, Park KC (2004) Terrein: a new melanogenesis inhibitor and its mechanism. Cell Mol Life Sci 61:2878–2885. doi:10.1007/s00018-004-4341-3.

41. Hosoe T, Moriyama H, Wakana D, Itabashi T, Kawai K (2009) Inhibitory effects of dihydroterrein and terrein isolated from Aspergillus novofumigatus on platelet aggregation. Mycotoxins 59:75–82. doi:10.2520/myco.59.75.

42. Kim DS, Lee HK, Park SH, Lee S, Ryoo IJ (2008) Terrein inhibits keratinocyte proliferation via ERK inactivation and G2/M cell cycle arrest. Exp Dermatol 17:312–317. doi:10.1111/j.1600-0625.2007.00646.x.

43. Macedo JFC, Porto ALM, Marzaioli AJ (2004) Terreinol: a novel metabolite from Aspergillus terreus: structure and C labeling. Tetrahedron Lett 45:53–55. doi:10.1016/j.tetlet.2003.10.128.

44. Lin T, Lu C, She Y (2009) Secondary metabolites of Aspergillus sp. F1, a commensal fungal strain of Trewia nudiflora. Nat Prod Res 23:77–85

45. Haritakun R, Rachtawee P, Chanthaket R, Boonyuen N, Isaka M (2010) Butyrolactones from the fungus Aspergillus terreus BCC 4651. Chem Pharm Bull 58:1545–1548. doi:10.1248/cpb.58.1545.

46. Ojima N, Takenaka S, Seto S (1975) Structures of pulvinone derivatives from Aspergillus terreus. Phytochemistry 14:573–576. doi:10.1016/0031-9422(75)85131-4.

47. Burkholder P, Burkholder IM, Almodovar LR (1960) Antibiotic activity of some marine algae of Puerto Rico. Botanica Marina 2:149–156. doi:10.1515/botm.1960.2.1-2.149.

48. Sajid I, Fondja YCB, Shaaban KA, Hasnain S, Laatsch H (2009) Antifungal and antibacterial activities of indigenous Streptomyces isolates from saline farmlands: prescreening, ribotyping and metabolic diversity. World J Microbiol Biotechnol 25:601–610. doi:10.1007/s11274-008-9928-7.

21

Phytochemical analysis and radical scavenging profile of juices of *Citrus sinensis, Citrus anrantifolia,* and *Citrus limonum*

Abdur Rauf*, Ghias Uddin and Jawad Ali

Abstract

Background: The aim of the current investigation was to identify bioactive secondary metabolites including phenols, tannins, flavonoids, terpinedes, and steroids and compare the phytochemical analysis and antioxidant profile of the juice extracted from the fruits of *Citrus sinensis, Citrus anrantifolia,* and *Citrus limonum.*

Results: Phytochemical screening is important for the isolation of new, novel, and rare secondary metabolites before bulk extraction. Phytochemical analysis of the desired plant fruits of family Rutaceae revealed the presence of phenols, flavonoids, reducing sugars, steroids, terpinedes and tannins. The fruits of *C. sinensis* and *C. anrantifolia* exhibited the presence of phenols, flavonoids, reducing sugars, steroids, terpinedes and tannins, while the fruits of *C. limonum* indicated the presence of phenols, flavonoids, reducing sugars, terpinedes, and tannins. The fruits of selected plants were also subjected to antioxidant potential by 2,2-diphenyl-1-picrylhydrazyl (DPPH) assay against ascorbic acid at various concentrations. Among the tested plants, *C. sinensis* showed promising antiradical effect (84.81%) which was followed by *C. Anrantifolia* (80.05%) at 100 µg/ml against ascorbic acid (96.36%). The *C. limonum* showed low antioxidant activity among the three selected plants of family Rutaceae.

Conclusions: The current finding is baseline information in the use of the fruits of selected plants as food supplement which may be due to the presence of antioxidant molecules in the family Rutaceae. Further research is needed in this area to isolate the phenolic constituents which possess ideal antiradical potential.

Keywords: Rutaceae; *Citrus sinensis; Citrus anrantifolia; Citrus limonum;* Phytochemical screening; Antioxidant activity

Background

Recently, there is keen biomedical interest in family Rutaceae (fruits) because their use as raw is mainly associated with low risk of gastric, colorectal, esophageal, and cancer diseases. Citrus is a promising source of vitamin C, folate, and flavonoids due to which citrus is used as a cancer preventing agent [1]. *Citrus sinensis* belong to the family Rutaceae, which is the most widely grown and commercialized species [2]. *C. sinensis* is a rich source of sugars, acids, polysaccharides, and many other phytochemicals such as vitamin C and carotenoids, which provided health benefits against various diseases including cardiovascular and cancer diseases [3,4].

Citrus anrantifolia belong to the family Rutaceae and is distributed in tropical and subtropical region. *C. anrantifolia* is commonly used in various traditional systems as an antihelmintic, mosquito repellent, and antiseptic and many other chronic diseases [5]. *Citrus limonum* is also a member of the family Rutaceae. *C. limonum* is a rich source of vitamin C, which is used as folk medicine for the treatment of stomachache, carminative, as antipneumonia, and also for the treatment of dysentery and diarrhea [6]. The current finding deals with the comparative phytochemical analysis for the identification of various classes of secondary metabolites and antioxidant profile of juices of *C. sinensis, C. anrantifolia,* and *C. limonum.*

Methods
Plant collection
The fresh fruits of *C. sinensis, C. anrantifolia,* and *C. limonum* were collected from the garden of Institute of

* Correspondence: mashaljcs@yahoo.com
Institute of Chemical Sciences, University of Peshawar, Peshawar KPK 25120, Pakistan

Chemical Sciences, University of Peshawar, Peshawar, Pakistan. The fruits of collected plants were stored in the refrigerator of Center of Phytomedicine natural product laboratory. The sample was identified and authenticated by Dr. Abdur Rashid, plants Taxonomist, the voucher no. (PUP714-716) was deposited at the Botany Department, University of Peshawar, Pakistan.

Place of study
The experimental work was carried out in the Centre for Phytomedicine and Medicinal Organic Chemistry Institute of Chemical Sciences, University of Peshawar, Peshawar, Pakistan.

Extraction
The fresh Juices of *C. sinensis*, *C. anrantifolia*, and *C. limonum* were extracted from the fresh fruits and freeze dried and stored in the refrigerator for further analysis.

Statistical analysis
Data were presented as mean and standard error of means. The statistical analysis was performed using Prism Graphed.

Chemical and reagents
The ascorbic acid, 2,2-diphenyl-1-picrylhydrazyl (DPPH), and analytical grade methanol were purchased from Merck, Darmstadt, Germany.

Phytochemical analysis
Chemical test was performed on the juices of *C. sinensis*, *C. anrantifolia*, and *C. limonum* to identify bioactive secondary metabolites according to standard assay procedure.

DPPH radical scavenging profile
The antioxidant activity of the juices of *C. sinensis*, *C. anrantifolia*, and *C. limonum* was performed by DPPH radical scavenging assay according to standard assay protocol [7]. The positive control used in the current finding was ascorbic acid. The hydrogen atom or electron donation capacities of the juices extracted from fruits and ascorbic acid were measured from the bleaching of the purple-colored methanol solution of DPPH. Experiments were carried out in triplicates. Briefly, a 1-mM solution of DPPH radical solution in methanol was prepared, and 1 ml of this solution was mixed with 3 ml of sample (juices) solutions in methanol (containing 10 to 100 µg) for various fractions (containing 10 to 100 µg) for pure compounds and control (without sample). The solution was allowed to stand for 30 min, in the dark, the absorbance was measured at 517 nm. Decreasing of the DPPH solution absorbance indicates an increase of the DPPH radical scavenging activity. Scavenging of free radicals by DPPH as

Table 1 Antioxidant effect of juices extracted from *C. sinensis*, *C. anrantifolia*, and *C. limonum*

Concentration	% DPPH C. sinensis	% DPPH C. anrantifolia	% DPPH of C. limonum	Ascorbic acid
10 µg/ml	49.69 ± 1.11	37.51 ± 1.00	25.47 ± 1.22	91.34 ± 1.22
20 µg/ml	58.46 ± 1.22	43.41 ± 1.90	28.60 ± 1.50	91.39 ± 1.28
30 µg/ml	62.48 ± 1.00	50.94 ± 1.89	34.12 ± 1.29	92.09 ± 1.38
40 µg/ml	65.74 ± 1.98	55.58 ± 1.00	38.51 ± 1.98	92.59 ± 1.99
50 µg/ml	68.13 ± 1.88	61.85 ± 1.24	40.90 ± 1.23	93.35 ± 1.24
60 µg/ml	74.78 ± 1.68	70.38 ± 1.23	50.06 ± 1.86	94.47 ± 1.90
80 µg/ml	81.93 ± 1.22	75.28 ± 1.55	55.45 ± 1.00	95.23 ± 1.98
100 µg/ml	84.81 ± 1.99	80.05 ± 1.90	63.73 ± 1.91	96.36 ± 1.78

percent radical scavenging activities (%RSA) was calculated as follows:

$$\% \, DPPH = (OD \, control\text{-}OD \, sample) \times 100/OD \, control$$

where OD control is the absorbance of the blank sample and OD sample is the absorbance of samples or standard sample.

Results and discussion
The phytochemical analysis of three selected plants of the family Rutaceae (*C. sinensis*, *C. anrantifolia*, *C. limonum*) are given in Table 1, while the antiradical effects are listed in Table 2.

Antioxidant effect
The effect of the different plants of the family Rutaceae juices at various concentrations against DPPH is presented in Table 1. All the tested plants (*C. sinensis*, *C. anrantifolia*, and *C. limonum*) exhibited promising antiradical activity as

Table 2 Phytochemical analysis of juices of *C. sinensis*, *C. anrantifolia*, and *C. limonum*

Chemical constituents	C. sinensis	C. anrantifolia	C. limonum
Alkaloids	−	−	−
Tannins	++	+++	++
Anthraquinones	−	−	−
Glycosides	−	−	−
Reducing sugar	+++	++	+
Saponins	−	−	−
Flavonoids	++	+	+
Phlobatanins	−	−	−
Steroids	++	+	−
Terpenoids	+	+	+
Phenol	+++	++	+

compared to the standard drug (ascorbic acid). *C. sinensis* showed 84.81% antiradical effect at 100 µg/ml which was followed by *C. anrantifolia* 80.05%, while *C. limonum* 63. 73%. The antioxidant effect of the tested juices was increase in dose-dependent mode.

Phytochemical screening is significant for the isolation of antioxidant natural product from medicinal plants. The fruits of the tested plants of the family Rutaceae exhibited the presence of phenols, flavonoids, reducing sugars, steroids, terpinedes, and tannins. The fruits of *C. sinensis* and *C. anrantifolia* showed the presence of phenols, flavonoids, reducing sugars, steroids, terpinedes, and tannins, while the fruits of *C. limonum* indicated the presence of phenols, flavonoids, reducing sugars, terpinedes, and tannins. Different reactive oxidative species (ROS) including superoxide radicals and hydroxyl (OH) radicals are natural products produced in living organisms [7]. Reactive oxidative species produced as by product play a key role in cell signaling. However, biomolecule oxidation produced excessive ROS which caused major damage to cell structure and resulted to different kinds of diseases such as cancer, stroke, and diabetes. Antioxidants are key inhibitors which produce lipid peroxidation not only for food protection but also as a defense mechanism of living cells against oxidative damage [8,9]. The juices extracted from the fruits of selected plants were also evaluated to antioxidant potential by DPPH assay against ascorbic acid at various concentrations (10 to 100 µg/ml). Among the tested plants, *C. sinensis* showed promising antiradical effect (84.81) which was followed by *C. Anrantifolia* (80.05) at 100 µg/ml against ascorbic acid (96.36). *C. limonum* showed low antioxidant activity among the three selected plants of the family Rutaceae.

Conclusions

The current finding suggests the use of the fruits of selected plants as food supplement which may be due to the desirable presence of antioxidant molecules in the family Rutaceae. The current finding directed the scientist to isolate new, rare, and novel antioxidant molecules from *C. sinensis*, *C. anrantifolia*, and *C. limonum*.

Competing interests
The authors declare that they have no competing interests.

References
1. Roussos PA (2011) Phytochemicals and antioxidant capacity of orange *Citrus sinensis* (l.) Osbeck cv. Salustiana) juice produced under organic and integrated farming system in Greece. Sci Hortic 129:253–258
2. Izquierdo L, Sendra JM (2003) Citrus fruits: composition and characterization. In: Caballero B, Trugo L, Finglas P (eds) Encyclopedia of food sci and nutri (Vol. 2). Academic Press, Oxford UK
3. Diplock AT (1994) Antioxidants and disease prevention. Mol Asp Med 15:293–376
4. Faulks M, Southon S (2001) Carotenoids, metabolism and disease. In: Wildman REC (ed) Handbook of nutraceuticals and functional foods. CRC press, Florida, USA
5. Pathan RK, Gali PR, Pathan P, Gowtham T, Pasupuleti S (2012) In vitro antimicrobial activity of *Citrus aurantifolia* and its phytochemical screening. Asi Pacif J Trop Dis :S328–S331
6. Kulkarni TR, Kothekar MA, Mateenuddin M (2005) Study of anti-fertility effect of lemon seeds (Citrus Limonum) in female albino mice. Indi J Phys and Pharmacol 49(3):305
7. Khan H, Saeed M, Muhammad N, Rauf A, Khan AZ, Ullah R (2013) Antioxidant profile of constituents isolated from polygonatum verticillatum rhizomes. Toxicol and indu health 0748233713498454,Oline
8. Rauf A, Khan R, Muhammad N (2013) Antioxidant studies of various solvent fractions and chemical constituents of Potentilla evestita Th. Wolf. Afr J Phar and Pharmacol 39:2707–2710
9. Rauf A, Uddin G, Arfan M, Muhammad N (2013) Chemical composition and biological screening of essential oils from *Pistacia integerrima*. Afr J Phar and Pharmacol 7(20):1220–1224

β-Keto esters from ketones and ethyl chloroformate: a rapid, general, efficient synthesis of pyrazolones and their antimicrobial, *in silico* and *in vitro* cytotoxicity studies

Ramasamy Venkat Ragavan[1], Kalavathi Murugan Kumar[2], Vijayaparthasarathi Vijayakumar[1*], Sundaramoorthy Sarveswari[1], Sudha Ramaiah[2], Anand Anbarasu[1,2], Sivashanmugam Karthikeyan[1,3], Periyasamy Giridharan[4] and Nalilu Suchetha Kumari[5]

Abstract

Background: Pyrazolones are traditionally synthesized by the reaction of β-keto esters with hydrazine and its derivatives. There are methods to synthesize β-keto esters from esters and aldehydes, but these methods have main limitation in varying the substituents. Often, there are a number of methods such as acylation of enolates in which a chelating effect has been employed to lock the enolate anion using lithium and magnesium salts; however, these methods suffer from inconsistent yields in the case of aliphatic acylation. There are methods to synthesize β-keto esters from ketones like caboxylation of ketone enolates using carbon dioxide and carbon monoxide sources in the presence of palladium or transition metal catalysts. Currently, the most general and simple method to synthesize β-keto ester is the reaction of dimethyl or ethyl carbonate with ketone in the presence of strong bases which also requires long reaction time, use of excessive amount of reagent and inconsistent yield. These factors lead us to develop a simple method to synthesize β-keto esters by changing the base and reagent.

Results: A series of β-keto esters were synthesized from ketones and ethyl chloroformate in the presence of base which in turn are converted to pyrazolones and then subjected to cytotoxicity studies towards various cancer cell lines and antimicrobial activity studies towards various bacterial and fungal strains.

Conclusion: The β-keto esters from ethyl chloroformate was successfully attempted, and the developed method is simple, fast and applicable to the ketones having the alkyl halogens, protecting groups like Boc and Cbz that were tolerated and proved to be useful in the synthesis of fused bicyclic and tricyclic pyrazolones efficiently using cyclic ketones. Since this method is successful for different ketones, it can be useful for the synthesis of pharmaceutically important pyrazolones also. The synthesized pyrazolones were subjected to antimicrobial, docking and cytotoxicity assay against ACHN (human renal cell carcinoma), Panc-1 (human pancreatic adenocarcinoma) and HCT-116 (human colon cancer) cell line, and lead molecules have been identified. Some of the compounds are found to have promising activity against different bacterial and fungal strains tested.

Keywords: β-keto esters; Ethyl chloroformate; Pyrazolones; Efficient synthesis; Anti-bacterial activity; Fungicidal activity; Cytotoxicity studies

* Correspondence: kvpsvijayakumar@gmail.com
[1]Centre for Organic and Medicinal Chemistry, VIT University, Vellore 632 014, India
Full list of author information is available at the end of the article

Background

Pyrazolones are important class of heterocyclic ring systems that have been used extensively in pharmaceutical industry [1,2] due to their numerous applications as analgesic, antipyretic, antiarthritic, uricosuric, anti-inflammatory and antiphlogistic properties. Especially, a pyrazolone derivative (edaravone) [3] acts as a radical scavenger to interrupt the peroxidative chain reactions and membrane disintegrations associated with ischemia [4-6]. Some of the aryloxypyrazolone derivatives are useful in the treatment of a variety of disorders caused by human immunodeficiency virus and other genetic ailments caused by retroviruses such as acquired immune deficiency syndrome [7]. In addition, these compounds are appropriate precursors for industrial preparation of herbicides [8], liquid crystals [9,10], dyes [11], thermally stable polymers [12] and colour photographical compounds [13]. Azadienophiles from the chemical oxidation of pyrazolones are acting as suitable substrates for hetero Diels-Alder reactions [14].

Pyrazolones are traditionally synthesized by the reaction of β-keto esters with hydrazine and its derivatives [15-21]. There are a number of alternative methods to synthesize pyrazolones which are documented in the literature [22-33] but tend to have serious drawbacks such as step-intensive, carbon monoxide usage and sensitive palladium catalysts. These factors revealed that using β-keto esters as an intermediate is the broadest and most efficient way to synthesize pyrazolones. There are methods to synthesize β-keto esters from esters [34-37] (Claisen condensation) and aldehydes [38,39], but these methods have main limitation in varying the substituents. Often, a number of methods such as acylation of enolates of malonates [40,41], acylation of Meldrum's acid [42-45], mixed malonate esters [46,47] and bistrimethylsilylmalonate [48,49] have a chelating effect employed to lock the enolate anion of malonate using lithium and magnesium salts [50,51]; however, these methods suffer from inconsistent yields in the case of aliphatic acylation. There are methods to synthesize β-keto esters from ketones like caboxylation of ketone enolates [52-54] using carbon dioxide and carbon monoxide sources in the presence of palladium or transition metal catalysts. Currently, the most general and simple method to synthesize β-keto ester is the reaction of dimethyl or ethyl carbonate with ketone in the presence of strong bases [55,56]. This method requires long reaction time, use of excessive amount of reagent and inconsistent yield. These factors lead us to develop a simple method to synthesize β-keto esters by changing the base and reagent.

Methods

Antibacterial study

The newly synthesized pyrazoles for their antibacterial activity against *Escherichia coli* (ATTC-25922),

Staphylococcus aureus (ATTC-25923), *Pseudomonas aeruginosa* (ATTC-27853) and *Klebsiella pneumonia* (recultured) bacterial strains by the disc diffusion method [57,58]. The discs measuring 6.25 mm in diameter were punched from Whatman No. 1 filter paper (GE Healthcare, Little Chalfont, UK). Batches of 100 discs were dispensed to each screw-capped bottle and sterilized by dry heat at 140°C for an hour. The test compounds were prepared with different concentrations using DMF. One milliliter containing 100 times the amount of chemical in each disc was added to each bottle, which contains 100 discs. The discs of each concentration were placed in triplicate in a nutrient agar medium separately seeded with fresh bacteria. The incubation was carried out at 37°C for 24 h. Solvent and growth controls were kept, and the zones of inhibition and minimum inhibitory concentrations (MIC) were noted. Results of these studies were given in Table 1 and compared with the standard ciprofloxacin.

Antifungal activity

Newly synthesized pyrazoles were screened for their antifungal activity against *Aspergillus flavus* (NCIM no. 524), *Aspergillus fumigates* (NCIM no. 902), *Penicillium marneffei* (recultured) and *Trichophyton mentagrophytes* (recultured) in dimethylsulfoxide (DMSO) by the serial plate dilution method [34-36]. Sabouraud agar media was prepared by dissolving peptone (1 g), D-glucose (4 g) and agar (2 g) in distilled water (100 mL), and the pH was adjusted to 5.7. Normal saline was used to make a suspension of spores of fungal strain for lawning. A loopful of particular fungal strain was transferred to 3 mL of saline to get a suspension of corresponding species. Agar media of 20 mL was poured into each Petri dish. An excess of suspension was decanted, and the plates were dried by placing them in an incubator at 37°C for 1 h. Using an agar, punch wells were made on these seeded agar plates, and 10 to 50 μg/mL of the test compounds in DMSO were added into each labelled well. A control was also prepared for plates in the same way using solvent DMSO. The Petri dishes were prepared in triplicate and maintained at 37°C for 3 to 4 days. Antifungal activity was determined by measuring the inhibition zone. The results of these studies were given in Table 2 and compared with the standard ciclopiroxolamine.

Docking studies

All the synthesized compounds **1** to **26** have been subjected to the docking studies against ACHN (human renal cell carcinoma), Panc-1 (human pancreatic adenocarcinoma) and HCT-116 (human colon cancer) and then subjected to WST-1 cytotoxicity assay. Based on the crystal structures of the target proteins and high-

Table 1 Antibacterial activity of the newly synthesized compounds

Compound number	S. aureus	E. coli	P. aeruginosa	K. pneumonia
1	21 (6.25)	17 (6.25)	18 (6.25)	20 (6.25)
2	20 (6.25)	18 (6.25)	19 (6.25)	21 (6.25)
3	23 (6.25)	19 (6.25)	20 (6.25)	22 (6.25)
4	20 (6.25)	17 (6.25)	18 (6.25)	19 (6.25)
5	16 (100)	17 (100)	12 (100)	14 (100)
6	17 (100)	17 (100)	11 (100)	15 (100)
7	26 (12.5)	23 (12.5)	21 (12.5)	20 (12.5)
8	19 (100)	23 (100)	22 (100)	16 (100)
9	26 (6.25)	23 (6.25)	21 (6.25)	20 (6.25)
10	22 (6.25)	18 (6.25)	19 (6.25)	21 (6.25)
11	17 (6.25)	21 (6.25)	20 (6.25)	21 (6.25)
13	28 (12.5)	22 (12.5)	25 (12.5)	23 (12.5)
14	29 (12.5)	25 (12.5)	22 (12.5)	21 (12.5)
15	23 (6.25)	20 (6.25)	21 (6.25)	22 (6.25)
17	31 (12.5)	25 (12.5)	27 (12.5)	20 (12.5)
19	18 (6.25)	19 (6.25)	22 (6.25)	20 (6.25)
20	24 (6.25)	25 (6.25)	26 (6.25)	26 (6.25)
21	30 (12.5)	24 (12.5)	25 (12.5)	22 (12.5)
23	24 (12.5)	27 (12.5)	24 (12.5)	23 (12.5)
24	16 (100)	17 (100)	12 (100)	14 (100)
25	21 (12.5)	24 (12.5)	26 (12.5)	22 (12.5)
26	21 (6.25)	23 (6.25)	22 (6.25)	20 (6.25)
Ciprofloxacin	23 (6.25)	32 (6.25)	28 (6.25)	24 (6.25)

Zone of inhibition (mm); MIC (µg/mL) given in parenthesis.

throughput molecular docking methods, four phases of Gemdock methods were used. These phases include target protein structure analysis, ligand optimization, molecular docking and post-docking analysis. The macro- and small-molecule optimization phase involved in editing the structural coordinates of the target protein and compounds. The third phase was molecular docking method to identify potential leads for the target protein; then, the fourth phase was post-docking analysis to identify best conformation of ligand molecule. In the present study, the coordinates of three cancer target proteins were selected and obtained from the Protein Data Bank (PDB) [59]. The PDB entry 1SVC (pancreatic cancer), 3B8Q (renal cancer) and 4FLH (colon cancer) were selected for structural analysis based on its high-resolution crystallographic structure. For docking studies, the PDB coordinates of obtained target proteins were edited by removing the co-crystallized ligand molecule. The crystallographic water molecules were eliminated from the atomic coordinate file, and the polar hydrogen atoms and Kollman united charges were added to each target protein, followed by

structure optimization and refinement using spdbv viewer [60]. The synthesized chemical compound structures were sketched with the help of ChemSketch [61]. A three-dimensional (3D) conversion and geometry optimization of all the compounds were performed using chimera [62] for flexible conformations of the compounds during the docking. To study the detailed intermolecular interactions between the target protein and the ligand molecule, automated docking program iGEMDOCK (a generic evolutionary method for molecular DOCKing) software was used [63]. iGEMDOCK integrated the virtual screening, molecular docking, post-screening analysis and visualization steps. We selected nuclear factor kappa b (NF-κb), vascular endothelial growth factor receptor-2 and human phosphoinositide 3-kinase (PI3K-gamma) (PDB ID: 1SVC, 3B8Q and 4FLH, respectively) as target proteins to carry out the docking analysis of our synthesized compounds. The 3D coordinates of each therapeutic target protein were implemented through the GEMDOCK graphical environment interface. Then, the default option

Table 2 Antifungal activities of the newly synthesized compounds

Compound number	Trichophyton	Penicillium	A. flavus	A. fumigates
1	25 (6.25)	23 (6.25)	26 (6.25)	27 (6.25)
2	24 (6.25)	25 (6.25)	24 (6.25)	26 (6.25)
3	29 (6.25)	26 (6.25)	27 (6.25)	28 (6.25)
4	21 (6.25)	22 (6.25)	26 (6.25)	22 (6.25)
5	16 (12.5)	17 (12.5)	12 (12.5)	14 (12.5)
6	17 (12.5)	17 (12.5)	11 (12.5)	15 (12.5)
7	24 (12.5)	21 (12.5)	21 (12.5)	20 (12.5)
8	26 (12.5)	24 (12.5)	27 (12.5)	23 (12.5)
9	27 (12.5)	25 (12.5)	28 (12.5)	22 (12.5)
10	20 (6.25)	22 (6.25)	17 (6.25)	22 (6.25)
11	21 (6.25)	21 (6.25)	23 (6.25)	21 (6.25)
13	22 (12.5)	25 (12.5)	27 (12.5)	23 (12.5)
14	30 (12.5)	22 (12.5)	26 (12.5)	24 (12.5)
15	26 (12.5)	23 (12.5)	27 (12.5)	23 (12.5)
17	31 (12.5)	25 (12.5)	28 (12.5)	23 (12.5)
19	25 (6.25)	24 (6.25)	27 (6.25)	24 (6.25)
20	28 (12.5)	29 (12.5)	25 (12.5)	25 (12.5)
21	31 (12.5)	28 (12.5)	27 (12.5)	24 (12.5)
23	29 (12.5)	27 (12.5)	26 (12.5)	21 (12.5)
24	23 (12.5)	26 (12.5)	23 (12.5)	25 (12.5)
25	21 (6.25)	20 (6.25)	21 (6.25)	23 (6.25)
26	25 (12.5)	22 (12.5)	27 (12.5)	28 (12.5)
Standard	27 (3.125)	23 (6.25)	27 (3.125)	26 (6.25)

Zone of inhibition (mm), MIC (µg/mL) given in parenthesis and ciclopiroxolamine as standard.

Table 3 Docking results of synthesized compounds in the binding site of nuclear factor kappa b

Compound number	Total energy	Z score	VDW
1	−74.15	−73.1	−73.15
2	−66.2304	−70.6	−56.7448
3	−78.2994	−90.8	−65.8385
4	−42.783	−45.93	−68.7026
5	−50.5602	−54.9	−50.366
6	−88.1508	−110.2	−70.312
7	−32.2859	−40.6	−55.3665
8	−49.5672	−50.8	−56.3479
9	−62.3895	−62.4	−50.3603
10	−74.4438	−72.3	−70.4519
11	−90.4298	−117.4	−80.5608
12	−83.3089	−90.4	−67.7796
13	−42.6816	−50.3	−60.7439
14	−91.9971	−119.9	−74.1695
15	−35.7564	−46.7	−68.4413
16	−72.932	−69.9	−60.4764
17	−60.4516	−60.2	−60.3893
18	−34.3128	−101.7	−53.5055
19	−41.0148	−50.9	−63.3827
20	−35.2375	−40.6	−87.3575
21	−79.2554	−85.2	−51.5586
22	−39.9575	−42.3	−67.6976
23	−32.1991	−42.3	−63.8354
24	−58.4277	−60.9	−67.0823
25	−58.424	−60.9	−53.7606
26	−30.0129	−44.6	−44.8782

was used to import the 3D coordinates of 27 synthesized compounds. Before docking, the output path was set. GEMDOCK default parameters included the population size (n = 200), generation (g = 70) and number of solutions (s = 10) to compute the probable binding conformation of synthesized compounds. Then, the docking run was started using GEMDOCK scoring function. After docking, the individual binding conformation of each ligand was observed, and their binding affinity with the target proteins was analyzed. The best binding pose and binding energy of each ligand was selected. In the post-docking analysis, van der Waals score, Z score and the details of interacted residues were saved in output folder. Protein-ligand binding site was analyzed and visualized using PyMOL [64]. The three-dimensional structures of NF-κb, vascular endothelial growth factor receptor-2 and human phosphoinositide 3-kinase are analyzed, and synthesized compounds 1 to 26 are optimized to have minimal potential energy using chimera. After minimization, all the ligands are docked into each target protein to study the molecular basis of interaction and binding affinity of

all the synthesized compounds. From the docking analysis, we listed best conformers based on total energy, Z score and van der Waals score (VDW) for each ligand molecule (Tables 3,4,5). The best docking poses for each ligand molecule into each target protein are determined, and the one having the lowest binding energy among the 20 different poses generated. The lower energy scores represent better protein-ligand binding affinity compared to higher energy values.

Cytotoxicity studies

The compounds **1** to **26** have been subjected to cyctotoxicity studies. Towards this, a panel of three cancer cells representing multiple cancers of clinical relevance were obtained from American Type Culture Collection (ATCC), namely ACHN (human renal cell carcinoma), Panc-1 (human pancreatic adenocarcinoma) and HCT-116 (human colon cancer). Cells were maintained in Dulbecco's modified Eagle's medium (DMEM) medium containing 10% heat-inactivated fetal bovine serum and

Table 4 Docking results of synthesized compounds in the binding site of vascular endothelial growth factor receptor-2

Compound number	Total energy	Z score	VDW
1	−75.0934	−72.2	−79.4166
2	−78.2062	−75.1	−69.6532
3	−70.5653	−95.6	−68.46
4	−78.7892	−72.3	−63.191
5	−65.564	−78.9	−59.3404
6	−86.6543	−105.7	−80.5888
7	−71.8927	−63.17	−59.0905
8	−95.9923	−120.5	−94.7849
9	−79.948	−71.9	−56.0692
10	−73.5766	−80	−86.6021
11	−72.3245	−73.6	−73.1902
12	−75.4277	−72.2	−70.7142
13	−85.3265	−94.6	−54.4274
14	−75.329	−75.3	−71.2839
15	−80.914	−75.1	−73.6739
16	−75.3033	−91.5	−63.0176
17	−68.7853	−74.3	−69.6841
18	−104.9856	−125.5	−105.697
19	−92.6464	−115.2	−87.8944
20	−74.3443	76.7	−70.902
21	−62.3597	−73.3	−50.6291
22	−60.2348	−78.2	−65.3015
23	−77.191	−75.6	−63.8723
24	−82.723	−77.2	−68.4238
25	−80.73	−75	−56.4072
26	−75.093	−104.3	−48.6469

Table 5 Docking results of synthesized compounds in the binding site of phosphoinositide 3-kinase

Compound number	Total energy	Z score	VDW
1	−119.541	−122.5	−78.0144
2	−67.4663	68.3	−53.8734
3	−105.3452	−90.9	−68.1224
4	−75.0481	−75	−70.3258
5	−77.1818	−77.2	−61.47
6	−101.23	−105.1	−55.6405
7	−96.8291	−110.9	−54.3328
8	−92.0488	−92	−61.893
9	−75.3184	−75.3	−62.0764
10	−119.421	−120.5	−76.7195
11	92.8443	−92.3	−62.324
12	−83.9072	−83.9	−85.1019
13	−80.5887	−80.6	−66.5004
14	−107.157	−102.2	−62.1177
15	−76.9716	−77	−70.2072
16	−94.8943	−106.4	−52.3224
17	−90.9786	−91.4	−66.5817
18	−110.067	−91	−80.4918
19	−83.2508	−83.3	−54.2574
20	−76.3532	−76.3	−86.3532
21	−82.2975	−82.3	−54.9572
22	−74.2083	−74.2	−71.0281
23	−81.0895	−81.1	−63.5472
24	−76.2358	−76.2	−58.7925
25	−67.4663	−67.5	−49.4389
26	−80.9917	−81.1	−48.6582

kept in humidified 5% CO_2 incubator at 37°C. Logarithmically, growing cells were plated at a density of 5×10^3 cells/well in a 96-well tissue culture grade micro-plate and allowed to recover overnight. The cells were challenged with varying concentrations of compounds for 48 h. Control cells received standard media containing dimethylsulfoxide vehicle at a concentration of 0.2%. After 48 h of incubation, cell toxicity was determined by the Cell Counting Kit-8 (CCK-8) reagent (Dojindo Molecular Technologies, Inc., Kumamoto, Japan); (WST-1 [2-(2-methoxy-4-nitrophenyl)-3-(4-nitrophenyl)-5-(2,4-disulfophenyl)]-2H-tetrazolium, monosodium salt assay). In accordance with the manufacturer's instructions [36], 5 μL/well CCK-8 reagent was added, and plates were incubated for 2 h. Cytotoxicity of all the compounds have been determined by measuring the absorbance on Tecan Sapphire multi-fluorescence micro-plate reader (Tecan GmbH, Crailsheim, Germany) at a wavelength of 450 nm corrected to 650 nm and normalized to controls. Each independent experiment was performed thrice and tabulated in Table 6.

Results and discussion

In continuation of our interest towards the synthesis of β-keto esters and pyrazolones [65-67], we made an attempt to synthesize β-keto esters from ethyl chloroformate in the presence of base which in turn are converted into pyrazolones *in situ* by the addition of either hydrazine or its derivatives, since we hypothesized that an enolate may react cleanly with highly electrophilic ethyl chloroformate to give β-keto esters. We tested our hypothesis in the synthesis of representative compound **12** by varying the solvents as well as bases (Scheme 1). The effects of base and solvent on the yield of **12** have been summarized and are given in Table 7.

The formation of β-keto ester was found to be in better yield when LiHMDS was used as a base. When other bases are used, the formation of β-keto ester intermediate from ketones was very slow, and the reactions were

Table 6 Cytotoxic activity of the newly synthesized compounds 1 to 26

Compound number	Concentration (μg/mL)	Percentage of cytotoxicity/ anti-proliferation		
		Panc1 (pancreas)	ACHN (renal)	HCT116 (colon)
1	10	−75	−7	−138
2	10	−64	5	1
3	10	−78	0	−16
4	10	−10	20	−12
5	10	−20	−3	6
6	10	−101	−25	−116
7	10	14	−16	−115
8	10	−15	−31	−107
9	10	−56	19	8
10	10	−75	−7	−138
11	10	−117	7	−107
12	10	−89	13	−70
13	10	−14	3	5
14	10	−118	−19	−123
15	10	12	5	17
16	10	−71	−10	−112
17	10	−51	4	−102
18	10	4	−41	−128
19	10	−10	−26	−80
20	10	71	73	79
21	10	−80	−5	−20
23	10	12	−7	−6
24	10	6	2	−103
25	10	−45	−18	−64
26	10	−7	−12	1
Tannase	10	17.3	12.4	9.7

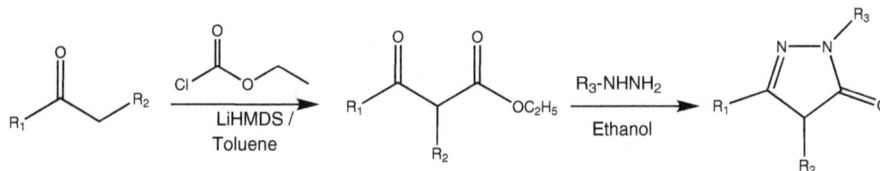

Scheme 1 Synthesis of β-keto esters from ethyl chloroformate and its conversion into pyrazolones.

also found to be incomplete even after 4 to 5 h of stirring at r.t. The addition of hydrazine hydrate to the latter reaction mixtures gave the desired product in low yield (Table 8), and the corresponding hydrazone of ketones was isolated as the major product. After finding the suitable base, the reaction conditions were optimized further by varying the solvents to improve the yield. It was found that the hydrocarbon solvent (toluene) produced better yield compared to the cyclic ether solvent (THF). This may be due to the possible destabilization of formed intermediate with charge in the case of hydrocarbon solvent like toluene, and hence, the formed enolate reacts with ethyl chloroformate smoothly.

After optimizing the reaction with the suitable base (LiHMDS) and solvent (toluene), the same conditions were employed for the synthesis of various β-keto esters which in turn are converted into their corresponding pyrazolones **1** to **21** and **23** to **26** *in situ* by the addition of either hydrazine or its derivatives to prove the generality of the reaction, and the results are tabulated in Table 8. The reactions have been monitored by thin layer chromatography (TLC), and the obtained crude products were purified by column chromatography. The β-keto esters were efficiently converted into their corresponding pyrazolones with good to excellent yields. All the synthesized compounds **1** to **21** and **23** to **26** have been characterized through IR, ^{1}H NMR, ^{13}C NMR and mass spectral data. The examination of the ^{1}H NMR spectrum of **26** clearly shows that the formation of doublet at δ 1.34 ppm with the coupling constant of 6.92 Hz integrating for six protons is due to the two methyl groups of isopropyl substituent at C3 of pyrazolone moiety. A multiplet between δ 2.79 and 2.49 ppm

integrating for one proton is due to the methine proton of *iso*-propyl substituent at C3 of pyrazolone moiety. The singlet at δ 3.33 ppm integrating for one proton is due to the proton at C4. Two broad singlets that appeared between δ 9.5 to 9.3 ppm and δ 11.2 to 11.1 ppm integrating for one proton each are due to -NH and -OH protons, respectively. This supports the ^{1}H NMR findings that pyrazolone moiety is in its enol rather than the keto form since the spectrum was recorded in deuterated DMSO solvent. Similarly, the examination of the ^{13}C NMR spectrum reveals the following points. The two signals that appeared at aliphatic regions 22.24 and 25.69 ppm are due to methyl and methine carbon, respectively, of the *iso*-propyl substituent at C3 of the pyrazolone moiety. The signal at 86.22 ppm is due to the C4. The two downfield signals appeared at 160.75 and 150.39 ppm. The relatively downfield signal has been assigned as C5, and the relatively upfield has been assigned as C3. The *m/z* observed at 126.9 in liquid chromatography-mass spectrometry (LC-MS) spectrum also supports the formation of compound **26**. In the similar way, the chemical shifts of all the other compounds have been assigned and are included in the experimental part. Some of the compounds **4, 7, 16, 21, 23** and **24** have been crystallized and subjected to the single crystal X-ray diffraction studies [68-75] and are available in the literature (Ortep plots are included in Additional file 1); particularly, sample **4** has been crystallized as both in keto form and enol form. All the above discussions clearly revealed the formation of the desired products. This method is very simple, fast and applicable to the ketones having the alkyl halogens, protecting groups like Boc and Cbz that were tolerated and proved to be useful in the synthesis of fused bicyclic and tricyclic

Table 7 Effect of solvent and base on the yield of 12

Base	Ketone (eq.)	Solvent	Temperature	Yield (%)[a]
LiHMDS (1.0M THF) (1 eq.)	3	THF	−78°C	68
LiHMDS (1.0M THF) (2 eq.)	3	Toluene	−78°C	56
KHMDS (3 eq.)	7	Toluene	−78°C	42
NaH (2 eq.)	50	THF	−78°C	17
NaOMe (2 eq.)	75	THF	Reflux	0
KOtBu (3 eq.)	10	THF	25°C	19
LiHMDS (1.0M THF) (3.5 eq.)	7	Toluene	−50°C to−30°C	92

[a]Isolated yield.

Table 8 Synthesis of β-keto esters by cross-Claisen condensation

Compound number	Ester	Product	Yield (%)
1			78
2			75
3			64
4			72
5			80
6			69
7			74
8			74
9			58
10			70
11			80
12			92

Table 8 Synthesis of β-keto esters by cross-Claisen condensation *(Continued)*

Compound number	Ester	Product	Yield (%)
13			72
14			77
15			84
16			78
17			65[a]
18			61
19			48
20			74
21			74
22			0[a]
23			81

Table 8 Synthesis of β-keto esters by cross-Claisen condensation *(Continued)*

24		78
25		81
26		79
27		0[a]

[a]Percentage of products in crude LC-MS.

pyrazolones efficiently using cyclic ketones. Since this method is successful for different ketones, it can also be useful for the synthesis of pharmaceutically important pyrazolones.

We have investigated the newly synthesized pyrazoles for their antibacterial activity against *E. coli* (ATTC-25922), *S. aureus* (ATTC-25923), *P. aeruginosa* (ATTC-27853) and *K. pneumonia* (recultured) bacterial strains by the disc diffusion method [57,58]. Results of these studies were given in Table 1 and compared with the standard ciprofloxacin. Most of the synthesized compounds exhibited very good bacterial activity; particularly, compounds 7, 13, 14, 23, 25 and 26 have shown very good inhibition against all the bacterial strains tested. Compounds 9 to 11, 13, 14, 19, 20 and 26 have shown a moderate to good inhibition against all the bacterial strains. Compounds 8 and 24 have poor bacterial

activity. The SAR studies on these compounds revealed that the aliphatic substituents (either cyclic or acyclic) on the main cage increase their biological activities. On the other hand, compounds bearing the aromatic substituents and the fused ring systems decrease their activity. Halogen substitution in alkyl group also reduces their activity. Some of the tested compounds are equipotent or more potent than the standards used.

Newly synthesized pyrazoles were screened for their antifungal activity against *A. flavus* (NCIM no. 524), *A. fumigates* (NCIM no. 902), *P. marneffei* (recultured) and *T. mentagrophytes* (recultured) in DMSO by the serial plate dilution method [34-36]. Most of the tested compounds exhibited good fungicidal activities; particularly, compounds 10, 11, 19 and 25 were found to be highly potent to all the four fungi tested. Compounds 1 to 9, 13 to 15, 17, 20, 21, 23, 25 and 26 were shown to have good to moderate activity to all the fungi tested.

All the synthesized compounds 1 to 26 have been subjected to the docking studies against ACHN (human renal cell carcinoma), Panc-1 (human pancreatic adenocarcinoma) and HCT-116 (human colon cancer) and then subjected to WST-1 cytotoxicity assay. Among the 26 synthesized compounds, compounds 14, 20 and 4 are found to have least binding energy value and Z score value. These compounds are more stable ligand-receptor complex amongst other compounds. Compound 14 shows the best binding conformation with nf-κb (total energy = −91.9971 kcal/mol, Z score = −119). The best binding mode of compound 14 at the NF-κb binding site and the residues involved in the interaction, corresponding two-dimensional (2D) interaction models, hydrogen bonds and bond distance are shown in Figure 1. Compound 14 binds to the binding sites and forms three hydrogen bonds with NF-κb involved in pancreatic cancer. It can be seen in Figure 1 that nitrogen atoms of compound 14 formed a hydrogen bond with Pro-65 and

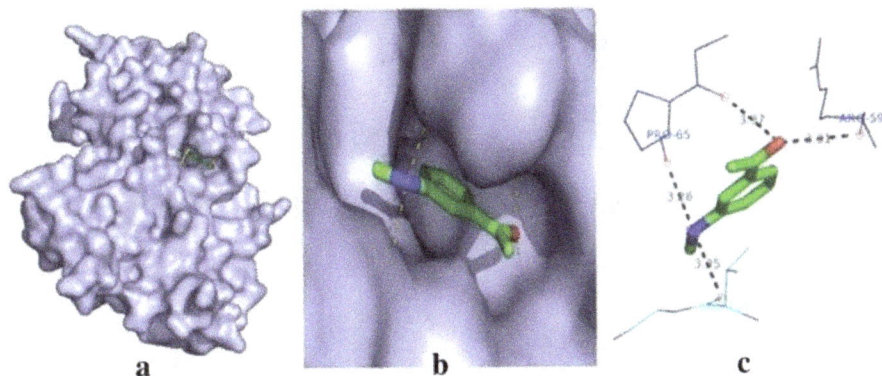

Figure 1 Molecular docking result of compound 14. (a) The docked poses of compound 14 at the site of nuclear factor kappa b; target protein is shown in the surface model, and the ligand is shown in the stick model. **(b)** A close-up view of the docked pose of compound 14. **(c)** The amino acid residue interaction, hydrogen bond networks in the binding pocket and the distance (in Angstrom units) of bonds are shown.

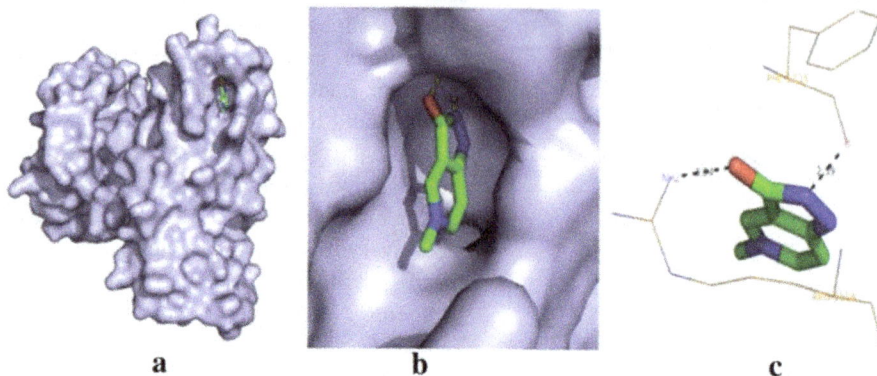

Figure 2 Molecular docking result of compound 18. (a) Binding pose of compound **18** in the vascular endothelial growth factor receptor-2. **(b)** A close-up view of the binding pose of compound **18**; protein structure is shown in the surface model, and the ligand is shown in the stick model. **(c)** H bond networks with protein residues are shown.

Val115. In addition, Arg59 has one H bond with the bond distance of 3.91 Å. The binding pose and inter-action mode of compound **14** are shown in Figure 1.

The post-docking analysis of compound **18** has shown higher affinity with VGFR2 which has key role in renal cancer development (total energy = −104.9856 kcal/mol, Z score = −125.5). Compound **18** binds to the VGFR2 and forms one H bond interaction with Arg118 and Phe115 residues. The best binding pose of compound **18** in the VGFR2 and corresponding 2D interaction models, hydrogen bonds and bond distance are depicted in Figure 2. Docking analysis of compound **1** has shown the best conformation with PI3K (total energy = −119.541 kcal/mol, Z score = −125.5). The binding affinity of compound **1** towards PI3K is investigated in detail. On analysis of the interaction and position of compound **1** in the PI3K binding site, it is observed that five H bonds are found, and the amino acid residues Asp654, Gln846, ARG649 and Trp201 participated in the interaction. The

surface of PI3K with compound **1** along with the main contact residues of PI3K is labelled, and hydro-gen bond distances are shown in Figure 3.

In continuation of the docking analysis, the com-pounds **1** to **26** have been subjected to the cyctotoxicity studies. Towards this, a panel of three cancer cells representing multiple cancers of clinical relevance were obtained from ATCC, namely ACHN (human renal cell carcinoma), Panc-1 (human pancreatic adenocarcinoma) and HCT-116 (human colon cancer). Cells were main-tained in DMEM containing 10% heat-inactivated fetal bovine serum and kept in humidified 5% CO_2 incubator at 37°C. Logarithmically growing cells were plated at a density of 5×10^3 cells/well in a 96-well tissue culture grade micro-plate and allowed to recover overnight. The cells were challenged with varying concentration of com-pounds for 48 h. Control cells received standard media containing dimethylsulfoxide vehicle at a concentration of 0.2%. After 48 h of incubation, cell toxicity was

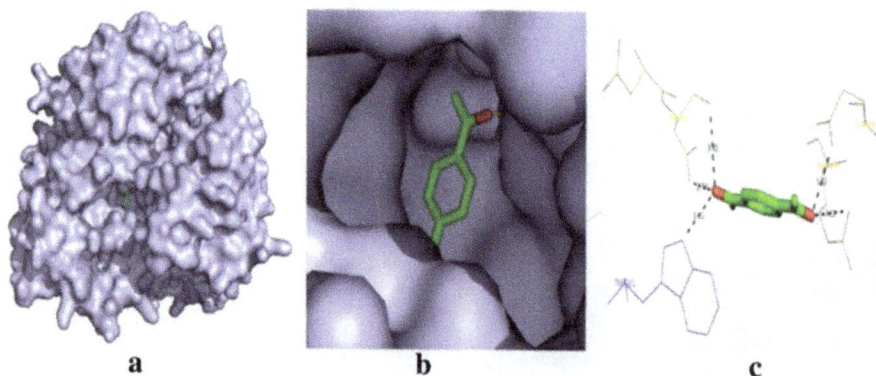

Figure 3 Molecular docking result of compound 1. (a) Docked poses of compound **1** in human phosphoinositide 3-kinase binding site. **(b)** A close-up view of the docked pose of compound **1**; protein structure is shown in the surface model, and the ligand is shown in the stick model (color by atom). **(c)** H bond networks and bond distance are shown.

determined by the CCK-8 reagent (Dojindo Molecular Technologies, Inc.); (WST-1 [2-(2-methoxy-4-nitrophenyl)-3-(4-nitrophenyl)-5-(2,4-disulfophenyl)]-2H-tetrazolium, monosodium salt assay). In accordance with the manufacturer's instructions [36], 5 µL/well CCK-8 reagent was added, and plates were incubated for 2 h. Cytotoxicity of all the compounds have been determined by measuring the absorbance on Tecan Sapphire multi-fluorescence micro-plate reader (Tecan GmbH, Germany) at a wavelength of 450 nm corrected to 650 nm and normalized to controls. Each independent experiment was performed thrice and tabulated in Table 6. The compound **18** was found to be inhibitive against only ACHN (human renal cell carcinoma) cell lines. The compounds **1** and **10** were found to be inhibitive against HCT-116 (human colon cancer) cell lines. The compound **14** was found to be inhibitive against Panc-1 (human pancreatic adenocarcinoma) as well as HCT-116 (human colon cancer) cell lines. The docking poses of the compounds **1**, **10**, **14** and **18** reveals that these molecules are having either more or strong hydrogen bonding interactions with the target molecules which may be due to the presence of either O-alkyl or O-aryl or cyanide groups in it, and hence, these molecules are found to have better activity.

Experimental

General

All the NMR spectra were recorded using Bruker AMX 400 or Bruker DPX 300 instrument (Billerica, MA, USA) with 5-mm PABBO BB-1H tubes. ^{1}H NMR spectra were recorded using approximately 0.03 M solutions in d_6-DMSO at 300 or 400 MHz with tetramethylsilane (TMS) as internal reference. ^{13}C NMR spectra were recorded using approximately 0.05 M solutions in d_6-DMSO at 75 or 100 MHz with TMS as internal reference. In many cases, pyrazolones were recorded in the enol form, whenever d_6-DMSO was used as solvent. Melting points were determined by Buchi B-545 apparatus (Golden Valley, MN, USA). LC-MS were obtained using Agilent 1200 series LC (Santa Clara, CA, USA) and MicromasszQ spectrometer (Manchester, UK).

All reagents were purchased from Sigma-Aldrich (St. Louis, MO, USA) and used as received. LiHMDS solutions were kept under nitrogen atmosphere after opening. Dry toluene, AcOH and EtOH were supplied by Spectrochem (Mumbai, India). All chemistry was performed under a nitrogen atmosphere using standard techniques. The chromatographic separations were performed over silica gel (230 to 400 mesh) using mixtures of EtOAc and methanol or EtOAc and hexane as eluent. Solvents were removed under reduced pressure on a rotovap. Organic extracts were dried with anhydrous Na$_2$SO$_4$. Visualization of spots on TLC plates was

effected by UV illumination, exposure to iodine vapor and heating the plates dipped in KMnO$_4$ stain.

General procedure to synthesize pyrazolones from ketones

LiHMDS (1.0 M solution in toluene, 11 mmol) was added quickly to a solution of ketone (10 mmol in toluene (15 mL) using a syringe at 0°C under stirring and stirred at this temperature for 10 min; then, ethyl chloroformate (11 mmol) was added quickly. Reaction mixture was slowly (10 min) brought to room temperature and stirred for 10 min; then, 2 mL of acetic acid, 15 mL of ethanol and hydrazine hydrate (30 mmol) were added and refluxed for 15 min. Reaction mixture was concentrated to dryness under reduced pressure and redissolved in ethyl acetate, the organic layer was washed with saturated brine solution, dried over Na$_2$SO$_4$ and evaporated under reduced pressure. Crude product was purified by recrystallisation using ethanol.

3-(4-Methoxyphenyl)-1H-pyrazol-5(4H)-one (1)

Purified by recrystallisation using ethanol (white solid), m.p: 221.0°C to 222.3°C, ^{1}H NMR (400 MHz, d_6-DMSO) δ_H: 3.76 (s, 3H, methyl protons of -OCH$_3$), 5.77 (s, 1H, proton at C-4), 6.95 (d, J = 8.80 Hz, 2 Hz, 2H, aryl protons), 7.57 (dd, J = 6.88 Hz and 1.92 Hz, 2H, aryl protons), 9.70 (bs, 1H, -NH proton), 11.90 (bs, 1H, -OH proton); ^{13}C NMR (100 MHz, d_6-DMSO): δ 55.19 (carbon at -OCH$_3$), 86.26 (C-3), 114.20, 123.15, 126.17, 143.09 (aryl carbons), 158.94 (C-4), 161.21 (C-5). MS calculated for C$_{10}$H$_{10}$N$_2$O$_2$: 190.19. Found: 189.0 (M-1).

3-(4-Chlorophenyl)-1H-pyrazol-5(4H)-one (2)

Purified by recrystallisation using ethanol (white solid), m.p: 243.5°C to 245.0°C, ^{1}H NMR (400 MHz, d_6-DMSO) δ_H: 5.93 (s, 1H, proton at C-4), 7.46 (d, J = 6.80 Hz, 2H, aryl protons), 7.69 (d, J = 8.40 Hz, 2H, aryl protons), 9.70 (bs, 1H, -NH proton), 12.15 (bs, 1H, -OH proton); ^{13}C NMR (100 MHz, d_6-DMSO): δ 86.82 (C-4), 126.44, 128.78, 132.10 (aryl carbons), 142.0 (C-3), 160.70 (C-5). MS calculated for C$_9$H$_7$ClN$_2$O: 194.61. Found: 195.0 (M + 1 for Cl^{35}) and 197.0 (M + 3 for Cl^{37}).

3-(4-Fluorophenyl)-1H-pyrazol-5-(4H)-one (3)

Purified by recrystallisation using ethanol (white solid), m.p: 240.0°C to 241.5°C, ^{1}H NMR (400 MHz, d_6-DMSO) δ_H: 5.86 (s, 1H, proton at C-4), 7.23 (t, J = 8.72 Hz, 2H, aryl protons), 7.69 (dd, J = 8.30 and 7.23 Hz, 2H, aryl protons), 9.70 (bs, 1H, -NH proton), 12.00 (bs, 1H, -OH proton); ^{13}C NMR (100 MHz, d_6-DMSO): δ 86.71 (C-4), 115.52, 115.74, 126.82, 126.74 (aryl carbons), 160.41 (C-4), 162.84 (C-5). MS calculated for C$_9$H$_7$FN$_2$O: 178.10. Found: 177.0 (M-1).

4-Methyl-3-phenyl-1H-pyrazol-5(4H)-one (4)

Purified by recrystallisation using ethanol (white solid), m.p: 218.5°C to 220.0°C, ^{1}H NMR (400 MHz, d_6-DMSO) δ_H: 1.99 (s, 3H, methyl protons at C-4), 7.34 (t, J = 7.20 Hz, 1H, *para* proton of aryl), 7.45 (t, J = 8.00 Hz, 2H, *meta* protons of aryl), 7.53 (d, J = 8.00 Hz, 2H, *ortho* protons of aryl), 9.50 (bs, 1H, -NH proton), 11.70 (bs, 1H, -OH proton); ^{13}C NMR (100 MHz, d_6-DMSO): δ 7.66 (methyl carbon at C-4), 95.98 (C-4), 126.31, 127.49, 128.78, 131.15 (aryl carbons), 139.54 (C-3), 160.28 (C-5). MS calculated for $C_{10}H_{10}N_2O$: 174.19. Found: 173.0 (M-1).

4,5,6,7-Tetrahydro-2H-indazol-3(3aH)-one (5)

Purified by recrystallisation using ethanol (white solid), m.p: 286.0°C to 288.0°C, ^{1}H NMR (400 MHz, d_6-DMSO) δ_H: 1.66 to 1.59 (m, 4H, four protons of cyclohexane fused ring), 2.21 (t, J = 5.20 Hz, 2H, two protons of cyclohexane fused ring), 2.42 (t, J = 6.0 Hz, 2H, two protons of cyclohexane fused ring), 9.95 (bs, 2H); ^{13}C NMR (100 MHz, d_6-DMSO): δ 19.35, 21.73, 22.74, 23.32 (carbons of fused cyclohexane part), 98.88 (C-3 of pyrazole ring), 140.19 (C-4 of pyrazole ring), 158.87 (C-5 of pyrazole ring). MS calculated for $C_7H_{10}N_2O$: 138.08. Found: 138.16 (M+).

3a,4,5,6,7,8-Hexahydrocyclohepta(e)pyrazol-3-(2H)-one (6)

Purified by recrystallisation using ethanol (white solid), m.p: 220.5°C to 221.8°C, ^{1}H NMR (400 MHz, d_6-DMSO) δ_H: 1.56 to 1.50 (m, 4H, four protons of fused cycloheptane), 1.71 (d, J = 5.52 Hz, 2H, two protons of fused cycloheptane), 2.29 (t, J = 5.60 Hz, 2H, two protons of fused cycloheptane), 2.50 (t, J = 3.28 Hz, 2H, two protons of fused cycloheptane), 9.20 (bs, 1H, -NH proton), 11.00 (bs, 1H, -OH proton); ^{13}C NMR (100 MHz, d_6-DMSO): δ 23.04, 27.68, 29.36, 32.01 (carbons of fused cycloheptane ring), 102.81 (C-4) 143.81 (C-3 of pyrazole ring), 159.25 (C-5). MS calculated for $C_8H_{12}N_2O$: 152.19. Found: 153.0 (M + 1).

4,5,6,7,8,9-Hexahydro-2H-cycloocta(c)pyraol-3(3aH)-one (7)

Purified by recrystallisation using ethanol (white solid), m.p: 221.6°C to 228.8°C, ^{1}H NMR (400 MHz, d_6-DMSO) δ_H: 1.40 (m, 4H, protons of fused cyclooctane ring), 1.51 (m, 2H, protons of fused cyclooctane ring), 1.58 (m, 2H, protons of fused cyclooctane ring), 2.34 (t, J = 6.2 Hz, 2H, protons of fused cyclooctane ring), 2.54 (t, J = 6.2 Hz, 2H, protons of fused cyclooctane ring), 9.03 (bs, 1H, -NH proton), 11.00 (bs, 1H, -OH proton); ^{13}C NMR (100 MHz, d_6-DMSO): δ 20.13, 24.27, 25.50, 25.76, 28.76, 28.94 (carbons of fused cyclooctane ring), 100.42 (C-4), 141.62 (C-3), 159.42 (C-5). MS calculated for $C_9H_{14}N_2O$: 166.20. Found: 167.0 (M + 1).

3-Cyclohexyl-1H-pyrazol-5(4H)-one (8)

Purified by recrystallisation using ethanol (white solid), m.p: 241.5°C to 243.0°C, ^{1}H NMR (400 MHz, d_6-DMSO) δ_H: 1.21 to 1.26 (m, 1H, proton of cyclohexyl ring), 1.29 to 1.34 (m, 4H, protons of cyclohexyl ring), 1.63 to 1.71 (m, 3H, protons of cyclohexyl ring), 1.84 to 1.90 (m, 2H, protons of cyclohexyl ring)), 2.44 to 2.50 (m, 1H, proton at C1′ of cyclohexyl ring), 5.20 (s, 1H, proton at C-4), 9.30 (bs, 1H, -NH proton), 11.00 (bs, 1H, -OH proton); ^{13}C NMR (100 MHz, d_6-DMSO) δ: 25.97, 26.08, 32.66, 35.60 (carbons of cyclohexyl ring), 86.74 (C-4), 149.83 (C-3), 161.17 (C-5). MS calculated for $C_9H_{14}N_2O$: 166.22. Found: 166.9 (M+).

3-(3-Chloropropyl)-1H-pyrazol-5(4H)-one (9)

Purified by recrystallisation using ethanol (white solid), m.p: 155.8°C to 156.5°C, ^{1}H NMR (400 MHz, d_6-DMSO) δ_H: 2.00 to 1.93 (m, 2H, methylene protons at C2′ of propyl), 2.57 (t, J = 7.36 Hz, 2H, methylene protons at C1′ of propyl), 3.62 (t, 6.40 Hz, 2H, methylene protons at C3′ of propyl), 5.25 (s, 1H), 9.50 (bs, 1H, -NH proton), 11.20 (bs, 1H, -OH proton); ^{13}C NMR (100 MHz, d_6-DMSO): δ 23.51 (C2′ of propyl), 37.18 (C1′ of propyl), 45.13 (C3′ of propyl), 88.56 (C-4), 143.39 (C-3), 161.20 (C-5). MS calculated for $C_6H_9ClN_2O$: 160.60. Found: 161.0 (M + 1 for Cl^{35}) and 163.60 (M + 3 for Cl^{37}).

7-Methoxy-4,5-dihydro-2H-benzo(g)indazol-23(3aH)-one (10)

Purified by recrystallisation using ethanol (white solid), m.p: 116.4°C to 118.2°C, ^{1}H NMR (400 MHz, d_6-DMSO) δ_H: 2.50 (t, J = 5.50 Hz, 2H, protons of cyclohexyl B ring), 2.82 (t, J = 5.6 Hz, 2H, protons of cyclohexyl B ring), 3.75 (s, 3H, protons of methoxy group), 6.80 (d, J = 7.0 Hz, 1H, aryl proton of C ring), 6.86 (s, 1H, aryl proton of C ring), 7.43 (d, J = 7.0 Hz, 1H, aryl proton of C ring), 9.50 (bs, 1H, -NH); ^{13}C NMR (100 MHz, d_6-DMSO): δ 17.91, 30.04, 30.52 (carbons of cyclohexyl B ring), 55.52 (methoxy carbon), 97.83 (C-4), 112.20, 114.59, 114.81, 120.61, 122.61, 138.18, 139.82, 157.82 (C-3), 158.97 (C-5). MS calculated for $C_{12}H_{12}N_2O_2$: 216.23. Found: 215.0 (M-1).

3-(2,3-Dihydrobenzofuran-5-yl)-1H-pyrazol-5(4H)-one (11)

Purified by recrystallisation using ethanol (white solid), m.p: 237.5°C to 239.0°C, ^{1}H NMR (400 MHz, d_6-DMSO) δ_H: 3.19 (t, J = 8.70 Hz, 2H, protons of benzofuran ring), 4.54 (t, J = 8.70 Hz, 2H, protons of benzofuran ring), 5.74 (s, 1H, proton at C-4), 6.67 (d, J = 8.28 Hz, 1H, aryl proton of benzofuran ring), 7.38 (dd, J = 8.28 Hz, 1.82 Hz, 1H, aryl proton of benzofuran ring), 7.51 (s, 1H, aryl proton of benzofuran ring), 9.65 (bs, 1H, -NH proton), 11.85 (bs, 1H, -OH proton); ^{13}C NMR (100 MHz, d_6-DMSO): δ 28.95 (C of benzofuran), 71.14 (C of benzofuran), 86.16 (C-3), 109.05, 121.84, 123.09, 124.77,

127.95 (carbons of benzofuran), 143.51 (C-3), 159.50 (carbon of benzofuran), 161.16 (C-5). MS calculated for $C_{11}H_{10}N_2O_2$: 202.20. Found: 203.0 (M + 1).

3-(Biphenyl-4-yl)-1H-pyrazol-5(4H)-one (12)

Purified by recrystallisation using ethanol (white solid), m.p: 236.5°C to 265.0°C, ^{1}H NMR (400 MHz, d_6-DMSO) δ_H: 5.94 (s, 1H, proton at C-4), 7.37 (t, J = 7.5 Hz, 1H, aryl proton), 7.47 (t, J = 7.5 Hz, 2H, aryl protons), 7.76 to 7.69 (m, 6H, aryl protons), 9.77 (bs, 1H, -NH proton), 12.13 (bs, 1H, -OH proton); ^{13}C NMR (100 MHz, d_6-DMSO): δ 86.88 (C-4), 125.26, 126.51, 126.97, 127.54, 128.96 (aryl carbons), 139.25 (C-3), 139.50 (C-5). MS calculated for $C_{15}H_{10}N_2O_2$: 236.26. Found: 235.0 (M-1).

3-(Thiophen-2-yl)-1H-pyrazol-5(4H)-one (13)

Purified by recrystallisation using ethanol (white solid), m.p: 204.0°C to 205.0°C, ^{1}H NMR (400 MHz, d_6-DMSO) δ_H: 5.67 (s, 1H, proton at C-4), 7.07 (bs, 1H, proton of thiophenyl ring), 7.32 (bs, 1H, proton of thiophenyl ring), 7.42 (bs, 1H, proton of thiophenyl ring), 9.67 (bs, 1H, -NH), 12.05 (bs, 1H, -OH). MS calculated for $C_7H_6N_2OS$: 166.20. Found: 167.0 (M + 1).

3-(5-Oxo-4,5-dihydro-1H-pyrazol-3-yl)benzonitrile (14)

Purified by recrystallisation using ethanol (white solid). ^{1}H NMR (400 MHz, d_6-DMSO) δ_H: 6.02 (s, 1H, proton at C-4), 7.59 (t, J = 10.4 Hz, 1H, aryl proton), 7.73 (d, J = 10.4 Hz, 1H, aryl proton), 7.99 (d, J = 10.4, 1H, aryl proton), 8.12 (s, 1H, aryl proton), 10.00 (bs, 1H, -NH proton), 12.02 (bs, 1H, -OH proton). MS calculated for $C_{10}H_7N_3O$: 185.18. Found: 184.0 (M-1).

Ethyl 3-oxo-2,3,3a,4,6,7-hexahydropyrazolo[4,3-c]pyridine-5-caboxylate (15)

Purified by recrystallisation using ethanol (white solid), m.p: 212.5°C to 213. 8°C, ^{1}H NMR (400 MHz, d_6-DMSO) δ_H: 1.90 (t, J = 7.08 Hz, 3H, methyl of ethyl group), 2.50 (m, 2H, protons of ring B), 3.56 (t, J = 5.7 Hz, 2H, protons of ring B), 4.04 (q, J = 7.08 Hz, 2H, methylene of ethyl group), 4.18 (s, 2H, protons of ring B), 9.80 (bs, 1H, -NH proton), 11.30 (bs, 1H, -OH proton); ^{13}C NMR (100 MHz, d_6-DMSO): δ 14.62 (methyl carbon of ethyl group), 21.62 (carbon of ring B), 21.92 (methylene carbon of ethyl group), 60.89, 96.06 (C-4 of pyrazole ring), 138.12, 155.08 (C-3 of pyrazole ring), 156.33 (C-5 of pyrazole ring). MS calculated for $C_9H_{13}N_3O_3$: 211.21. Found: 212.0 (M + 1).

Tert-butyl 3-oxo-2,3,3a,4,6,7-hexahydropyrazolo[4,3-c]pyridine-5-carboxylate (16)

Purified by recrystallisation using ethanol (white solid), m.p: 225.5°C to 227.5°C, ^{1}H NMR (400 MHz, d_6-DMSO) δ_H: 1.40 (s, 9H, methyl protons of Boc), 2.49 (t, q = 1.77 Hz, 2H, protons of ring B), 3.51 (t, J = 5.72 Hz, 2H, protons of ring B), 4.13 (s, 2H, protons of ring B); ^{13}C NMR (100 MHz, d_6-DMSO): δ 21.75 (carbons of B ring), (28.08 methyl carbons of Boc group), 59.77 (carbon of B ring), 78.94 (quaternary carbon of Boc), 96.21 (C-4 of pyrazole ring), 138.24 (C-3 carbon of pyrazole ring), 154.19 (C-5 carbon of pyrazole ring), 156.37 (carbonyl carbon of Boc). MS calculated for $C_{11}H_{17}N_3O_3$: 239.27. Found: 239.8 (M+).

3-(2,5-Dimethylfuran-3-yl)-1H-pyrazol-5(4H)-one (17)

Purified by recrystallisation using ethanol (white solid), ^{1}H NMR (400 MHz, d_6-DMSO) δ_H: 2.21 (s, 3H, methyl proton of furan ring), 2.32 (s, 3H, methyl proton of furan ring), 5.51 (s, 1H, proton at C-4) 6.27 (s, 1H, proton of furan ring), 9.60 (bs, 1H, -NH proton), 11.62 (bs, 1H, -OH proton). MS calculated for $C_9H_{10}N_2O_2$: 178.18. Found: 179. 0 (M + 1).

Benzyl 3-oxo-2,3,3a,4,6,7-hexahydropyrazolo[4,3-c]pyridine-5-carboxylate (18)

Purified by recrystallisation using ethanol (white solid), m.p: 225.4°C to 226.1°C, ^{1}H NMR (400 MHz, d_6-DMSO) δ_H: 2.50 to 2.56 (m, 2H, protons of ring B), 3.61 (s, 2H, protons of ring B), 4.23 (d, J = 10.80 Hz, 2H, protons of ring B), 5.10 (s, 2H, protons of methylene of Cbz group), 7.38 to 7.30 (m, 5H, aryl protons of Cbz), 9.88 (bs, 1H, -NH proton), 11.16 (bs, 1H, -OH proton); ^{13}C NMR (100 MHz, d_6-DMSO): δ 41.27, 42.77, 66.39 (carbons of ring B), 86.72 (C-4), 127.69, 127.01, 128.46 (aryl carbons), 136.90 (C-3), 157.72 (C-5). MS calculated for $C_{14}H_{15}N_3O_3$: 273.28. Found: 273.8 (M+).

5-Tert-butyl-4,5,6,7-tetrahydro-2H-indazol-3(3aH)-one (19)

Purified by recrystallisation using ethanol (white solid), m.p: 243.5°C to 244.8°C, ^{1}H NMR (400 MHz, d_6-DMSO) δ_H: 0.89 (s, 9H, protons of three methyl groups), 1.18 to 1.25 (m, 2H, protons of ring B), 1.85 to 1.92 (m, 2H, protons of ring B), 2.39 to 2.29 (m, 2H, protons of ring B), 2.55 (m, 1H, proton of ring B); ^{13}C NMR (100 MHz, d_6-DMSO): δ 20.73 (carbons of methyl groups of tertiary group), 22.54, 24.48, 27.81, 27.85, 32.70, 45.50 (quaternary carbon of tertiary group), 99.42 (C-4 of pyrazole ring), 140.46 (C-3 of pyrazole ring), 158.88 (C-5 of pyrazole ring). MS calculated for $C_{11}H_{18}N_2O$: 194.21. Found: 194.8 (M+).

3-(Biphenyl-4-yl)-1-(4-fluorophenyl)-1H-pyrazol-5(4H)-one (20)

Purified by recrystallisation using ethanol (white solid), m.p: 156.2°C to 157.5°C, ^{1}H NMR (400 MHz, d_6-DMSO) δ_H: 6.07 (s, 1H at C-4), 7.31 to 7.40 (m, 3H, aryl protons), 7.48 (t, J = 8.0 Hz, 2H, aryl protons), 7.07 to 7.33 (m, 4H, aryl protons), 7.83 to 7.93 (m, 4H, aryl protons), 11.94 (bs, 1H, -OH proton at C-5); ^{13}C NMR (100 MHz,

d_6-DMSO): δ 85.57 (C-4), 116.01, 116.24, 123.52, 123.60, 126.10, 126.96, 127.25, 127.94, 129.42, 132.92, 135.74, 139.91, 140.17 (aryl carbons), 149.69 (C-3), 154.18, 159.05 (aryl carbons), 161.46 (C-5). MS calculated for $C_{21}H_{15}FN_2O$: 330.55. Found: 329.0 (M-1).

3-Ethyl-4-methyl-1H-pyrazol-5(4H)-one (21)

Purified by recrystallisation using ethanol (white solid), m.p: 233.4°C to 234.1°C, ^{1}H NMR (400 MHz, d_6-DMSO) δ_H: 1.07 (t, J = 7.64 Hz, 3H, methyl protons of ethyl group), 1.72 (s, 3H, methyl at C-4), 2.40 (q, J = 7.6 Hz, 2H, methylene protons of ethyl group), 9.50 (bs, 1H, -OH proton), 10.05 (bs, 1H, -OH proton); ^{13}C NMR (100 MHz, d_6-DMSO): δ 11.34 (methyl carbon of ethyl group), 18.35 (methyl group at C-4), 22.99 (methylene carbon of ethyl group), 99.73 (C-4), 147.27 (C-3), 164.86 (C-5). MS calculated for $C_6H_{10}N_2O$: 126.15. Found: 128.0 (M + 2).

4-Ethyl-3-phenyl-1H-pyrazol-5(4H)-one (23)

Purified by recrystallisation using ethanol (white solid), m.p: 88.3°C to 89.1°C. ^{1}H NMR (400 MHz, d_6-DMSO) δ_H: 1.15 (t, J = 7.6 Hz, 3H, protons of methyl group), 2.64 (q, J = 7.6 Hz, 2H, protons of methylene group), 7.17 to 7.13 (m, 1H), 7.41 to 7.32 (m, 3H), 10.00 (bs, 2H, -OH and -NH protons); ^{13}C NMR (100 MHz, d_6-DMSO): δ 13.57 (methyl carbon of ethyl group), 19.10 (methylene carbon of ethyl group), 102.27 (C-4), 125.34 (ipso), 128.12 (ortho), 128.60 (meta), 133.88 (para), 142.49 (C-3), 159.20 (C-5). MS calculated for $C_{11}H_{12}N_2O$: 188.22. Found: 188.8 (M+).

3-Cyclohexyl-4-methyl-1H-pyrazol-5(4H)-one (24)

Purified by recrystallisation using ethanol (white solid), m.p: 205.4°C to 206.2°C. ^{1}H NMR (400 MHz, d_6-DMSO) δ_H: 1.25 to 1.28 (m, 1H, proton of cyclohexyl ring) 1.32 to 1.40 (m, 4H, protons of cyclohexyl ring), 1.66 to 1.76 (m, 8H, 5 protons of cyclohexyl ring and protons of methyl group), 2.40 to 2.50 (m, 1H, proton of cyclohexyl ring), 9.50 (bs, 1H, -NH proton) 10.52 (bs, 1H, -OH proton); ^{13}C NMR (100 MHz, d_6-DMSO): δ 6.91 (carbon of methyl group), 26.01, 26.53, 31.91, 36.42 (carbons of cyclohexyl ring), 94.38 (C-4), 145.71 (C-3), 160.12 (C-5). MS calculated for $C_{10}H_{16}N_2O_2$: 180.24. Found: 180.8 (M+).

3-Cyclopropyl-1H-pyrazol-5(4H)-one (25)

Purified by recrystallisation using ethanol, m.p: 215.5°C to 216.8°C (white solid). ^{1}H NMR (400 MHz, d_6-DMSO) δ_H: 0.58 to 0.55 (m, 2H, protons of cyclopropyl), 0.85 to 0.81 (m, 2H, protons of cyclopropyl), 1.75 to 1.68 (m, 1H, proton of cyclopropyl), 9.50 (bs, 1H, -NH proton), 11.52 (bs, 1H, -OH proton); ^{13}C NMR (100 MHz, d_6-DMSO): δ 7.27 (C-1′ of cyclopropyl ring), 7.59 (C-2′, 3′ of cyclopropyl

ring), 85.78 (C-4), 146.75 (C-3), 160.78 (C-5). MS calculated for $C_6H_8N_2O$: 124.14. Found: 124.9 (M+).

3-Isopropyl-1H-pyrazol-5(4H)-one (26)

Purified by recrystallisation using ethanol, m.p: 198.2°C to 199.4°C (white solid). ^{1}H NMR (400 MHz, d_6-DMSO) δ_H: 1.13 (d, J = 6.92 Hz, 6H), 2.79 to 2.72 (m, 1H), 5.20 (s, 1H), 9.32 (bs, 1H, -NH proton), 11.50 (bs, 1H, -OH proton); ^{13}C NMR (100 MHz, d_6-DMSO): δ 22.24 (carbon of two CH_3 of iso-propyl), 25.69 (methine carbon of iso-propyl), 86.22 (C-4), 150.39 (C-3), 160.75 (C-5). MS calculated for $C_6H_{10}N_2O$: 126.15. Found: 126.9 (M+).

Conclusions

The β-keto esters from ethyl chloroformate was successfully attempted, and the developed method is simple, fast and applicable to the ketones having the alkyl halogens, protecting groups like Boc and Cbz that were tolerated and proved to be useful in the synthesis of fused bicyclic and tricyclic pyrazolones efficiently using cyclic ketones. Since this method is successful for different ketones, it can be useful for the synthesis of pharmaceutically important pyrazolones also. All the new pyrazolones were subjected to antimicrobial, docking and cytotoxicity assay against ACHN (human renal cell carcinoma), Panc-1 (human pancreatic adenocarcinoma) and HCT-116 (human colon cancer) cell line. Most of them were found to be active against different bacterial and fungal strains tested, and some of them were found to have promising activity. The in silico and cytotoxicity studies reveal that compound **18** was found to be inhibitive against only ACHN (human renal cell carcinoma) cell lines. The compounds **1** and **10** were found to be inhibitive against HCT-116 (human colon cancer) cell lines. The compound **14** was found to be inhibitive against Panc-1 (human pancreatic adenocarcinoma) as well as HCT-116 (human colon cancer) cell lines, and hence, further investigations are in need in these promising lead molecules.

Additional file

Additional file 1: Spectral evidences. A copy of original ^{1}H NMR and ^{13}C NMR spectra of the compounds **1** to **26** has been included.

Competing interests

The authors declare that they have no competing interests.

Acknowledgements

The authors are grateful to Syngene International Pvt. Ltd., Bengaluru for providing spectral facilities. They are also thankful to the VIT management for their generous support and facilities.

Author details

^{1}Centre for Organic and Medicinal Chemistry, VIT University, Vellore 632 014, India. ^{2}Medical and Biological Computing Laboratory, School of Biosciences and Technology, VIT University, Vellore 632 014, India. ^{3}Industrial

Biotechnology Division, School of Bio Sciences and Technology, VIT University, Vellore 632 014, India. [4]Department of Oncology, HCS & HTS, Piramal Life Sciences Ltd. Guregaon (E), Mumbai 400063, India. [5]Department of Biochemistry, K.S. Hegde Medical Academy, Deralakatte 574 162, India.

References

1. Ueda TH, Mase N, Oda II (1981) Synthesis of pyrazolone derivatives. XXXIX. Synthesis and analgesic activity of pyrano[2,3,-c]pyrazoles. Chem Pharm Bull 29:3522–3528

2. Hukki J, Laitinen P, Alberty JE (1968) Preparation and pharmacological activity of pyrazole derivatives with potential antihistaminic properties II. An attempted synthesis of 1-phenyl and 1-benzyl-3-methyl-5-pyrazolones aminoalkylated at position 2. Pharm Acta Helv 43:704–712

3. Nakagawa H, Ohyama R, Kimata A, Suzuki T, Miyata N (2006) Hydroxyl radical scavenging by edaravone derivatives: efficient scavenging by 3-methyl-1-(pyridine-2-yl)-5-pyrazolone with an intramolecular base. Bioorg Med Chem Lett 16:5939–5942

4. Kawai H, Nakai H, Suga M, Yuki S, Watanabe T, Saito KI (1997) Effects of a novel free radical scavenger, MCI-186, on ischemic brain damage in the rat distal middle cerebral artery occlusion model. J Pharmacol Exp Ther 281:921–927

5. Watanabe T, Yuki S, Egawa M, Nishi H (1984) Protective effects of MCI-186 on cerebral ischemia: possible involvement of free radical scavenging and antioxidant actions. J Pharmacol Exp Ther 268:1597–1604

6. Wu TW, Zeng LH, Wu J, Fung KP (2002) Myocardial protection of MCI-186 in rabbit ischemia-reperfusion. Life Sci 71:2249–2255

7. Barba O, Jones LH (2004) Pyrazole derivatives as reverse transcriptase inhibitors.. WO Patent 029042 A1, 8 Apr 2004

8. Plath P, Rohr W, Wuerzer B (1980) Herbicides containing 3-aryl-5-methylpyrazole-4-carboxylic acid esters. Ger Offen. DE 2920933 A1 1801204, 4 Dec 1980

9. Cativiela C, Serrano JL, Zurbano MM (1995) Synthesis of 3-substituted pentene-2,4-diones: valuable intermediates for liquid crystals. J Org Chem 60:3074–3083

10. Sugiura S, Ohno S, Ohtani O, Izumi K, Kitamikado T, Asai H, Kato K, Hori M, Fujimura H (1977) Synthesis and antiinflammatory and hypnotic activity of 5-alkoxy-3-(N-substituted carbomoyl)-1-phenyl pyrazoles. J Med Chem 20:80–85

11. Sabaa MW, Oraby FH, Abdel-Naby AS, Mohamed RR (2006) Organic thermal stabilizers for rigid poly(vinylchloride). Part XII: N-phenyl-3-substituted-5-pyrazolone derivatives. Polym Degrad Stab 91:911–923

12. Kendall JD, Duffin GF (1955) Production of 3-pyrazolidones. US Patent: 2,704,762. Chem Abstr 50:2680f

13. Reynolds GA (1955) Photographic developer composition. US Patent: 2,688,548. Chem Abstr 49:596

14. Johnson MP, Moody CJ (1985) Azodienophiles. Diels-Alder reactions of 4-phenyl-1,2,4-triazole-3,5-dione and 5-phenylpyrazole-3-one with functionalised diones. J Chem Soc Perkin Trans 1:71–74

15. Hiremath SP, Saundane AR, Mruthyunjayaswamy BHM (1993) A new method for the synthesis of 6H,11H-indolo[3,2-c]-isoquinolin-5-ones/thiones and their reactions. J Heterocycl Chem 30:603–609

16. Duffy KJ, Darcy MG, Delorme E, Dillon SB, Eppley DF, Miller CE, Giampa L, Hopson CB, Huang Y, Keenan RM, Lamb P, Leong L, Liu N, Miller SG, Price AT, Rosen J, Shaw TN, Smith H, Stark KC, Tain SS, Tyree C, Wiggall KJ, Zhang L, Luengo JI (2001) Hydrazinonapthalene and azonapthalene thrombopoietin mimics are nonpeptidyl promoters of megakaryocytopoiesis. J Med Chem 44:3730–3745

17. Jonathan FM, David JB, Kelvin C, John PM, Mark HS (1995) Novel antagonists of platelet-activating factor. 2. Synthesis and structure-activity relationships of potent and long-acting heterofused[1,5]benzodiazepine and [1,4]diazepine derivatives of 1-phenyl-2-methyl imidazo[4,5-c]pyridine. J Med Chem 38:3524–3535

18. Darin EK, Miller RB, Mark JK (1999) Fused pyrazoloheterocycles: intramolecular [3 + 2]-nitrile oxide cycloadditions applied to syntheses of pyrazolo [3,4-g] [2,1] dihydrobenzoisoxazol(in)es. Tetrahedron Lett 40:3535–3538

19. Janja M, Vinko S (1995) Preparation of homologous pyrazolonedicarboxylates. Heterocycles 41:1207–1218

20. Tietze LF, Steinmetz A (1996) A general and expedient method for the solid-phase synthesis of structurally diverse 1-phenylpyrazolone derivatives. Synlett:667–668

21. Kuo S, Huang L, Nakamura K (1984) Studies on heterocyclic compounds. 6. Synthesis and analgesic and anti-inflammatory activities of 3,4-dimethylpyrano[2,3-c] pyrazol-6-one. J Med Chem 27:539–544

22. Boeckman RK, Jr, Reed JE, Ge P (2001) A novel route to 2,3-pyrazol-1 (5H)-ones via palladium-catalyzed carbonylation of 1,2-diaza-1,3-butadienes. Org Lett 3:3651–3653

23. Hans N, Gernot K, Juergen DH (1985) Hydrazidine, IV. Reaktion von Hydrazidinenmit 1,2-bifunktionellen Verbindungen. Liebigs Ann Chem GE 1:78–89

24. Habi A, Gravel D (1994) Efficient 1,3 ester shift in α-disubstituted β-keto ester enolates. Remarkable influence of the metal counterion on the rate of reaction. Tetrahedron Lett 35:4315–4318

25. Gavrilenko BB, Miller SI (1975) Synthesis and properties of 3-amino-3-pyrazolin-5-ones. J Org Chem 40:2720–2724

26. Hu Q, Guan H, Hu C (1995) Synthesis of 3-hydrox-5-per(poly) fluoroalkylpyrazoles. J Fluorine Chem 75:51–54

27. Al-Jallo HN, Al-Khashab A, Sallomi IG (1972) Reactions of unsaturated tetra and tri-esters with hydrazine hydrate and semicarbazide hydrochloride. J Chem Soc Perkin Trans 1:1022–1023

28. Zhang Q, Lu L (2000) A novel synthetic route to ethyl 3-substituted-trans-2,3-difluoro-2-acrylates and their reactions with nucleophiles. Tetrahedron Lett 41:8545–8548

29. Omar MT, Sherif FA (1981) New synthetic route to 3-oxo-5-phenyl-2, 3-dihydro-pyrazoles. Synthesis:742–743

30. Tietze LT, Evers H, Hippe T, Steinmetz A, Topkin E (2001) Solid-phase synthesis of substituted pyrazolones from polymer-bound beta-ketoesters. Eur J Org Chem 2001(9):1631–1634

31. Kobayashi S, Furuta T, Sugaita K, Oyamada H (1998) Use of acyl hydrazones as electrophiles in Mannich-type reactions, β-lactam, pyrazolidinone, and pyrazolone synthesis. Synlett:1019–1021

32. Oyamada H, Kobayashi S (1998) Rare earth triflate-catalyzed addition reactions of acylhydrazones with silyl enolates. A facile synthesis of pyrazole derivatives. Synlett:249–250

33. Kobayashi S, Furuta T, Sugita D, Okitsu O, Oyamada H (1999) Polymer-supported acylhydrazones. Use of Sc(OTf)₃-catalyzed Mannich-type reactions providing an efficient method for the preparation of diverse pyrazolone derivatives. Tetrahedron Lett 40:1341–1344

34. Adkins H, Elofson RM, Rossow AG, Robinson CC (1949) The oxidation potentials of aldehydes and ketones. J Am Chem Soc 71:3622–3629

35. Pratt DD, Robinson R (1925) A synthesis of pyrylium salts of anthocyanidin type. Part V. The synthesis of cyanidin chloride and of delphinidin chloride. J Chem Soc Trans 127:166–175

36. Stahler G, Waltersdorfer A (1984) 1-Alkyl-3-alkoxymethyl-4-alkoxy-5-dialkyl carbamethoxypyrazoles and use as aphicides. US Patent: 4447444 A. Chem Abstr 101:151840

37. Petersen JM, Hauser CR (1949) Acylation of certain α-alkoxy and α-aryloxy ketones and esters. J Am Chem Soc 71:770–773

38. Hiroaki M, Haruro I, Masakazu I (2008) Selective synthesis of α-substituted β-ketoesters from aldehydes and diazoesters on memoporous silica catalysts. Tetrahedron Lett 49:4788–4791

39. Yadav JS, Subba Reddy BV, Eeshwaraiah B, Reddy PN (2005) Niobium (V) chloride-catalyzed C-H insertion reactions of α-diazoesters: synthesis of α-ketoesters. Tetrahedron 61:875–878

40. Barbieri G, Seonane G, Trabazo JL, Riva A, Umpierrez F, Radesca L, Tubio R, Kart LD, Hudicky T (1987) General method of synthesis for natural long-chain β-diketones. J Nat Products 50:646–649

41. Maibaum J, Rich DH (1988) A facile synthesis of statine and analogs by reduction of β-keto esters from Boc-protected amino acids. HPLC analyses of their enantiomeric purity. J Org Chem 53:869–873

42. Schmidt HW, Kalde M (1988) A convenient synthesis of β-ketodiesters. Org Prep Proced Int 20:184–187

43. Mills FD, Mills GD, Brown RT (1989) Synthesis of methylene-linked pyrethroids. J Agr Food Chem 37:501–507

44. Oikawa Y, Sugano K, Yonemitsu O (1978) Meldrum's acid in organic synthesis. 2. A general and versatile synthesis of beta keto esters. J Org Chem 43:2087–2088

45. Khoukhi N, Vaultier M, Carrie R (1987) Synthesis and reactivity of methyl γ-azido and ethyl σ-azidovalarates and of the corresponding acid chlorides as useful reagents for the aminoalkylation. Tetrahedron 43:1811–1822

46. Chu DTW, Maleczka RE (1987) Synthesis of 4-oxo-4H-quino[2,3,4-i, j] [1,4] benoxazine-5-carboxylic acid derivatives. J Heterocycl Chem 24:453–456

47. Mansour TS, Evans CA (1990) Decarboxylative carbon acylation of malonates with aminoacylimidazoles mediated by lewis acids. Synthetic Commun 20:773–781

48. Rathke M, Nowak MA (1985) Synthesis of beta-keto acids and methyl ketones using bis(trimethylsilyl) malonate and triethylamine in the presence of lithium or magnesium halides. Synthetic Commun 15:1039–1049

49. Taylor EC, Turchi I (1978) A convenient synthesis of β-ketoesters. Org Prep Proced Int 10:221–224

50. Mellow DS, Baumgarten E, Hauser CR (1994) A new synthesis of beta-ketoesters of the type RCOCH$_2$COOC$_2$H$_5$. J Am Chem Soc 66:1286

51. Banerji A, Jones RB, Mellows G, Phillips L, Sim KY (1976) Fusicoccin. Part 6. Biosynthesis of fusicoccin from [3-^{13}C] and (4R)-[4-^{3}H]-mevalonic acid. J Chem Soc Perkin Trans 1:2221–2228

52. Tetsuo T, Yoshiki C, Takeo S (1980) A copper(I)-bicarbonato complex. A water-stable reversible carbon dioxide carrier. J Am Chem Soc 102:431–433

53. Hamed O, El-Qisairi A, Patrick MH (2000) Palladium(II) catalyzed carbonylation of ketones. Tetrahedron Lett 41:3021–3024

54. Mori H, Satake Y (1985) Carboxylation of cyclohexanone with carbon dioxide and potassium phenoxide. Dependence of the reaction upon the amount of carbon dioxide complexed with potassium phenoxide. Chem Pharm Bull 33:3469–3472

55. Robert L, Charles RH (1944) The carbethoxylation and carbonylation of ketones using sodium amide. Synthesis of β-ketoester. J Am Chem Soc 66:1768–1770

56. Wallingford Jones H (1941) Alkyl carbonatres in synthetic chemistry. Condensation with ketones. Synthesis of β-ketoesters. J Am Chem Soc 63:2252–2254

57. Cruickshank R, Duguid JP, Marmion BP, Swain RHA (1975) Medicinal microbiology, 12th edn, vol 2. Churchill Livingstone, London, p 196

58. Collins AH (1976) Ed., Microbiological Methods, 2nd edition. Butterworth, London

59. Berman HM, Westbrook J, Feng Z, Gilliland G, Bhat TN, Weissig H, Shindyalov IN, Bourne PE (2000) The Protein Data Bank. Nucleic Acids Res 28:235–242

60. Guex N, Peitsch MC (1997) SWISS-MODEL and the Swiss-Pdb Viewer: an environment for comparative protein modeling. Electrophoresis 18:2714–2723

61. Li Z, Wan H, Shi Y, Ouyang P (2004) Personal experience with four kinds of chemical structure drawing software: review on ChemDraw, ChemWindow, ISIS/Draw, and ChemSketch. J Chem Inf Comput Sci 44(5):1886–1890

62. Pettersen EF, Goddard TD, Huang CC, Couch GS, Greenblatt DM (2004) UCSF Chimera—a visualization system for exploratory research and analysis. J Comput Chem 5:1605–1612

63. Yang J-M, Chen C-C (2004) GEMDOCK: a generic evolutionary method for molecular docking. Proteins: Structure, Function and Bioinformatics 55:288–304

64. Seeliger D, de Groot BL (2010) Ligand docking and binding site analysis with PyMOL and Autodock/Vina. J Comput Aided Mol Des 24(5):417–422

65. Venkat Ragavan R, Vijayakumar V, Sucheta Kumari N (2009) Synthesis of some novel bioactive 4-oxy/thio substituted-1H-pyrazol-5(4H)-ones via efficient cross-Claisen condensation. Eur J Med Chem 44:3852–3857

66. Venkat Ragavan R, Vijayakumar V, Sucheta Kumari N (2010) Synthesis and antimicrobial activities of novel 1,5-diaryl pyrazoles. Eur J Med Chem 45:1173–1180

67. Venkat Ragavan R, Vijayakumar V (2010) A novel route to 4-oxy/thio substituted-1H-pyrazol-5(4H)-ones via efficient cross-Claisen condensation. J Heterocyclic Chem 48:323–330

68. Loh WS, Fun HK, Venkat Ragavan R, Vijayakumar V, Sarveswari S (2011) 4-Methyl-5-phenyl-1H-pyrazol-3(2H)-one. Acta Cryst E67:o151–o152

69. Shahani T, Fun HK, Venkat Ragavan R, Vijayakumar V, Sarveswari S (2010) 4-Methyl-5-phenyl-1H-pyrazol-3-ol. Acta Cryst E66:o1697–o1698

70. Fun HK, Yeap CS, Venkat Ragavan R, Vijayakumar V, Sarveswari S (2010) 4,5,6,7,8,9-Hexahydro-2H-cycloocta-[c]pyrazol-1-ium-3-olate. Acta Cryst E66:o3019

71. Shahani T, Fun HK, Venkat Ragavan R, Vijayakumar V, Sarveswari S (2010) Tert-butyl 3-oxo-2,3,4,5,6,7-hexahydro-1H-pyrazolo[4,3-c]pyridine-5-carboxylate. Acta Cryst E66:o142–o143

72. Shahani T, Fun HK, Venkat Ragavan R, Vijayakumar V, Sarveswari S (2010) 5-Ethyl-4-methyl-1H-pyrazol-3(2H)-one. Acta Cryst E66:o1357–o1358

73. Rathore RS, Narasimhamurthy T, Venkat Ragavan R, Vijayakumar V, Sarveswari S (2011) 3-Ethyl-4-methyl-1H-pyrazol-2-ium-5-olate. Acta Cryst E67:o2129

74. Loh WS, Fun HK, Venkat Ragavan R, Vijayakumar V, Venkatesh M (2011) 5-Ethyl-4-phenyl-1H-pyrazol-3(2H)-one. Acta Cryst E67:o403–o404

75. Shahani T, Fun HK, Venkat Ragavan R, Vijayakumar V, Sarveswari S (2010) 5-Cyclohexyl-4-methyl-1H-pyrazol-3(2H)-one monohydrate. Acta Cryst E66:o2760–o2761

23

Synthesis and screening of antibacterial and antifungal activity of 5-chloro-1,3-benzoxazol-2 (3 h)-one derivatives

Priya R Modiya* and Chhaganbhai N Patel

Abstract

Background: An antibacterial is a substance that either kills bacteria or slows their growth. Antifungal are the agents that use drugs for treatment of fungal infections. 5-Chloro-1,3-benzoxazol-2(3 H)-one (5-Chloro Benzoxazolinone) contains an azole ring structure. Numbers of azole compounds are reported as antibacterial and antifungal agents. Benzoxazolinones naturally occur in plants. They play a role as defense compounds against bacteria, fungi, and insects.

Results: In this article, synthesis of six Benzoxazolinone derivatives with various substituents is presented. Benzoxazolinone substituted with *p*-aminobenzoic acids and sulphanilamide derivatives. The above both substituents are reported as potent antimicrobial agents. Attachment with azole leads to increase its potency. The other substituents are 2,4-dichlorobezylchloride. The same rings are found in miconazole and this may lead to increase its antifungal activity. Fluconazole also contains triazole moiety and triazole is having other numbers of activity like antimicrobial, anti-inflammatory, local anesthetic, antiviral, anticancer, antimalarial, etc. Here, there is a substitution for azole ring at 5-Chloro position which might increase antibacterial and antifungal activity. The synthesis and interpretation of six final compounds and three intermediates are presented in this article. Synthesis of 5-Chloro Benzoxazolinone derivatives substituted with Halogenated rings, sulfonated and benzylated derivatives and azole derivatives. There is a synthesis of P2A, P2B, P4A, P4B, P5A, and P6A compounds and their structures were characterized by UV–Visible, IR, MASS spectroscopy, and NMR spectroscopy.

Conclusions: The antibacterial activity of all six compounds is measured against various Gram-positive and Gram-negative bacteria and against fungi. Compounds P4A and P4B have good antibacterial and antifungal activity, half of the Ampicillin and Cephalexin. P4A, P4B, P6A have good activity against *Staphylococcus aureus* and *Escherichia coli*. Compound P2B has good antifungal activity, half of the Miconazole against *Candida albicans*. P2A, P2B, P5A, P6A have almost equal antibacterial activity.

Keywords: Antibacterial, Antifungal, Benzoxazolinone, *p*-aminobenzoic acid, Sulfanilamide, Triazole

Background

An antibacterial is a substance that either kills bacteria or slows their growth. An antifungal drug is a medication used to treat fungal infection such as athlete's foot, ring worm, candidiasis (thrust), serious systemic infections such as *cryptococcal meningitis* and other. The benzoxazolinone ring is having number of activities.

Benzoxazolinone derivatives naturally occur in plants. It has natural defense mechanism in plants against bacteria, fungi, and insects. Antibiotics Qustinamycin and *N*-acetyl Quistinamycin belong to this group. As described in literature review, it has potential as antibacterial and antifungal agents. A number of azoles are used in fungi and bacterial infection. So, here we are going to synthesize various derivatives of benzoxazolinone with various substituents.

---

* Correspondence: modiyapriya@gmail.com
Department of Pharmaceutical Chemistry, Shri Sarvajanik Pharmacy College,
Gujarat Technological University, Arvind Baug, Mehsana 384001, Gujarat, India

Methods

5-Chloro-2(3 H)-benzoxazolinone-3-acetyl-2-(*p*-substituted benzalhydrazone) and 5-chloro-2(3 H)-benzoxazolinone-3-acetyl-2-(*p*-substituted acetophenone) hydrazone derivatives were synthesized (Figure 1). Among them, the analytical data of five original compounds were given. In this study, the microwave synthesis method and antimicrobial evaluation of all the compounds were also reported for the first time. The minimum inhibition concentration (MIC) values of the compounds were determined by the Microdilution method using two Gram-positive bacteria (*Staphylococcus aureus, Bacillus subtilis*), two Gram-negative bacteria (*Pseudomonas aeruginosa, Escherichia coli*), and two yeast-like fungi (*Candida albicans, Candida parapsilosis*) [1]. Fang et al. [2] have reported *N*-(2-(1 H-1,2,4-triazol-1-yl) ethyl)-*N*-(2,4-difluorobenzyl)-2-(1 H-1,2,4-triazol-1-yl)ethanamine hydrochloride, *N*-(2-(1 H-1,2,4-triazol-1-yl)ethyl)-*N*-(2,4-dichlorobenzyl)-2-(1 H-1,2,4-triazol-1-yl)ethanamine hydrochloride, *N*-(2-(1 H-1,2,4-triazol-1-yl)ethyl)-*N*-(3,4-dichlorobenzyl)-2-(1 H-1,2,4-triazol-1-yl)ethanamine hydrochloride and number of other compounds having potent antibacterial and antifungal activity (Figure 2). Miconazole contains two 2,4-dichlorobenzyl ring and imidazole as azole. As per the SAR study of the above compounds, the halogenated ring is responsible for the antifungal activity potential and azoles are also present. So, we will attach the halogenated ring to benzoxazolinone and synthesize the P2A and P2B compounds. A series of novel benzoxazole benzenesulfonamides was synthesized (Figure 3) as inhibitors of fructose-1,6-bisphosphatase (FBPase-1), and they are proved as antibacterial agents [3]. The sulfanilamide derivatives and *p*-aminobenzoic acid are very good

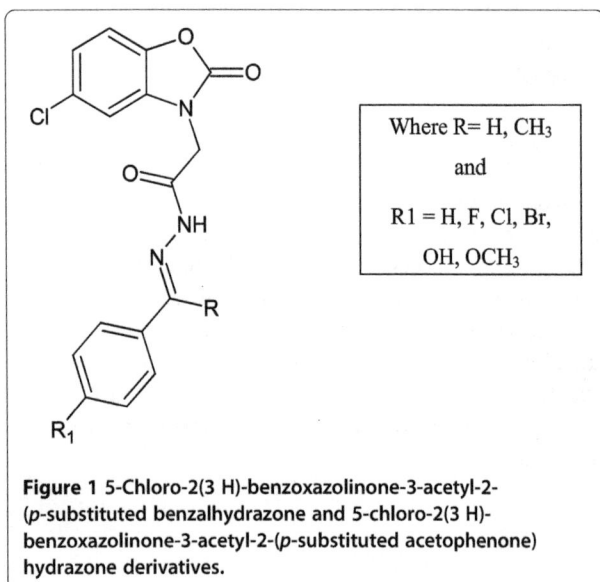

Where Az= Triazole, Imidazole, benzimidazole

Compound code	X1	X2	X3
3a	F	H	F
3b	Cl	H	Cl
3c	H	Cl	Cl
3d	Cl	H	H
7a	F	H	F
7b	Cl	H	Cl
7c	H	Cl	Cl

Figure 2 *N*-(2-(1 H-1,2,4-triazol-1-yl)ethyl)-*N*-(2,4-difluorobenzyl)-2-(1 H-1,2,4-triazol-1-yl)ethanamine hydrochloride, *N*-(2-(1 H-1,2,4-triazol-1-yl)ethyl)-*N*-(2,4-dichlorobenzyl)-2-(1 H-1,2,4-triazol-1-yl)ethanamine hydrochloride, *N*-(2-(1 H-1,2,4-triazol-1-yl)ethyl)-*N*-(3,4-dichlorobenzyl)-2-(1 H-1,2,4-triazol-1-yl) ethanamine hydrochloride.

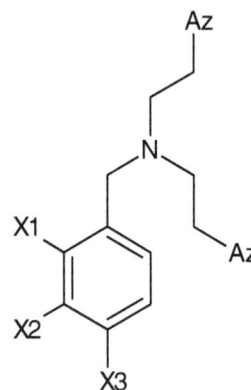

Where R= H, CH₃
and
R1 = H, F, Cl, Br, OH, OCH₃

Figure 1 5-Chloro-2(3 H)-benzoxazolinone-3-acetyl-2-(*p*-substituted benzalhydrazone and 5-chloro-2(3 H)-benzoxazolinone-3-acetyl-2-(*p*-substituted acetophenone) hydrazone derivatives.

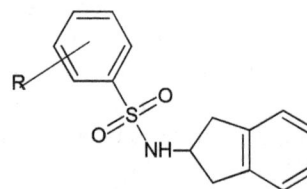

Where R = H, 2-Br, 2-CN, 2-Ph, 3-Cl, 3-NO₂, 3-Ph, 4-F, 4-Me, 4-Ph, 2-Cl, 6-Me

Figure 3 Benzoxazole benzenesulfonamide derivatives.

antimicrobial agents as per traditional drug review. So, here we will attach the sulfanilamide and *p*-aminobenzoic acid with benzoxazolinone. Triazole derivatives are having number of activities. Moreover, fluconazole is having two triazole ring and 2,4-difluorobenzyl ring. Wang et al. [4] have reported triazole substituted with sulfanilamide as potent antimicrobial agent (Figure 4) compounds such as 4-amino-*N*-((1-pentyl-1 H-1,2,3-triazol-4-yl)methyl) benzenesulfonamide, 4-amino-*N*-((1-hexyl-1 H-1,2, 3-triazol-4-yl)methyl)benzenesulfonamide and other compounds [4].

Results and discussion

Antibacterial screening

The microbiological assay is based upon a comparison of inhibition of growth of micro-organisms by measured concentrations of test compounds with that produced by known concentration of a standard antibiotic. Two methods generally employed are *turbidometric (tube-dilution) method* and *cylinder plate (cup-plate) method*. In the turbidometric method, inhibition of growth of microbial culture in a uniform solution of antibiotic in a fluid medium is measured. It is compared with the synthesized compounds. Here, the presence or absence of growth is measured. The cylinder plate method depends upon diffusion of antibiotic from a vertical cylinder through a solidified agar layer in a Petridish or plate to an extent such that growth of added micro-organisms is prevented entirely in a zone around the cylinder containing solution of the antibiotics. The cup-plate method is simple and measurement of inhibition of microorganisms is also easy. Here, we have use this method for antibacterial screening of the test

compounds. The media was prepared from nutrient agar 2%, peptone 1%, beef extract 1%, sodium chloride 0.5%, and distilled water up to 100 mL. All the ingredients were weighed and added to water. This solution was heated on water bath for about one and half-hour till it became clear. This nutrient media was sterilized by autoclave. The antibacterial and antifungal activity was measured against *Bacillus subtillis* (MTCC-212), *Staphylococcus aureus* (MTCC-737) were used as Gram-positive bacteria, *Escherichia coli* (NCLM-2066) were used as Gram-negative bacteria and *Candida albicans* (MTCC-227) was used as fungi for this study. The master culture was prepared on agar slant of the above nutrient media and kept in refrigerator. The working culture was prepared from it by weekly transferred in nutrient agar medium [5,6].

Preparation of inoculums

In the aseptic condition from the working culture, small amount of culture was transferred to about 10–15 mL of sterile normal saline (0.9% NaCl solution). This solution was gently mixed and used for the antibacterial activity. About 0.5 mL of inoculum was added to the sterilized Petridish and melted agar cooled to 45°C was added, mixed gently, and allowed to solidify. Then, Watmann filter paper disk was kept in each plate which was soaked in test drug solutions. The solution was allowed to diffuse for a period of 90 min. The Petri dishes were then incubated at 37°C for 24 h after which zone of inhibition was measured.

Preparation of test solution

Specified quantity of the compound was weighed and dissolved in 5 mL of DMSO and further dilution was made to get the concentration of 500, 1000, and 1500 µg/mL. Similarly, the standard drugs Ampicillin, Cephalexin, and Miconazole were dissolved in appropriate quantity of water to obtain the concentration of 500, 1000, and 1500 µg/mL each. The images of zone of inhibition are given in Figures 5, 6, 7, and 8, and the results are shown in Table 1, and the histogram of antibacterial and antifungal activity is given in Figure 9.

MIC

MIC is the lowest concentration of an antimicrobial that will inhibit the visible growth of a microorganism after overnight incubation. MIC values can be determined by a number of standard test procedures. The most commonly employed methods are the tube dilution and agar dilution methods. Serial dilutions are made of the products in bacterial growth media. The test organisms are then added to the dilutions of the products, incubated, and scored for growth. This procedure is a standard

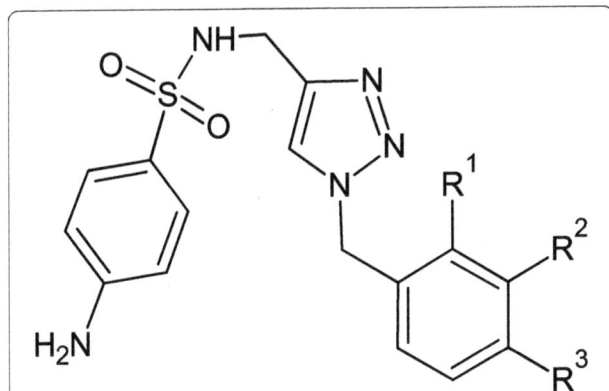

Where $R^1, R^2, R^3 =$ H, F, Cl, NO_2, CH_3

Figure 4 4-Amino-*N*-((1-pentyl-1 H-1,2,3-triazol-4-yl)methyl) benzenesulfonamide, 4-amino-*N*-((1-hexyl-1 H-1,2,3-triazol-4-yl) methyl)benzenesulfonamide.

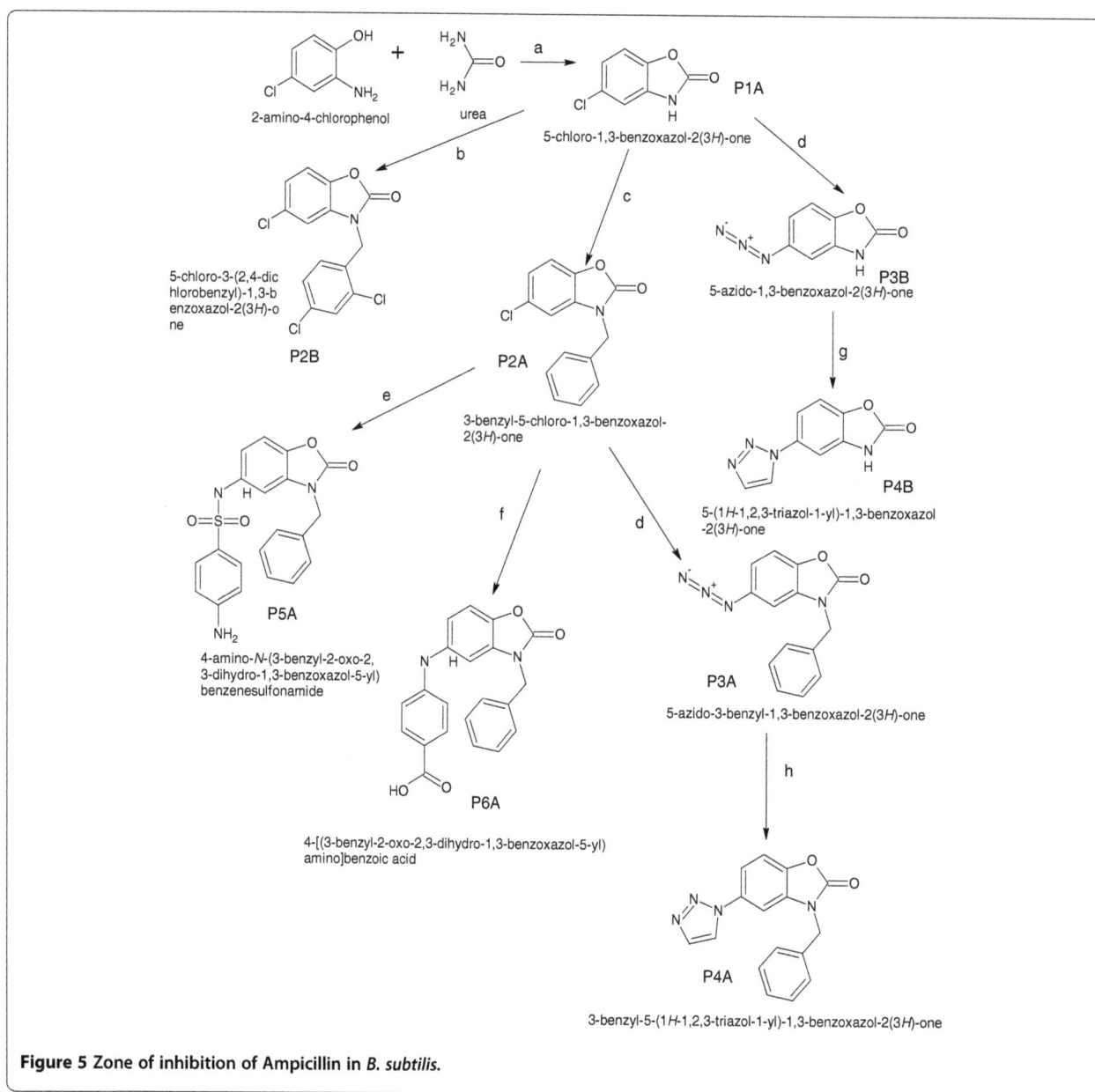

Figure 5 Zone of inhibition of Ampicillin in *B. subtilis*.

assay for antimicrobials. Minimum inhibitory concentrations are important in diagnostic laboratories to confirm resistance of microorganisms to an antimicrobial agent and also to monitor the activity of new antimicrobial agents. A MIC is generally regarded as the most basic laboratory measurement of the activity of an antimicrobial agent against an organism. The data derived from the test can be corrected with the knowledge of expected or measured compound level *in vivo* to predict the efficacy of compound. In this study, MIC was determined using "Serial tube dilution technique". In this technique, the tubes of broth medium, containing graded doses of compounds, are inoculated with the test organisms. After suitable incubation, growth will occur

in those tubes where the concentration of compound is below the inhibitory level and the culture will become turbid (cloudy). Therefore, growth will not occur above the inhibitory level and the tube will remain clear. Results are shown in Table 2 [7].

Procedure

- Twelve test tubes were taken, nine of which were marked 1, 2, 3, 4, 5, 6, 7, 8, 9, and the rest three were assigned as T_M (medium), T_{MC} (medium + compound), and T_{MI} (medium + inoculum).
- 2 mL of nutrient broth medium was poured to each of the 12 test tubes.

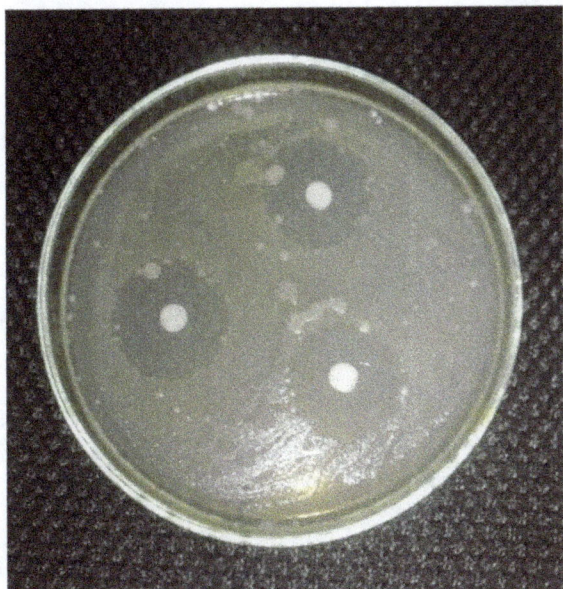

Figure 6 Zone of inhibition of Cephalexin in *E. coli.*

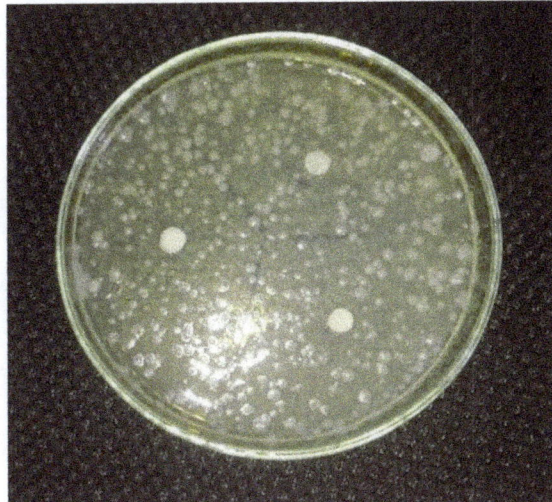

Figure 8 Zone of inhibition of P2B in *C. albicans.*

- These test tubes were cotton plugged and sterilized in an autoclave for 15 lbs/sq. inch pressure.
- After cool 2 mL of the sample solution (5 mg/mL) was added to the first test tube and mixed well and then 2 mL of this content was transferred to the second test tube.
- The content of the second test tube was mixed well and again 2 mL of this mixture was transferred to the third test tube. This process of serial dilution was continued up to the ninth test tube.

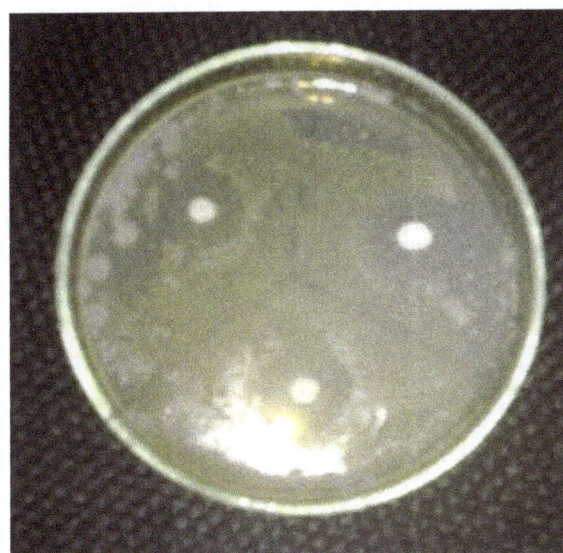

Figure 7 Zone of inhibition of P4B in *S. ureu.*

- *l* of properly diluted inoculum was added to each of nine test tubes and mixed well.
- To the control test tube T_{MC}, 2 mL of the sample was added, mixed well and 2 mL of this mixed content was discarded to check the clarity of the medium in presence of diluted solution of the compound.
- 10 µL of the inoculum was added to the control test tube T_{MI}, observed the growth of the organism in the medium used.
- The control test tube T_M, containing medium only was used to confirm the sterility of the medium.
- All the test tubes were incubated at 37°C for 18 h.
- The resultant concentration in all the nine test tubes will be 2.5 mg/mL, 1.25 mg/mL, 625, 312.5, 156.25, 78.1, 39.06, 19.53, 9.76 µg/mL.

Experimental

All the chemicals used for the synthesis of title compounds were procured from Himedia Laboratories Pvt. Ltd., Mumbai, S. D. Fine Chem. Ltd., Mumbai, Finar Chemicals Ltd., Ahmedabad, Loba chemie Pvt. Ltd., Mumbai, Chemdyes Corporation, Ahmedabad, Spectrochem Pvt. Ltd., Mumbai. The scheme of synthesis is given in Scheme 1. The chemicals were used without further purification. All the melting points were determined in open capillaries and are uncorrected. Thin layer chromatography was performed on microscopic slides (2×7.5 cm^2) coated with silica-Gel-G and spots were visualized under UV light. UV spectra were recorded in U.V-1700 Shimadzu spectrophotometer. IR spectra of all the compounds were recorded in KBr on FT-IR 8400 S Shimadzu

Table 1 Zone of inhibition antibacterial activity of synthesized compounds

Compound code/name	Concentration (mg/ml)	Zone of inhibition (mm)			
		B. subtilis	S. aureus	E. coli	C. albicans
P2A	0.5	2	1	–	2
	1.0	4	3	2	4
	1.5	6	5	4	7
P2B	0.5	–	–	–	–
	1.0	1	2	3	3
	1.5	3	3	5	6
P4A	0.5	–	5	–	–
	1.0	6	7	2	3
	1.5	7	8	3	5
P4B	0.5	–	3	1	3
	1.0	4	5	3	4
	1.5	7	6	4	7
P5A	0.5	1	–	–	2
	1.0	5	3	–	5
	1.5	6	5	3	7
P6A	0.5	4	3	–	–
	1.0	6	5	2	4
	1.5	7	7	5	6
Ampicillin	0.5	10	11	8	–
	1.0	12	12	10	–
	1.5	14	14	12	–
Cephalexin	0.5	7	7	5	–
	1.0	9	8	8	–
	1.5	11	10	9	–
Miconazole	0.5	–	–	–	6
	1.0	–	–	–	7
	1.5	–	–	–	9

spectrophotometer using KBr. Mass spectra were obtained using 2010EV LCMS Shimadzu instrument. The ^{1}H NMR was recorded on Bruker advanced–II NMR-400 MHz instruments using CDCl3/DMSO-d6 as solvent and tetramethylsilane as internal standard, chemical shifts were expressed as δvalues (ppm).

Preparation of 5-chloro-1,3-benzoxazol-2(3 H)-one (P1A)

(7.15 g, 0.05 mol) 2-amino-4 chlorophenol was dissolved in 10 mL of Dimethyl formamide. (3 g, 0.05 mol) of urea was added in this mixture. The whole mixture was reflux for 3 h at 60°C till all the ammonia gas is liberated. Then, pour this mixture in ice-cold water with constant stirring and collect the precipitates. The product was recrystallized from Rectified ethanol. The compound was characterized by TLC, UV, IR, and melting point

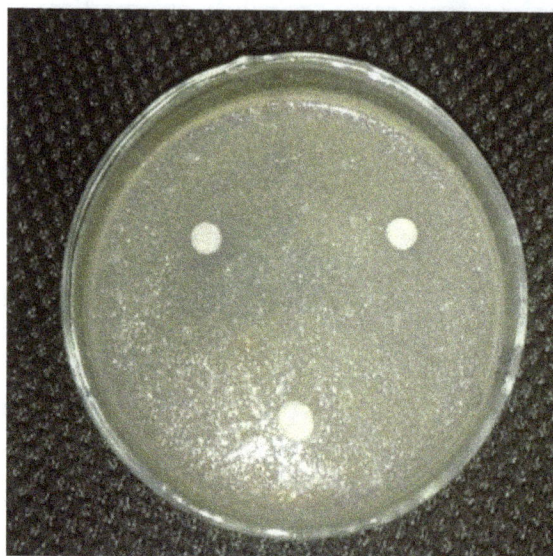

Figure 9 Histogram of antibacterial/antifungal act.

determination (Tables 3 and 4). Mobile phase of TLC was hexane:ethylacetate (3:2) [1] Scheme 2.

Preparation of 3-benzyl-5-chloro-1,3-benzoxazol-2 (3 H)-one (P2A)

(1.69 g, 0.010 mol) of P1A was added in 5 mL of acetonitrile in a round bottom flask. To this mixture, (1.26 g, 0.01 mol) of benzyl chloride (density 1.100 g/cm^3) was added. The whole solution was reflux for 3 h at 60°C. Then, this solution was added in cold water with constant stirring. Product was collected and recrystallized from rectified ethanol. The compounds were characterized by TLC, UV, IR, MASS, and melting point determination (Tables 3 and 4). Mobile phase of TLC was hexane:ethyl acetate (3:2) [2] Scheme 3.

Table 2 MIC of synthesized compounds

Compound code/name	Concentration (µg/mL)			
	B. subtilis	S. aureus	E. coli	C. albicans
P2A	>312	>312	>312	>312
P2B	>312	>312	>312	>156
P4A	>156	>156	>156	>156
P4B	>156	>156	>156	>156
P5A	>312	>312	>312	>156
P6A	>312	>156	>312	>312
Ampicillin	>39	>78.1	>1250	–
Cephalexin	>39	>78.1	>78.1	–
Miconazole	–	–	–	>78.1

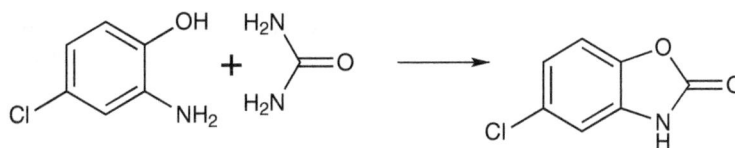

Scheme 1 Synthesis of 5-chloro-1,3-benzoxazol-2(3 *H*)-one (P1A).

Preparation of 5-chloro-3-(2,4-dichlorobenzyl)-1, 3-benzoxazol-2(3 H)-one (P2B)

(1.69 g, 0.01 mol) of P1A was added to the 5 ml of acetonitrile in a round bottom flask. To this mixture, (1.365 g, 0.01 mol) of 2,4-dichlorobenzyl chloride (density 1.386 g/cm^3) was added. The whole mixture was refluxed for 4 h at 60°C and reaction was monitored by TLC. Then, resultant mixture was added in cold water with constant stirring. The product was collected and recrystallized from rectified ethanol. The compound was characterized by TLC, UV, IR, MASS, NMR, and melting point determination (Tables 3 and 4). Mobile phase of TLC was hexane: ethyl acetate (3:2) [2].

Preparation of 5-azido-3-benzyl-1,3-benzoxazol-2(3 H)-one (P3A)

(2.59 g, 0.01 mol) of P2A was dissolved in 5 mL of dimethyl formamide in a conical flask. (0.21 g, 0.01 mol) of sodium azide and 0.5 g of zinc chloride were added. Then, 5 mL of carbon disulfide was added and mixed well. The mixture was kept at room temperature for 10–12 h. Then, the mixture was added in ice-cold water. The azide product was collected and used for further reaction. The compound was characterized by TLC, UV, IR, and melting point determination (Tables 3 and 4). Mobile phase of TLC was hexane:ethyl acetate (3:2) [4] Scheme 4.

Table 3 Physical data of compounds

Compound code	Molecular formula	Molecular weight (g/mol)	Melting point (°C)	Yield (%w/w)	R_f value
P1A	C$_7$H$_4$ClNO$_2$	169.565	158	70.1	0.73
P2A	C$_{14}$H$_{10}$ClNO$_2$	259.68	169	78.4	0.84
P2B	C$_{14}$H$_8$Cl$_3$NO$_2$	328.577	176	56.9	0.68
P3A	C$_{14}$H$_{10}$N$_4$O$_2$	266.25	176	70.17	0.78
P3B	C$_7$H$_4$N$_4$O$_2$	176.13	168–172	94.23	0.74
P4A	C$_{16}$H$_{12}$N$_4$O$_2$	292.29	135	37.03	0.87
P4B	C$_9$H$_6$N$_4$O$_2$	202.169	179–183	42.15	0.54
P5A	C$_{20}$H$_{17}$N$_3$O$_4$S	395.43	195–200	65.79	0.71
P6A	C$_{21}$H$_{16}$N$_2$O$_4$	360.36	182	54.02	0.72

Preparation of 5-azido-1,3-benzoxazol-2(3 H)-one (P3B)

(1.69 g, 0.01 mol) of P1A was dissolved in 5 mL of dimethyl formamide in a conical flask. (0.21 g, 0.01 mol) of sodium azide and 0.5 g of zinc chloride were added in the above solution. Then, 5 mL of carbon disulfide was added and kept the mixture at room temperature for 10–12 h. Then, the mixture was added in ice-cold water. The azide product was collected and used for further reaction. The compound was characterized by TLC, UV, IR, and melting point determination (Tables 3 and 4). Mobile phase of TLC was hexane:ethyl acetate (3:2) [4].

Preparation of 3-benzyl-5-(1 H-1,2,3-triazol-1-yl)-1,3-benzoxazol-2(3 H)-one (P4A)

(2.66 g, 0.01 mol) of P3A was dissolved in 10 mL of absolute ethanol and it was refluxed with (0.86 g, 0.01 mol) of vinyl acetate (density 0.93 g/cm^3) for 8 h. The reaction was monitored by TLC. Mobile phase was hexane:ethyl acetate (2:1). Then, the product was collected from ice-cold water and recrystallized from rectified ethanol. The compound was characterized by TLC, UV, IR, MASS, NMR, and melting point determination [8].

Preparation of 5-(1 H-1,2,3-triazol-1-yl)-1,3-benzoxazol-2 (3 H)-one (P4B)

(1.76 g, 0.01 mol) of P3B was dissolved in 10 mL of absolute ethanol and it was refluxed with (0.86 g, 0.01 mol) of vinyl acetate (density 0.93 g/cm^3) for 6 h. The reaction was monitored by TLC. Mobile phase was hexane:ethyl acetate (3.5:1.5). Then, the product was collected from ice-cold water and recrystallized from rectified ethanol. The compound was characterized by TLC, UV, IR, MASS, NMR, and melting point determination [8].

Preparation of 4-amino-N-(3-benzyl-2-oxo-2,3-dihydro-1, 3-benzoxazol-5-yl)benzenesulfonamide (P5A)

(2.59 g, 0.010 mol) of P2A was dissolved in 10 mL of absolute ethanol. Equal weight of potassium carbonate (anhydrous) and (1.72 g, 0.010 mol) of sulfanilamide was added and the whole mixture was refluxed for 3 h and the reaction was monitored by TLC. Mobile phase was hexane:ethyl acetate (3.5:1.5). Then, add the mixture in water and reprecipitate the

Table 4 Spectral data of compounds

Compound code	UV λ-max (cm)	IR KBr (cm^{-1})	Mass m/z (abundance)	H^1 NMR (CDCl$_3$) signals, δ, multiplicity, J value (Hz)
P1A	283.0	3055.03 (−NH−CO−),	–	–
		800−400(Ar−Cl),		
		1481.23(Cyclic Ester),		
		1600−1400 (C = C)		
		1782.10 (C = O)		
P2A	282.0	3051.18 (=N−CO−),	259(M$^-$),	7.1 (s, 5H, Ar−<u>H</u>),
		800−400(Ar−Cl),	168(91),	4.2 (s, 2H, −C<u>H</u>$_2$−),
		1481.23(Cyclic Ester),	223(35),	7.1, 7.0 (m, 2 H, −^{3}C<u>H</u>−
		1600−1400 (C = C)	186(73),	^{4}C<u>H</u>−),
		713.0 & 694.33 (Mono Substituted benzene ring)	113(164)	7.3, 7.2 (m, 1 H, −^{6}C<u>H</u>)
		1774.39 (C = O)		
P2B	282.5	3055.03 (−NH−CO−),	326(M$^-$),	–
		800−400(Ar−Cl),	168(158),	
		1620.09−1778.25 (1,2,4-trisubstituted benzene ring),	292.9(35),	
		1477.37(Cyclic Ester),	258.9(70),	
		1600−1450 (C = C),	218(105),	
		3050−3010 (−C−H str.),	181(146),	
		1778.25 (C = O)	159(167)	
P3A	282.0	3039.09 (=N−CO−),	–	–
		713.1 & 698.18 (Mono substituted benzene ring),		
		1481.23(Cyclic Ester),		
		1600−1400 (C = C),		
		3050−3010 (−C−H str),		
		1782.10 (C = O)		
P3B	282.0	3055.03 (−NH−CO−),	–	–
		1485.09(Cyclic Ester),		
		1600−1450 (C = C),		
		3050−3010 (−C−H str),		
		1782.10 (C = O)		
P4A	282.0	3058.89 (=N−CO−),	292(M$^-$),	7.02 (s, 5 H, Ar−<u>H</u>),
		1485.09(Cyclic Ester),	168(106),	4.02 (s, 2 H, −C<u>H</u>$_2$−),
		1600−1450 (C = C),	224(68),	7.8 (s, 1 H, ^{6}C<u>H</u>),
		713.61 & 690.47 (Mono substituted benzene ring),	201(91),	7.36, 7.35 (m, 2 H, −^{3}C<u>H</u>−^{4}C<u>H</u>−),
		3050−3010 (−C−H str)	133(159)	7.1, 7.0 (d, 2 H, −C<u>H</u> = C<u>H</u>− in triazole)
		1762.82 (C = O)		
P4B	282.0	3055.03 (−NH−CO−),	202(M$^-$),	
		1481.23(Cyclic Ester),	168(34),	
		1600−1400 (C = C),	134(68)	
		3050−3010 (−C−H str),		
		1782.10 (C = O)		
P5A	281.0 & 218.0	1261.36 & 1149.50 (−SO$_2$NH−),	395(M$^-$),	–

Table 4 Spectral data of compounds *(Continued)*

		3055.03 (=N–CO–),	167.9(227),	
		1620.09 (–NH$_2$),	224(171)	
		1299.93 & 1149.50 (–S = O),	304(91)	
		1477.37(Cyclic Ester),	133(262)	
		1782.10 (C = O)		
P6A	282.0 & 219.0	1782.10 (–COOH),	360(M$^-$),	7.02 (s, 5 H, Ar–H̲),
		3058.89 (=N–CO–),	310.8(49),	7.01,7.00 (d, 4 H, CH̲ in PABA),
		713.60 & 694.33 (Mono substituted benzene ring),	168(192),	5.01 (s, 1 H, NH̲),
		1481.23(Cyclic Ester),	223.9(136),	11.51 (s, 1 H, –COOH̲),
		1600–1400 (C = C)	132(227)	4.3 (s, 2 H, –CH̲$_2$–),
		1616.24 (C = O)		7.24, 7.22 (m, 1 H, ^{6}CH̲),
				7.76,7.74 (m, 2 H, –^{3}CH̲–^{4}CH̲–)

product by acidifying with conc. HCl. Collect the crude P5A and recrystalize byrectified ethanol. The compound was characterized by TLC, UV, IR, MASS, and melting point determination [4,8].

Preparation of 4-[(3-benzyl-2-oxo-2,3-dihydro-1, 3-benzoxazol-5-yl)amino]benzoic acid (P6A)

(2.59 g, 0.010 mol) of P2A was dissolved in 10 mL of absolute ethanol. Equal weight of potassium carbonate (anhydrous) and (1.37 g, 0.010 mol) of *p*-aminobenzoic acid was added and the whole mixture was refluxed for 3 h and the reaction was monitored by TLC. Mobile phase was hexane:ethyl acetate (3.5:1.5). Then, add the mixture in water and reprecipitate the product by acidifying with conc. HCl. Collect the crude P6A and recrystalize by rectified ethanol. The compound was characterized by TLC, UV, IR, MASS, and melting point determination [4,8].

Conclusions

Benzoxazole was reported as naturally occurring plant product and considered responsible for antibacterial activity in plant protection. We have synthesized and concluded its other synthetic derivatives. Compounds P4A and P4B have good antibacterial and antifungal activity, half of the Ampicillin and Cephalexin. P4A, P4B, P6A have good activity against *S. aureus* and *E. coli*. Compound P2B has good antifungal activity, half of the Miconazole against *C. albicans*. P2A, P2B, P5A, P6A have almost equal antibacterial activity.

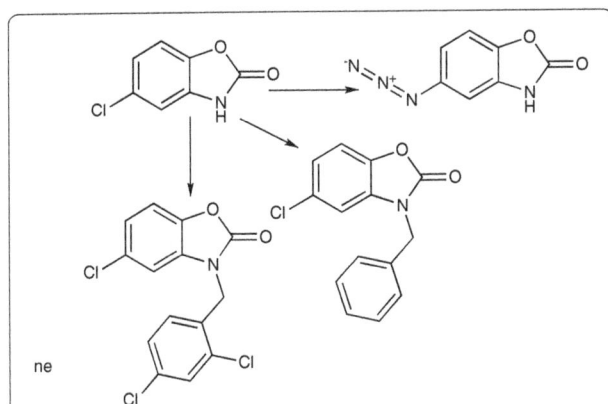

Scheme 2 Synthesis of 3-benzyl-5-chloro-1,3-benzoxazol-2(3 *H*)-one (P2A), 5-chloro-3-(2,4-dichlorobenzyl)-1,3-benzoxazol-2(3 *H*)-one (P2B), 5-azido-1,3-benzoxazol-2(3 *H*)-one (P3B).

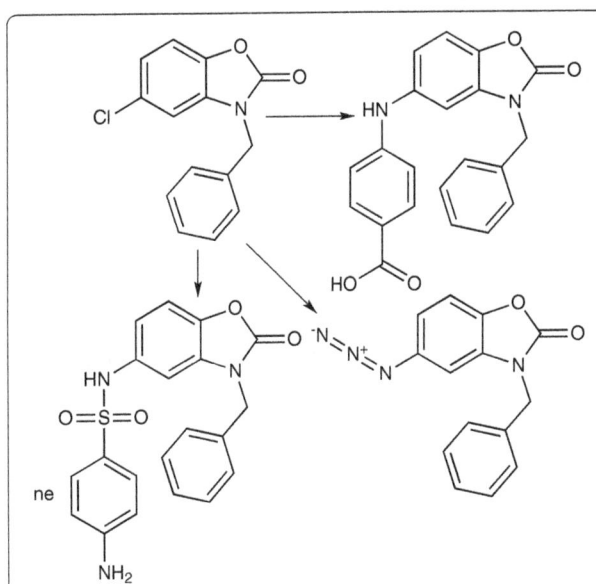

Scheme 3 Synthesis of 5-azido-3-benzyl-1,3-benzoxazol-2(3*H*)-one(P3A), 4-amino-*N*-(3-benzyl-2-oxo-2,3-dihydro-1,3-benzoxazol-5-yl)benzenesulfonamide (P5A), 4-[(3-benzyl-2-oxo-2,3-dihydro-1,3-benzoxazol-5-yl)amino]benzoic acid (P6A).

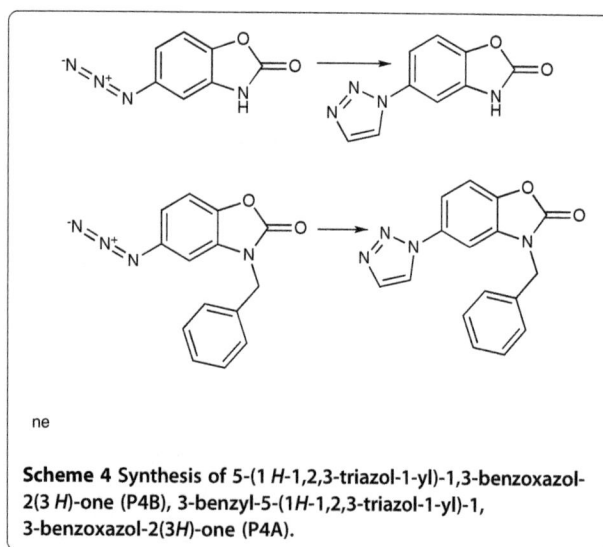

ne

Scheme 4 Synthesis of 5-(1 *H*-1,2,3-triazol-1-yl)-1,3-benzoxazol-2(3 *H*)-one (P4B), 3-benzyl-5-(1*H*-1,2,3-triazol-1-yl)-1,3-benzoxazol-2(3*H*)-one (P4A).

Competing interests
The authors declare that they have no competing interests.

Authors' contributions
The CN Patel has guided this project. Both authors read and approved final manuscript.

Acknowledgment
The authors thank Sophisticated Analytical Instrument Laboratory, Chandigarh, for ^{1}H NMR spectra and Oxygen Healthcare Pvt. Ltd., for MASS analysis data.

References

1. Onkol T, Mehtap Gokce Ah, Tosun U, Polat S, Mehmet S, Serin ST (2008) Microwave synthesis and antimicrobial evaluation of 5-Chloro-2(3 h) benzoxazolinone-3- acetyl-2-(p-substituted benzal)hydrazone and 5-Chloro-2 (3 h)-benzoxazolinone-3-acetyl-2-(p-substituted acetophenone) hydrazone derivative. Turk J Pharm Sci 5(3):155–166
2. Fang B, Cheng-He Z, Rao X-C (2010) Synthesis and biological activities of novel amine-derived bis-azoles as potential antibacterial and antifungal agents. Eur J Med Chem. doi:10.10.ejmech.2010.06.012
3. Lai C, Rebecca J, Gum MD, Fry EH, Hutchins C (2006) Benzoxazole benzenesulfonamides as allosteric inhibitors of fructose-1,6-bisphosphatase. Bioorg Med Chem Lett 16:1807–18104
4. Wang XL, Wan K, Zhou CH (2010) Synthesis of novel sulfanilamide-derived 1,2,3-triazoles and their evaluation for antibacterial and antifungal activities. Eur J Med Chem. doi:10.1016/j.ejmech.2010.07.031
5. Pelczar MJ, Chan ES, Pelczar JR, Krieg NR (1997) Text Book of Microbiology, Vol 5. Tata McGraw-Hill Education, New York, pp 73–98
6. Chakraborty PA (2005) Text Book of Microbiology, Vol 2. New Central Book Agency (P) Ltd, Kolkata, pp 9–-24, 57–64
7. Andrews JM (2001) Determination of minimum inhibitory concentrations. J Antimicrob Chemother 48:5–16
8. Slamova K, Marhol P, Bezouska K, Lindkvist L, Signe G, Hansen VK, Jensen HH (2010) Synthesis and biological activity of glycosyl-1H-1,2,3-triazoles. Bioorg Med Chem Lett 20:4263–4265

24

Two new aliphatic lactones from the fruits of *Coriandrum sativum* L.

Kamran J Naquvi, Mohammed Ali* and Javed Ahmad

Abstract

Background: The present paper describes the isolation and characterization of two new aliphatic δ-lactones along with three glycerides and n-nonadecanyl cetoleate from the fruits of *Coriandrum sativum* L. (Apiaceae). The structures of all the isolated phytoconstituents have been established on the basis of spectral data analysis and chemical reactions.

Results: Phytochemical investigation of the methanolic extract of *C. sativum* L. (Apiaceae) fruits resulted in the isolation of two new aliphatic δ-lactones characterized as 2α-n-heptatriacont-(Z)-3-en-1,5-olide (1) (coriander lactone) and 2α-n-tetracont-(Z,Z)-3,26-dien-18α-ol-1,5-olide (2) (hydroxy coriander lactone) together with glyceryl-1,2-dioctadec-9,12-dienoate-3-octadec-9-enoate (3); glyceryl-1,2,3-trioctadecanoate (4); n-nonadecanyl-n-docos-11-enoate (5) and oleiyl glucoside (6).

Conclusions: Phytochemical investigation of the methanolic extract of *C. sativum* gave coriander lactone and hydroxy coriander lactone as the new phytoconstituents.

Keywords: *Coriandrum sativum*, Apiaceae, Aliphatic δ-lactones, Fatty acid glycerides

Background

Coriandrum sativum L. is an annual and herbaceous plant belonging to the Apiaceae family. It is a medicinal plant, native of southern Europe and western Mediterranean region and is cultivated worldwide [1]. India is the largest producer of coriander in the world. Major production centers are Rajasthan, Maharastra, Gujarat, and Karnataka [2]. The whole plant and especially the unripe fruits are characterized by a strong disagreeable odor, hence the name coriander, giving characteristic aroma when rubbed [3]. The most important constituents of coriander seeds are the essential oil and the fatty oil. The dried coriander seeds contain an essential oil (0.03% to 2.6%) with linalool as main component [4,5], phenolics, flavonoides [6], and isocoumarin compounds [7]. It has traditionally been referred to as antidiabetic [8] and cholesterol lowering drug [9,10]. This paper describes the isolation and characterization of two new aliphatic δ-lactones along with fatty acid glycerides, ester, and glucoside from the fruits of *C. sativum* of Delhi region of India.

Methods

General

Melting points were determined on a Perfit melting apparatus (Ambala, Haryana, and India) and are uncorrected. UV spectra were measured with a Lambda Bio 20 spectrophotometer (Perkin-Elmer-Rotkreuz, Switzerland) in methanol. Infrared spectra were recorded on Bio-Rad FTIR 5000 (FTS 135, Kowloon, Hong Kong) spectrophotometer using KBr pellets; γ_{max} values are given in cm^{-1}. ^{1}H nuclear magnetic resonance (NMR) and ^{13}C NMR spectra were screened on Bruker spectrospin 300 and 75 MHz, respectively, instruments (Karlesruthe, Germany) using $CDCl_3$ and TMS as an internal standard. Mass spectra were measured by effecting fast atom bombardment (FAB) ionization at 70 eV on a JEOL-JMS-DX 303 spectrometer (JEOL, Japan) equipped with direct inlet probe system. Column chromatography was performed on silica gel (60 to 120 mesh; Qualigen, Mumbai, India). TLC was run on silica gel G (Qualigen, Carlsbad, CA). Spots were visualized by exposing to iodine vapors, UV radiation, and spraying with ceric sulphate.

* Correspondence: maliphyto@gmail.com
Department of Pharmacognosy and Phytochemistry, Faculty of Pharmacy, Jamia Hamdard, New Delhi 110062, India

Results and discussion

Compound 1, named coriander lactone (Scheme 1), was obtained as a pale yellow crystalline mass from petroleum ether eluents. Its IR spectrum showed characteristic absorption bands for δ-lactone group (1738 cm^{-1}), unsaturation (1621 cm^{-1}), and long aliphatic chain (806, 721 cm^{-1}). On the basis of FAB mass spectrum, its molecular weight was established at m/z 546 consistent with the molecular formula of an unsaturated lactone, $C_{37}H_{70}O_2$. It indicated three double bond equivalents; two of them were adjusted in the lactone ring and remaining one in the vinylic linkage. The prominent ion peaks arising at m/z 97 [C_2-C_6 fission, $C_5H_5O_2$]$^+$ and 449 [M-97, $(CH_2)_{31}$ CH_3]$^+$ suggested that δ lactone was attached to the C-32 aliphatic chain. The ^{1}H NMR spectrum of 1 showed a one-proton double doublet at δ 5.36 (J = 6.6, 7.2 Hz) and a one-proton multiplet at δ 5.32 assigned to (Z)-vinylic H-3 and H-4 protons, respectively. A two-proton doublet at δ 4.14 (J = 7.2 Hz) was ascribed to oxygenated methylene H_2-5 protons. A one-proton broad multiplet at δ 2.78 with half width of 6.1 Hz was attributed to β-oriented H-2 methine proton. A two-proton multiplet at δ 2.30, two four-proton multiplets at δ 2.05 and 1.59, and a broad signal at δ 1.26 integrating for 52 protons were associated with the methylene protons. A three-proton triplet at δ 0.90 (J = 6.3) was accounted to C-37 primary methyl protons. The ^{13}C NMR spectrum of 1 displayed signals for lactone carbon at δ 173.56 (C-1), vinylic carbons at δ 130.15 (C-3) and 127.91 (C-4), oxygenated methylene carbon δ 66.83 (C-5), methine carbon at δ 34.21 (C-2), methylene carbons between δ 31.91 and 22.64, and methyl carbon at δ 14.03 (C-37). The ^{1}H-^{1}H correlation spectroscopy (COSY) spectrum of 1 showed correlations of H_2-5 with H-4 and H-3; and H-2 with H-3, H-4 and H_2-6. The heteronuclear multiple bond correlation (HMBC) spectrum of 1 exhibited interactions of C-1 with H-2, H-3 and H_2-6; and C-5 with H-4 and H-3. On the basis of the foregoing account, the structure of 1 has been established as 2-α-n-heptatriacont-(Z)-3-en-1,5-olide. This is a new δ-lactone isolated from a plant source [see Additional file 1].

Compound 2, named hydroxy coriander lactone, was obtained as a pale yellow crystalline mass from chloroform eluents (Scheme 2). Its IR spectrum showed distinctive absorption bands for a hydroxy group (3463 cm^{-1}), lactone ring (1743 cm^{-1}), unsaturation (1645 cm^{-1}), and long aliphatic chain (722 cm^{-1}). Its FAB mass spectrum had a molecular ion peak at m/z 603 [M + H]$^+$ corresponding to a long chain hydroxylated aliphatic lactone, $C_{40}H_{75}O_3$. It showed four degrees of unsaturation; two each of them were adjusted in the lactone ring and two in vinylic linkages. The prominent ion peaks arising at m/z 97 [C_2-C_6 fission, $C_5H_5O_2$]$^+$, 265 [C_{17}-C_{18} fission, $C_5H_5O_2(CH_2)_{12}$]$^+$,

337 [M-265, $HOCH(CH_2)_7CH = CH(CH_2)_{12}CH_3$]$^+$, 295 [$C_{18}$-$C_{19}$ fission, $C_5H_5O_2(CH_2)_{12}CHOH$]$^+$ suggested the presence of one of the vinylic linkage in the lactone ring and the hydroxyl group at C-18. The ion peak forming at m/z 393 [C_{25}-C_{26} fission, $C_5H_5O_2(CH_2)_{12}CHOH(CH_2)_7$]$^+$ indicated the location of another vinylic linkage at C-26. The ^{1}H NMR spectrum of 2 showed a one-proton double doublet at δ 5.34 (6.8, 7.5 Hz) and four multiplets at 5.26, 5.17 ($w_{1/2}$ = 8.5 Hz), and 5.11 ($w_{1/2}$ = 9.5 Hz) assigned correspondingly to cis-oriented H-4, H-3, H-26, and H-27 vinylic protons, respectively. Two one-proton doublets at δ 4.32 (J = 7.5 Hz) and 4.28 (J = 7.5 Hz) were attributed to the oxygenated methylene H_2-5. A one-proton broad multiplets at δ 4.16 with half width of 5.7 Hz was ascribed to β-oriented H-18 carbinol proton. A one-proton multiplet at δ 2.76 ($w_{1/2}$ = 6.8 Hz) was accounted to β-oriented H-2 methine protons. Two multiplets at δ 2.30 and 2.02 integrating for two protons each were due to methylene H_2-25 and H_2-28 protons located nearby the C-26 and C-27 vinylic carbons. The remaining methylene protons resonated between δ 1.98 and 1.26. A three-proton triplet at δ 0.87 (J = 6.5 Hz) was associated with the C-40 primary methyl protons. The ^{13}C NMR spectrum of 2 displayed signals for lactone carbon at δ 172.78 (C-1), vinylic carbons at δ 130.34 (C-4), 129.78 (C-3), 128.78 (C-26), and 127.96 (C-27), carbinol carbon at δ 68.83 (C-18), oxygenated methylene carbon at δ 65.95 (C-5), methine carbon at δ 42.03 (C-2), methylene carbons between δ 33.76 and 22.55, and methyl carbon at δ 13.94 (C-40). The ^{1}H-^{1}H COSY spectrum of 2 showed correlations of H_2-5 with H-4 and H-3; H-2 with H-3, H-4, and H_2-6; H-18 with H_2-17 and H_2-19; H-26 with H_2-25, H-27, and H_2-28; and H_3-40 with H_2-39. The HMBC spectrum of 2 exhibited interactions of C-1 with H-2; C-3 with H-2, H_2-6, and H-4; C-4 with H_2-5 and H-3; C-18 with H_2-17 and H_2-19; and C-26 with H-27 and H_2-25. These evidences led to formulate the structure of 2 as 2α-n-tetracont-(Z,Z)-3, 26-dien-18α-ol-1,5-olide. This is a new δ-lactone isolated from a plant source.

Earlier δ-lactonic constituents have been isolated from the root bark of *Capparis deciduas* [11], hulls of *Oryza sativa* [12], and seeds of *Althea officinalis* [13]. The compound 3 to 6 were the known phytoconstituents identified as glyceryl-1,2-dioctadec-9,12-dienoate-3-octadec-9,12-dienoate, glyceryl-1,2,3-trioctadecanoate, n-nonadecanyl-n-docos-1-enoate, and n-octadec-9-enyl-β-D-glucopyranoside, respectively.

Experimental

Plant material

The fruits of *C. sativum* were collected from the herbal garden of Jamia Hamdard, New Delhi. The plant material was identified by Prof. MP Sharma, Taxonomist, Department of Botany, Faculty of Science, Jamia Hamdard, New Delhi. A voucher specimen (PRL/JH/07/27) of drug is

Two new aliphatic lactones from the fruits of Coriandrum sativum L.

165

preserved in the Phytochemistry Research Laboratory, Department of Pharmacognosy and Phytochemistry, Faculty of Pharmacy, Jamia Hamdard, New Delhi.

Extraction

C. sativum fruits (1.6 kg) were dried in air and then in an oven at 45°C temperature. The material was coarsely powdered. Exhaustive extraction of powdered drug was carried out in a Soxhlet apparatus using methanol as extracting solvent. The methanolic extract was concentrated under reduced pressure to yield a dark brown viscous mass, 187 g (11.68%).

Isolation of phytoconstituents

The methanolic extract (85 g) was dissolved in a minimum amount of methanol and adsorbed on silica gel (60 to 120 mesh) for preparation of slurry. The air-dried slurry was chromatographed over the silica gel column packed in petroleum ether (60 to 80°C). The column was eluted with petroleum ether (60 to 80°C), chloroform, and methanol in order of increasing polarity to isolate the following compounds:

Coriander lactone (1)

Elution of the column with petroleum ether furnished pale yellow crystals of **1**, recrystallized from acetone, 76 mg (0.089% yield); R_f value, 0.9 (petroleum ether); m.p, 110 to 111°C; UV λ_{max} (MeOH), 206 nm (log ϵ 4.9); IR γ_{max} (KBr), 2924, 2854, 1738, 1621, 1460, 1260, 1064, 806, 721 cm^{-1}; ^{1}H NMR (CDCl$_3$), δ 5.36 (1 H, dd, J = 6.6, 7.2, H-3), 5.32 (1 H, m, H-4), 4.14 (2 H, d, J = 7.2 Hz), 2.78 (1 H, brm, w$_{1/2}$ = 6.1 Hz, H-2β), 2.30 (2 H, m, H$_2$-6), 2.05 (4 H, m, 2 × CH$_2$), 1.59 (4 H, m, 2 × CH$_2$), 1.28 (52 H, brs, 26 × CH$_2$), 0.90 (3 H, t, J = 6.3, Me-37); ^{13}C NMR (CDCl$_3$), δ 173.56 (C-1), 130.15 (C-3), 127.91 (C-4), 66.83 (C-5), 34.21 (C-2), 31.90 (CH$_2$), 29.65 (21 × CH$_2$), 29.33 (4 × CH$_2$), 27.19 (CH$_2$), 25.61 (CH$_2$), 24.90 (CH$_2$), 22.64 (CH$_2$), 14.03 (Me-37); +ve ion FAB MS *m/z* (*rel. int.*), 546 [M]$^+$ (C$_{37}$H$_{70}$O$_2$) (19.7), 449 (31.8), 97 (71.0).

Hydroxy coriander lactone (2)

Elution of the column with chloroform afforded pale yellow crystals of **2**, recrystallized from acetone, 102 mg (0.12% yield); R$_f$ value, 0.73 (chloroform); m.p., 95 to 96°C; UV λ_{max} (MeOH), 205 nm (log ϵ 5.1); IR γ_{max} (KBr), 3463, 2921, 2852, 1743, 1645, 1463, 1379, 1145, 1092, 1019, 722 cm^{-1}; ^{1}H NMR (CDCl$_3$), δ 5.34 (1 H, dd, J = 6.8, 7.5 Hz, H-3), 5.30 (1 H, m, H-4), 5.17 (1 H, brm, w$_{1/2}$ = 8.5 Hz, H-26), 5.11 (1 H, brm, w$_{1/2}$ = 9.5, H-27), 4.32 (1 H, d, J = 7.5 Hz, H-5a), 4.28 (1 H, d, J = 7.5 Hz, H$_2$-5b), 4.16 (1 H, brm, w$_{1/2}$ = 5.7 Hz, H-18β), δ 2.76 (1 H, m, w$_{1/2}$ = 6.8 Hz, H-2β), 2.30 (2 H, m, H$_2$-25), δ 2.02 (2 H, m, H$_2$-28), 1.98 (2 H, m, CH$_2$), 1.68 (2 H, m, CH$_2$), 1.62 (2 H, m, CH$_2$). 1.60 (2 H, m, CH$_2$), 1.26 (50 H, brs, 25 × CH$_2$), 0.87

(3 H, t, J = 6.5 Hz, Me-40); ^{13}C NMR (CDCl$_3$), δ 172.78 (C-1), 130.34 (C-4), 129.78 (C-3), 128.78 (C-26), 127.96 (C-27), 68.83 (C-18), 65.95 (C-5), 42.03 (C-2), 33.76 (CH$_2$), 31.79 (CH$_2$), 31.68 (CH$_2$), 29.54 (11 × CH$_2$), 29.21 (5 × CH$_2$), 29.02 (5 × CH$_2$), 27.67 (CH$_2$), 27.11 (CH$_2$), 26.66 (CH$_2$), 25.50 (CH$_2$), 24.73 (CH$_2$), 24.34 (CH$_2$), 22.55 (CH$_2$), 13.94 (Me-40); +ve ion FAB MS *m/z* (*rel. int.*), 603[M + H]$^+$ (C$_{40}$H$_{75}$O$_3$) (100), 559 (3.7), 503 (6.1), 461 (3.6), 405 (3.8), 393 (18.0), 337 (18.2), 295 (14.1), 265 (39.8), 97 (37.9).

Glyceryl-1,2-dioctadec-9,12-dienoate-3-octadec-9-enoate (3)

Elution of column with chloroform-methanol (19:1) afforded light green resinous mass of **3**, crystallized from acetone, 82 mg (0.096% yield); R$_f$ value, 0.6 (chloroform-methanol, 19: 1); m.p., 65 to 66°C; UV λ_{max} (MeOH), 206 nm (log ϵ 4.6); IR γ_{max} (KBr), 2925, 2855, 1743, 17251640, 1460, 1375, 1167, 723 cm^{-1}; ^{1}H NMR (CDCl$_3$), δ 5.34 (4 H, m, H-9′, H-13′, H-9′′, H-13′′), 5.32 (4 H, m, H-10′, H-12′, H-10′′, H-12′′), 5.27 (2 H, m, H- 9′′′, H-10′′′), 4.33 (1 H, d, J = 1.7 Hz, H-2), 4.14 (2 H, m, H$_2$-1), 4.11 (2 H, m, H$_2$-3), 2.31 (1 H, d, J = 3.0 Hz, H$_2$-2′a), δ 2.30 (1 H, d, J = 3.0 Hz, H$_2$-2′b), 2.20 (1 H, d, J = 6.3 Hz, H$_2$-2′′a), δ 2.18 (1 H, d, J = 6.3 Hz, H$_2$-2′′b), 2.16 (1 H, d, J = 7.5 Hz, H$_2$-2′′′ a), 2.14 (1 H, d, J = 7.5 Hz, H$_2$-2′′′b), 1.85 (2 H, m, H$_2$-11′). 1.81 (2 H, m, H$_2$-11′′), 1.79 (4 H, m, H$_2$-8′, H-8′′), 1.77 (4 H, m, H2-14′, H$_2$-14′′), 1.61 (4 H, m, H$_2$-8′′′, H$_2$-11′′′), 1.26 (48 H, brs, 24 × CH$_2$), 1.16 (4 H, m, 2 × CH$_2$), 0.87 (9 H, m, H$_3$-18′, H$_3$- 18′′, H$_3$-18′′′); ^{13}C NMR (CDCl$_3$) δ 173.37 (C-1′), 172.80 (C-1′′), 172.49 (C-1′′′), 130.22 (C-10′, C-10′′), 129.83 (C-12′), 129.66 (C-12′′), 128.68 (C-9′′′, C-10′′′), 128.68 (C-9′, C-9′′) 127.82 (C-13′), 127.68 (C-13′′), 68.77 (C-2), 64.72 (C-1), 61.87 (C-3), 56.93 (C-2′), 56.62 (C-2′′), 56.31 (C-2′′′), 33.84 (C-11′), 33.81 (C-11′′), 31.68 (2 × CH$_2$), 31.28 (CH$_2$), 29.42 (10 × CH$_2$), 29.09 (5 × CH$_2$), 28.91 (5 × CH$_2$), 27.54 (CH$_2$), 26.96 (CH$_2$), 26.55 (CH$_2$), 25.94 (CH$_2$), 25.38 (CH$_2$), 28.58 (CH$_2$), 24.23 (CH$_2$), 22.42 (3 × CH$_2$), 13.80 (Me-18′, Me-18′′, Me-18′′′); +ve ion FAB MS *m/z* (*rel. int.*), 880 [M]$^+$ (C$_{57}$H$_{100}$ O$_6$) (1.5), 617 (29.8), 602 (37.0), 339 (71.8), 337 (31.1), 281 (21.5), 279 (31.6), 265 (24.8), 137 (26.2), 111 (39.9).

Glyceryl-1,2,3-trioctadecanoate (4)

Elution of column with chloroform-methanol (97: 3) furnished a colorless resinous mass of **4**, crystallized from from acetone, 132 mg (0.155% yielded); R$_f$ value, 0.23 (chloroform-methanol, 22: 3); m.p. 86 to 88°C; UV λ_{max} (MeOH), 207 nm (log ϵ 4.6); IR γ_{max} (KBr), 2924, 2854, 1725, 1721, 1459, 1373, 1265, 1170, 723 cm^{-1}; ^{1}H NMR (DMSO-d6), δ 3.63 (1 H, m, H-2), 3.50 (2 H, m, H$_2$-1), 3.23 (2 H, m, H$_2$-3), 2.49 (2 H, brs, H$_2$-2′′), 2.25 (2 H, brs, H$_2$-2′), 2.18 (2 H, brs, H$_2$-2′′′), 2.05 (2 H, m, CH$_2$), 1.98 (4 H, m, 2 × CH$_2$), 1.70 (2 H, m, CH$_2$), 1.61 (4 H, m, 2 × CH$_2$), 1.49 (6 H, m, 3 × CH$_2$), 1.31 (8 H, brs, 4 × CH$_2$), 1.22 (20 H, brs, 10 × CH$_2$), 1.20 (18 H, brs, 9 × CH$_2$), 1.18

(18 H, brs, $9 \times CH_2$), 1.16 (8 H, brs, $4 \times CH_2$), 0.84 (9 H, brs, $3 \times CH_3$); ^{13}C NMR (DMSO-d6), δ 174.51 (C-1''), 173.80 (C-1'), 172.72 (C-1'''), 71.40 (C-2), 69.89 (C-1), 64.81 (C-3), 56.67 (C-1''), 56.67 (C-1'), 51.35 (C-1'''), 33.73 (CH$_2$), 32.62 (CH$_2$), 29.19 ($20 \times CH_2$), 28.87 ($16 \times CH_2$), 27.73 (CH$_2$), 26.70 (CH$_2$), 25.21 (CH$_2$), 24.55 (CH$_2$), 22.20 ($3 \times CH_2$); +ve ion FAB MS m/z (rel. int.), 890[M]$^+$ ($C_{57}H_{110}O_6$) (1.5), 283 (15.1), 267 (18.3).

n-nonadecanyl-n-docos-11-enoate (5)

Elution of column with chloroform-methanol (91:9) afforded light brown mass resinous mass of **5**, crystallized from acetone, 112 mg (0.131% yield); R_f value, 0.44 (chloroform-methanol, 22: 3); m.p., 71 to 73°C; UV λ_{max} (MeOH), 207 nm (log ϵ 4.3); IR γ_{max} (KBr), 2924, 2854, 1721, 1459, 1373, 1265, 1170, 723 cm^{-1}; ^{1}H NMR (CDCl$_3$), δ 5.34 (2 H, m, H-11. H-12), 3.79 (1 H, d, $J = 9.9$ Hz, H$_2$-1'a), 3.75 (1 H, d, $J = 9.9$ Hz, H$_2$-1'b), 2.62 (2 H, brs, H$_2$-2), 2.30 (2 H, m, H$_2$-10), 2.03 (2 H, m, H$_2$-13), 1.60 (4 H, m, $2\times$ CH$_2$), 1.25 (60 H, brs, $30 \times CH_2$), 0.87 (3 H, t, $J = 6.3$ Hz, Me-22), 0.84 (3 H, t, $J = 6.1$ Hz, Me-19'); ^{13}C NMR (CDCl$_3$), δ 172.51 (C-1), 130.01 (C-11), 116.02 (C-12), 65.16 (C-1'), 51.74 (C-2), 32.88 (CH$_2$), 31.76 (CH$_2$), 29.53 ($20 \times CH_2$), 29.20 ($9 \times CH_2$), 27.07 (CH$_2$), 24.53 (CH$_2$), 22.52 (CH$_2$), 13.94 (Me- 22, Me- 19'); +ve ion FAB MS m/z (rel. int.), 604[M]$^+$ ($C_{41}H_{80}O_2$) (23.1), 337 (31.0), 267 (22.5).

Oleyl glycoside (6)

Elution of column with chloroform-methanol (22: 3) afforded colorless mass of **6**, crystallized from acetone, 145 mg (0.170% yield); R_f value, 0.2 (chloroform-methanol, 17: 3); m.p., 60 to 62°C; UV λ_{max} (MeOH), 209 nm (log ϵ 5.3); IR γ_{max} (KBr), 3410, 3360, 2925, 2855, 1733, 1640, 1457, 1261, 1091, 801 cm^{-1}; ^{1}H NMR (CDCl$_3$), δ 5.31 (2 H, m, H-9, H-10), 5.25 (1 H, brs, H-1'), 4.41 (1 H, m, H-5'), 4.19 (1 H, m, H-2'), 3.61 (1 H, m, H-3'), 3.58 (1 H, m, H-4'), 3.27 (2 H, brs, H$_2$-6'), 2.67 (2 H, m, H$_2$-2), 2.18 (2 H, m, H$_2$-8), 1.93 (2 H, m, H$_2$-11), 1.48 (4 H, brs, $2 \times CH_2$), 1.16 (18 H, brs, $9 \times CH_2$), 0.77 (3 H, t, $J = 6.1$ Hz, Me-18) . ^{13}C NMR (CDCl$_3$), δ 173.67 (C-1), 129.85 (C-9), 127.71 (C-10), 103.15 (C-1'), 80.23 (C-5'), 69.83 (C- 2'), 68.06 (C-3'), 67.08 (C-4'), 61.05 (C-6'), 55.67 (C-2), 52.27 (CH$_2$), 38.55 (CH$_2$), 33.74 (CH$_2$), 31.57 (CH$_2$), 29.34 ($3 \times CH_2$), 29.02 ($2 \times CH_2$), 26.89 (CH$_2$), 25.31 (CH$_2$), 24.55 (CH$_2$), 22.34 (CH$_2$), 13.78 (Me-18); +ve ion FAB MS m/z (rel. int.), 445[M + H]$^+$ ($C_{24}H_{45}O_7$) (35.6), 265 (28.3), 180 (26.7).

Conclusions

Phytochemical investigation of fruits of *C. sativum* led to isolate new aliphatic δ-lactones which may be used as chromatographic markers for quality control of the drugs.

Additional file

Additional file 1: Showing spectrum of ^{1}H NMR and ^{13}C NMR of coriander lactone and hydroxy coriander lactone and mass spectrum of hydroxy coriander lactone. The file contains ^{1}H NMR, ^{13}C NMR, and mass spectrum of coriander lactone and hydroxyl coriander lactone.

Competing interests

The authors declare that they have no competing interests.

Acknowledgments

The authors are thankful to the Head, Sophisticated Instrumentation Analytical Facility, Central Drug Research Institute, Lucknow, for recording the mass spectra of the compounds.

References

1. Innocent BX, Fathima MSA, Dhanalakshmi (2011) Studies on the immouostimulant activity of *Coriandrum sativum* and resistance to *Aeromonas hydrophila* in *Catla catla*. J Appl Pharmaceut Sci 1(7):132–135
2. Anonymous (2001) Wealth of India, aw aterial. National Institute of Science Communication, CSIR, New Delhi, pp 203–206, 2
3. Pathak NL, Kasture SB, Bhatt NM, Rathod JD (2011) Phytopharmacological properties of *Coriander sativum* as a potential medicinal tree: an overview. J Appl Pharmaceut Sci 1(4):20–25
4. Coskuner Y, Karababa E (2007) Physical properties of coriander seed (*Coriandrum sativum* L.). J Food Eng 80(2):408–416
5. Eikani MH, Golmohammad F, Rowshanzamir S (2007) Supercritical water extraction of essential oils from coriander seeds (*Corinadrum sativum* L.). J Food Eng 80(2):735–740
6. Helle W, Anne BS, Karl EM (2004) Antioxidant activity in extracts from coriander. Food Chem 88(2):293–297
7. Taniguchi M, Yanai M, Xiao YQ, Kido T, Baba K (1996) Three isocoumarins from *Coriandrum sativum*. Phytochemistry 42(3):843–846
8. Gray AM, Flatt PR (1999) Insulin-releasing and insulin-like activity of the traditional anti-diabetic plant *Coriandrum sativum* (coriander). Br J Nutr 81(3):203–209
9. Chithra V, Leelamma S (1997) Hypolipidemic effect of coriander seeds (*Coriandrum sativum*): mechanism of action. Plant Foods Hum Nutr 51(2):167–172
10. Lal AA, Kumar T, Murthy PB, Pillai KS (2004) Hypolipidemic effect of *Coriandrum sativum* L. in triton-induced hyperlipidemic rats. Indian J Exp Biol 42(9):909–912
11. Gupta J, Ali M (1997) Oxygenated heterocyclic constituents from *Capparis deciduas* root barks. Indian J Heterocyclic Chem 6(4):295–302
12. Chung IM, Ali M, Chun S-C, Lee O-K, Ahmad A (2007) Sativalanosteronyl glycoside and oryzatriacontolide constituents from the Hulls of *Oryza sativa*. Asian J Chem 19(2):1535–1543
13. Reni S, Khan SA, Ali M (2010) Phytochemical investigation of the seeds of *Althea officinalis* L. Nat Prod Res 24(14):1358–1364

25

Application of different fertilizers on morphological traits of dill (*Anethum graveolens* L.)

Fatemeh Nejatzadeh-Barandozi[1*] and Fathollah Gholami-Borujeni[2]

Abstract

Background: The aim of this study was to evaluate the effects of nitroxin biofertilizer and chemical fertilizer on the growth, yield, and essential oil composition of dill. The experiment was conducted under field condition in randomized complete block design with three replications and two factors.

Results: The first factor was the concentrations of nitroxin biofertilizer (0%, 50%, and 100%) of the recommended amount (1 l of biological fertilizer for 30 kg of seed). The second factor was the following chemical fertilizer treatments: no fertilizer (control) and 50 and 100 kg ha^{-1} urea along with 300 kg ha^{-1} ammonium phosphate. Different characteristics such as plant height, number of umbel per plant, number of umbellet per umbel, number of grain per umbellet, 1,000 seed weight, grain yield, biological yield, and oil percentage were recorded. According to the results, the highest height, biological yield, and grain yield components (except harvest index) were obtained on biological fertilizer. The results showed the highest essential oil content detected in biological fertilizer and chemical fertilizer. Identification of essential oil composition showed that the content of carvone increased with the application of biofertilizers and chemical fertilizers. The results indicated that the application of biofertilizers enhanced yield and other plant criteria in this plant.

Conclusions: Generally, it seems that the use of biofertilizers or combinations of biofertilizer and chemical fertilizer could improve dill performance in addition to reduction of environmental pollution.

Keywords: *Anethum graveolens*; Nitroxin; Biofertilizer; Chemical fertilizer; Essential oil

Background

Plant nutrients are essential for the production of crops and healthy food for the world's expanding population. The use of chemical fertilizer, organic fertilizer, or biofertilizer has its advantages and disadvantages in the context of nutrient supply, crop growth, and environmental quality. The advantages need to be integrated in order to make optimum use of each type of fertilizer and achieve balanced nutrient management for crop growth [1].

Biological fertilizers are complex of some microorganisms that mobilize main nutrients from unavailable form to available form and can improve root system and seed germination. Presently, these fertilizers are considered as a replacement for chemical fertilizers to improve soil fertility and crop production in sustainable agriculture which is based on ecological principles [2]. Regarding

the importance of medicinal plants and their role in human health, it is imperative to increase their biomass without the application of harmful chemical fertilizers, pesticides, and herbicides. The most important advantages of growth-promoting bacteria include production of growth-inducing and growth-regulating hormones, development of root system, improving water and nutrient uptake [3], improving seed germination and generation of plantlets [4], interaction effect with rhizobiums, improving availability of phosphorous to the plants, biological fixation of nitrogen [5], generation of ionophores especially siderophores, and production of some antibiotic compounds such as bacteriocins to control infections [4]. The application of biofertilizers *Azospirillum* and *Azotobacter* in the medicinal plant *Salvia officinalis* was reported to increase plant height and shoot dry and wet weights [6]. Also, a study by Ratti et al. [7] showed that simultaneous application of mycorrhiza fungus with *Azospirillum* and *Bacillus* increased biomass in the medicinal plant *Cymbopogon maritinii*. Moreover, in *Thymus*

* Correspondence: fnejatzadeh@yahoo.com
[1]Department of Horticulture, Faculty of Agriculture, Islamic Azad University, Khoy Branch, P.O. Box 58168-44799, Khoy, Iran
Full list of author information is available at the end of the article

Table 1 Soil chemical characteristics of the experimental area at 0- to 20-cm depth (Tabriz, 2012/2013)

pH$_{CaCl_2}$	P (mg dm^{-3})	O.M. (%)	Ca (cmolc dm^{-3})	K	N (%)	Ec (ds/m)	C.C.C.	V(%)
7.77	9.52	1.14	1.40	0.46	18	2.85	7.02	33.21

O.M., organic matter; C.C.C., cationic change capacity; Ec, electrical conductivity; V, basis saturation.

vulgaris, the application of biological fertilizers made a significant increase in the plant growth [8].

Dill (*Anethum graveolens* L.) is an aromatic annual grassy plant belonging to the Umbelliferae family that originally comes from Eastern Mediterranean. The entire vegetative organ contains essence. The most important essential oil compounds in this plant are d-carrone and phellandrene, and the most important compounds from the fully grown seeds are d-carrone and limenene. Combined application of organic fertilizer and urea fertilizer or the combination of urea fertilizer and polyamines significantly increases yield, vegetative growth, and evaluations on the chlorophyll index [9]. The aim of the present study was to investigate the effects of biofertilizers and chemical fertilizers on the growth characteristics and yield of *A. graveolens* L. and, consequently, reducing the application of chemical fertilizers.

Methods

This experiment was conducted at an Agriculture Research farm in Tabriz (46° 39′ E, 38° 36′ N) during 2012. The soil texture was sandy clay and results of the soil analysis are shown in Table 1. The first factor tested three levels of nitroxin biofertilizer 0%, 50%, and 100% of the recommended amount (1 l of biofertilizer for 30 kg of seed). The second factor tested the following levels of chemical fertilizer: no fertilizer (control) and 50 and 100 kg ha^{-1} urea recommended along with 300 kg ha^{-1} ammonium phosphates. The field was prepared by cultivating and twice perpendicular disc harrowing followed by smoothing with leveler and then making furrows in March. Locally available seeds of dill were then sown in 4 × 2 plots of six rows in mid-April. Potassium fertilizer was applied to the land evenly into the soil base at 100 kg of potassium sulfate per hectare. Nitrogen was distributed evenly in the respective plots as follows: one third at the 5 to 4 leaf stage and another third at the emergence of the inflorescence emergence and then pre-respective irrigated plots were broadcast between rows. Seeds inoculated with

nitroxin biofertilizer were stored in a black plastic in a cool place until planting time. The maximum time between inoculation of seeds and planting was about 5 h, and irrigated cultivation took place 1 week after emergence on 20 June. The sowing was done in 4 × 2 plots with six rows in each plot. The rows were set 30 cm apart from each other, and thinning was done when plants were in 4 leaf stage so that in each row, the plants were 20 cm apart. During the experiment, no herbicides, pesticides, or fungicides were applied. In order to supply the plants with nutrients, recommended amount of manure (rotten manure, 10 tons per hectare) and phosphate fertilizers prepared in triple phosphate (50 kg per hectare) were applied to the field. Weeding was done at two stages, 20 and 45 days after sowing. Flooding irrigation was done every 7 days.

In order to measure the dry weight of the plants, samples were harvested and put into numbered paper bags to be sent to the laboratory. Samples were oven-dried at 50°C for 72 h and then weighed with a digital scale with ±0.01 g error of measurement. In order to observe yield compounds before harvesting, the marginal rows in each plot and also plants grown up to 50 cm from the ends of each row were set aside, and ten plants were randomly selected from each plot. The number of seeds in each spike, number of spikes per plant, number of spike in each florescence, dry and wet weights of the plants, seed performance in each plant, and weight of 1,000 seeds were recorded. Finally, statistical analysis was carried out using SPSS software and the relevant graphs were prepared using Excel. Means were compared using Duncan test ($p \leq 0.05$).

Results

Plant height

The findings are displayed in Table 2. Comparison of the means for various treatments suggests that nitroxin and nitroxin × nitrogen resulted in significant effect in the plant height, and the highest plants were observed in the samples treated with nitroxin biofertilizers (Table 3).

Table 2 Duncan's multiple range tests analysis for evaluated traits

Treatments	Height of plant	Biological yield	Seed yield	Number of umbel per plant	Number of umbellet per umbel	Number of grain per umbellet	Thousand seed weight	Harvest index	Essential oil percentage	Essential oil yield
Control	55.00 c	3,033 c	1,005 c	10.67 c	7.00 c	13.00 a	3.02 c	33.10 b	2.96 c	29.74 c
Nitroxin	79.67 a	3,475 a	1,320 a	20.03 a	13.03 a	16.00 a	3.00 a	36.00 a	3.96 a	52.27 a
Nitrogen	70.09 b	3,215 b	1,140 b	14.30 b	10.11 b	14.00 a	3.09 b	35.02 ab	3.59 b	40.92 b
Nitroxin × nitrogen	77.43 a	33.70 a	1,270 a	17.30 a	10.56 b	15.00 a	3.09 b	37.01 a	4.01 a	50.92 a

Different letters indicate statistically significant differences.

Application of different fertilizers on morphological traits of dill (Anethum graveolens L.)

169

Table 3 Variance analysis of nitrogen and nitroxin on evaluated traits of (*Anethum graveolens* L.)

	df	Height of plant	Biological yield	Seed yield	Number of umbel per plant	Number of umbellet per umbel	Number of grain per umbellet	Thousand seed weight	Harvest index	Oil percentage	Oil yield
Block	2	0.037	403.862	383.861**	0.106	0.005	0.26	0.0005	0.446*	0.004	3,649.354
Nitroxin	3	68.826**	91,422.843**	11,110.33**	191.16**	10.061**	91.378**	0.001**	0.99	1.77**	1,525,732.09**
Nitrogen	2	3.919**	2,381.861**	481.361**	0.679	0.880**	1.48**	0.0000076	0.256	0.121**	96,287.921**
Nitroxin × nitrogen	6	1.489*	394.231	63.694	0.286	0.098**	0.875**	0.00033	0.059	0.014	8,716.477
Error	22	0.411	300.376	63.740	0.209	0.014	0.029	0.00018	0.087	0.009	5,306.168
CV%		0.78	0.81	1.10	1.15	0.80	0.85	7.35	0.87	3.75	3.89

*Significant at 5% level of probability; **significant at 1% level of probability.

Biological yield

Comparison of the means of different treatments showed nitroxin and nitroxin × nitrogen resulted in significant effect in the biological yield of *A. graveolens* L. The highest and lowest biological yields were obtained with nitroxin and control plants, respectively (Table 2).

Seed yield

Comparison of the means of different treatments showed nitroxin and nitroxin × nitrogen resulted in significant effect in the seed yield of *A. graveolens* L. The highest and lowest seed yields were obtained with nitroxin and control plants, respectively (Table 2).

Number of umbel per plant and number of umbellet per umbel

Analysis of variance showed that nitroxin had significant effect on the number of umbel per plant and number of umbellet per umbel (Table 2).

Number of grain per umbellet

There is no significant effect between treatments in this trait (Table 2).

1,000 seed weight

The results of analysis of variance showed that the trait of seed weight under treatments of biofertilizer, chemicals, and their interactions was very significant (Table 2). The results showed that evaluations for seed weight increased with increasing concentrations of biological and chemical fertilizers. The highest evaluation for seed weight was achieved from the application of nitroxin biofertilizer (Table 2). The results of treatments comparing organic fertilizer and chemical fertilizer showed that the highest evaluation for weight of seeds was obtained by integrating biofertilizer treatment.

Harvest index

Analysis of variance showed that the effect of combined chemical fertilizer and biofertilizer and nitroxin had significant effect on the harvest index (Table 2).

Essential oil percentage and essential oil yield

The results showed the highest essential oil content detected in nitroxin fertilizer and nitroxin × nitrogen fertilizers. Identification of essential oil composition showed that the content of carvone increased with the application of biofertilizers and chemical fertilizers. The results indicated that the application of biofertilizers enhanced yield and other plant criteria in this plant (Table 4).

Discussion

Favorable result for the effect of *Azospirillum* and *Azotobacter* and also phosphate-solubilizing bacteria on the medicinal plant *Majorana hortensis* was reported by [10]. Improvement in germination indexes such as percentage and speed of germination, viability, and also the length of roots and stems of *Ocimum sanctum* and *Withania somniferum* treated with *Azospirillum* and *Azotobacter* biofertilizers, phosphate-solubilizing bacteria, nitrogen-fixing bacteria, and a combination of these fertilizers was reported by [11].

Many research studies have mentioned the positive effect of microorganisms on improving the growth and performance of medicinal plants. In addition to nitrogen fixation, *Azospirillum* improves root growth through generation of stimulating compounds, and these results in an increase in water and nutrient uptake and the general performance of the plant [12]. The most important growth-stimulating bacteria are *Azospirillum*, *Azotobacter*, and *Pseudomonas* which, in addition to biological fixation

Table 4 Oil composition of dill seeds affected by different fertilizers

Compound (%)	Nitroxin × nitrogen	Nitrogen	Nitroxin	Control
Carvone	56.34 a	54.00 b	56.00 a	54.31 b
Limonene	26.10 c	28.00 b	31.30 a	31.04 a
α-Phellandrene	3.31 b	3.01 b	4.21 a	2.22 c
Dill ether	2.00 a	1.01 b	2.02 a	1.01 b
trans-Dihydrocarvone	4.00 b	4.01 b	4.02 b	5.01 a

Different letters indicate statistically significant differences.

of nitrogen and solubilization of soil phosphate, considerably affect plant growth regulators especially auxin, gibberellin, and cytokinin and hence improve the plant performance. *Azotobacter* is able to produce antifungal compounds that fight plant diseases and improve viability and germination of the plantlets and, as a result, improve the overall plant growth [1].

The results of the present study are in agreement with [13] who reported that the application of biological fertilizers in *Calendula officinallis* L. and *Matricaria recutita* L. improved the performance of the shoots in these medicinal plants. Also, there is an increase in plant height and dry and wet weights of the shoots in the first and second harvest [8,14].

Conclusions

The findings of the present study suggest that the application of biological fertilizers had promising effects on dill, and this is in agreement with infrequent research studies on the effect of these fertilizers on medicinal plants. Therefore, it is recommended that the mineral nitrogen and phosphate fertilizers be replaced with biofertilizers to reduce production costs and stop damages to the environment due to the use of chemical fertilizers especially nitrogen as nitrate. The application of biofertilizer combined with growth hormones such as auxin, gibberellin, and cytokines promoted root growth that improved crop yields. Generally, it seems that the use of biofertilizers or combinations of biofertilizer and chemical fertilizer could improve dill performance in addition to reduction of environmental pollution.

Competing interests
The authors declare that they have no competing interests.

Author details
[1]Department of Horticulture, Faculty of Agriculture, Islamic Azad University, Khoy Branch, P.O. Box 58168-44799, Khoy, Iran. [2]Social Determinants of Health Research Center and Environmental Health Engineering, School of Health, Urmia University of Medical Science, Urmia, Iran.

References
1. Chen J (2006) The combined use of chemical and organic fertilizers and or biofertilizer for crop growth and soil fertility. International workshop on sustained management of the soil-rhizosphere system for efficient crop production and fertilizer use, Thailand, pp 16–26
2. Elsen TV (2000) Species diversity as a task for organic agriculture in Europe. Agri Ecosystem Environ 77:101–109
3. Kravchenko LV, Lenova El, Tikhonovich IA (1994) Effect of root exudates of non-legume plants on the response of auxin production by associated diazotrophs. Micro Release 2:267–271
4. Kloepper JW, Lifshitz K, Schroth MN (1998) *Pseudomonas* inoculants to benefit plant production. Plant Sci 1:60–64
5. Ishizuka L (2002) Trends in biological nitrogen fixation research and application. Plant & Soil 11:197–209
6. Vessey JK (2003) Plant growth promoting rhizobacteria as biofertilizers. Plant & Soil 255:571–586
7. Ratti N, Kumar S, Verma HN, Gautams SP (2001) Improvement in bioavailability of tricalcium phosphate to *Cymbopogon martini* var. *motia* by rhizobacteria, AMF and *Azospirillum* inoculation. Microbiol Rese 156:145–149
8. Youssef AA, Edri AE, Gomma AM (2004) A comparative study between some plant growth regulators and certain growth hormones producing microorganisms on growth and essential oil composition of *Salvia officinalis* L. Plant Annl Agric Sci 49:299–311
9. Zeid IM (2008) Effect of arginine and urea on polyamines content and growth of bean under salinity stress. Acta Physiol Plant 28:44–49
10. Fatma EM, El-zamik I, Tomader T, El-Hadidy HE, Abd El-Fattah L, Seham Salem H (2006) Efficiency of biofertilizers, organic and inorganic amendments application on growth and essential oil of marjoram (*Majorana hortensis* L.) plant grown in sandy and calcareous. Agric. Microbiology Dept., Faculty of Agric, Zayazig University and Soil Fertility and Microbiology Dept., Desert Research Center, Cairo, Egypt
11. Krishna A, Patil CR, Raghavendra SM, Jakati MD (2008) Effect of bio-fertilizers on seed germination and seedling quality of medicinal plants. Karnataka J Agric Sci 21(4):588–590
12. Joshee N, Mentreddy SR, Yadav K (2007) Mycorhizal fungi and growth and development of micropropagated *Scutelleria integrifolia* plants. Ind Crops &Prod 25:169–177
13. Leithy S, EL-meseiry TA, Abdallah EF (2006) Effect of biofertilizer, cell stabilizer and irrigation regime on rosemary herbage oil yield and quality. J Appl Res 2:773–779
14. Kapoor R, Giri B, Mukerji KG (2002) *Glomus macrocarpum*: a potential bioinoculant to improve essential oil quality and concentration in dill (*Anethum graveolens* L.) and carum (*Trachyspermum ammi* (Linn.) Sprague). World J Microbiol & Biotechnol 18:459–463

26

Synthesis of some novel 4-arylidene pyrazoles as potential antimicrobial agents

Poonam Khloya[1], Pawan Kumar[1], Arpana Mittal[2], Neeraj K Aggarwal[2] and Pawan K Sharma[1*]

Abstract

Background: Pyrazole and pyrazolone motifs are well known for their wide range of biological activities such as antimicrobial, anti-inflammatory, and antitumor activities. The incorporation of more than one pharmacophore in a single scaffold is a well known approach for the development of more potent drugs. In the present investigation, a series of differently substituted 4-arylidene pyrazole derivatives bearing pyrazole and pyrazolone pharmacophores in a single scaffold was synthesized.

Results: The synthesis of novel 4-arylidene pyrazole compounds is achieved through Knovenagel condensation between 1,3-diaryl-4-formylpyrazoles and 3-methyl-1-phenyl-1*H*-pyrazol-5-(4*H*)-ones in good yields. All compounds were evaluated for their *in vitro* antimicrobial activity.

Conclusions: A series of 4-arylidene pyrazole derivatives was evaluated for their *in vitro* antimicrobial activity against two Gram-positive (*Bacillus subtilis* and *Staphylococcus aureus*) and two Gram-negative bacteria (*Pseudomonas fluorescens* and *Escherichia coli*), as well as two pathogenic fungal strains (*Candida albicans* and *Saccharomyces cerevisiae*). The majority of the compounds displayed excellent antimicrobial profile against the Gram-positive (*B. subtilis* and *S. aureus*), and some of them are even more potent than the reference drug ciprofloxacin.

Keywords: Pyrazole; Pyrazolone; Antibacterial activity; Antifungal activity; Sulfonamide

Background

Over the years, excessive use of antimicrobial drugs has led to a worldwide phenomenon of antibacterial resistance. This has resulted into an increase in morbidity and mortality, and has become a worldwide health issue. As a consequence, the development of new antimicrobial agents is in constant demand. The compounds bearing pyrazole nucleus are well known to exhibit versatile range of biological activities such as antimicrobial [1-4], anti-inflammatory [5-7], antidepressant [8], antiviral [9], and antitumor activities [10]. Among these, 4-functionalized pyrazoles occupy a unique position in medicinal chemistry because of their association with antimicrobial [11], anti-inflammatory [12], antiparasitic [13], and antitumor activities [14]. Pyrazol-5-(4*H*)-one also constitutes the core scaffold of various biologically active synthetic heterocyclic compounds which have been associated with some interesting pharmaceutical properties, including analgesic [15], antimicrobial [16,17], anti-inflammatory [18], antitumor

[19], and cytotoxicity [20] properties. Understanding that the incorporation of both pyrazole and pyrazolone together in the same scaffold could provide novel compounds with interesting biological activities coupled with our continuing research interest in the field of 4-functionalized pyrazole derivatives [12,21-23] and other biologically active synthetic heterocyclic compounds [24-27], we set out to undertake the synthesis of some novel 4-arylidene pyrazole derivatives bearing benzenesulfonamide moiety at the N1-position of the pyrazole ring (Scheme 1) as potential antimicrobial agents.

Methods

In vitro antibacterial activity

The agar well diffusion method [28] was used for the determination of antimicrobial activity of all the synthesized compounds. Overnight broth culture of the respective bacterial strains was adjusted to approximately 10^8 colony forming units (CFU/mL) with sterile distilled water, and 100 μL of diluted inoculum was spread over the petriplates containing 25 mL of nutrient agar media. Eight wells (8 mm in diameter) were made

* Correspondence: pksharma@kuk.ac.in
[1]Department of Chemistry, Kurukshetra University, Kurukshetra 136119, India
Full list of author information is available at the end of the article

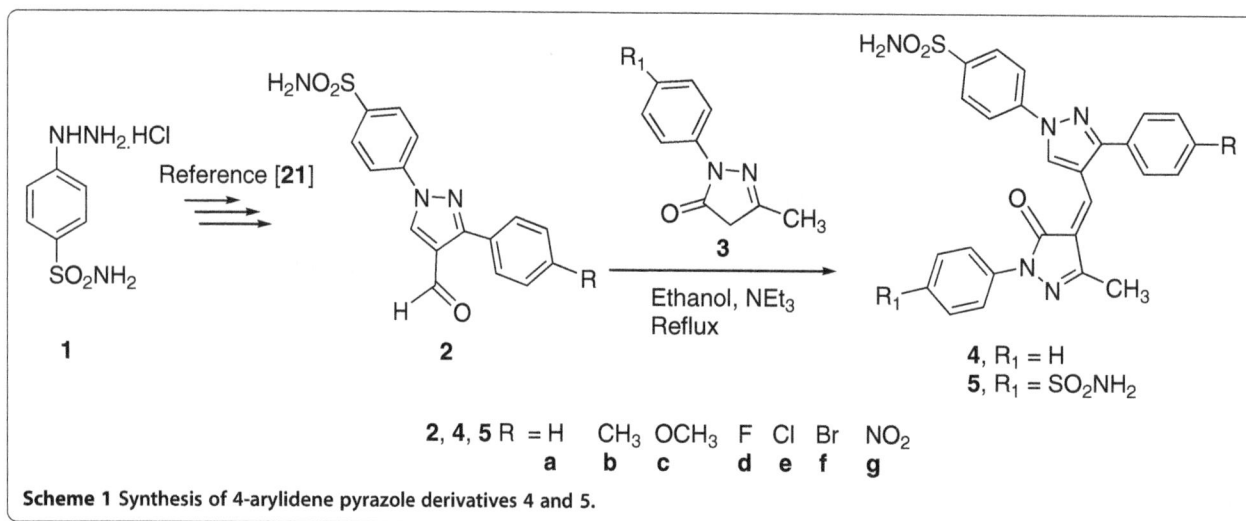

Scheme 1 Synthesis of 4-arylidene pyrazole derivatives 4 and 5.

equidistant with each of the plates using a sterile cork borer. The test compounds were dissolved in dimethyl-sulfoxide (DMSO) and then the antimicrobial effect of the synthesized compounds was evaluated. The wells were filled with 100 μL of the test compound having a concentration of 4.0 mg/mL. The plates were incubated at 37°C for 48 h. The antimicrobial activity was evaluated by measuring the zone of growth inhibition of bacteria surrounding the wells after 24 and 48 h. Ciprofloxacin (4.0 mg/mL) served as the antibacterial control. DMSO was taken as the negative control which did not produce any significant zone of inhibition.

Determination of minimum inhibitory concentration

The minimum inhibitory concentration (MIC) against the tested bacteria was determined using the macrodilution tube method [29] as recommended by NCCLS (2000). The MIC is the lowest concentration of an antimicrobial compound, which will inhibit the visible growth of a microorganism after an overnight incubation. The MIC of each compound giving an inhibitory zone at a concentration of 4 mg/mL was also tested with the agar well diffusion method. Different concentrations (4,000 to 0.004 μg/mL) of a single compound were applied to the number of wells in the agar plates. The determinations were performed in triplicates, and the results were averaged.

In vitro antifungal activity

The agar well diffusion method was used for the determination of antimicrobial activity of the compounds. Overnight broth culture of the respective fungal strains was adjusted to approximately 10^8 CFU/mL with sterile distilled water, and 100 μL of diluted inoculum was spread over the petriplates containing 25 mL of Sabouraud's dextrose agar media (pH 5.6). Eight wells (8 mm in diameter) were made equidistant with each of the plates using a sterile cork borer. The test compounds were dissolved in

DMSO and then the antimicrobial effect of the test compounds was tested. The wells were filled with 100 μL of the test compound having a concentration 4 mg/mL. The plates were incubated at 30°C for 48 to 72 h. The antimicrobial activity was evaluated by measuring the zone of growth inhibition of fungi surrounding the wells after 48 and 72 h. Fluconazole (4 mg/mL) served as the antifungal control. DMSO was taken as the negative control which did not produce any significant zone of inhibition. The experiments were performed in triplicates. The diameter of the fungal colonies was measured.

Results and discussion
Chemistry

The synthetic route used to synthesize the target 4-arylidene pyrazole derivatives (4 and 5) is outlined in Scheme 1. 4-Formyl pyrazoles (2) were synthesized using our earlier reported procedure [21], while 3-methyl-1-aryl-1H-pyrazol-5-(4H)-ones (3) was prepared by condensation of ethylacetoacetate with appropriate hydrazine [30,31]. Finally, base-catalyzed Knoevenagel condensation of appropriately substituted pyrazol-5-(4H)-ones (3) with various substituted 4-formylpyrazoles (2) in ethanol containing catalytic amount of triethylamine afforded the target 4-arylidene pyrazole derivatives (4 and 5) in good yield. Spectral data (IR, ^{1}H NMR, and mass) of the newly synthesized compounds 4a-g and 5a-g were in full agreement with the proposed structures. In the ^{1}H NMR spectra of 4 and 5, the C=CH proton displayed more downfield signal in the range δ 10.18 to 10.25. Besides this, C_5-H of the pyrazole ring resonates at around δ 7.51 to 7.63. The IR spectra of 4 and 5 showed a characteristic absorption band around 1,674 to 1,682 cm^{-1} that was assigned to the C=O stretching, while the two absorptions bands around 1,304 to 1,335 and 1,149 to 1,165 cm^{-1} which further supported the proposed structures of newly synthesized compounds displayed the SO$_2$ stretchings.

Biological evaluation

In vitro antibacterial activity

All the synthesized compounds (**4** and **5**) were screened for their *in vitro* antibacterial activity against the four pathogenic bacteria, *Bacillus subtilis* (microbial-type culture collection (MTCC) 121) and *Staphylococcus aureus* (MTCC 96) representing the Gram-positive bacteria, and *Pseudomonas fluorescens* (MTCC 1749) and *Escherichia coli* (MTCC 1652) representing the Gram-negative bacteria (Table 1), by agar well diffusion method [28] using ciprofloxacin as the reference drug. The MIC measurements were performed using a macrodilution method [29] (Table 1).

The results revealed that all the tested compounds showed variable antibacterial activity against the Gram-positive as well as the Gram-negative bacteria. Among the tested compounds, the antibacterial activity of compounds **4a** and **5a** with a zone of inhibition of 28 mm (MIC 0.04 µg/mL) was found to be better than that of the reference drug ciprofloxacin with a zone of inhibition of 26 mm (MIC 0.4 µg/mL) against *B. subtilis*. Compounds **4f** and **5d** also displayed appreciable activity with a zone of inhibition of 24 mm (MIC 0.4 µg/mL) and 22 mm (MIC 4.0 µg/mL), respectively, against *B. subtilis*. Compound **5a** with two sulfonamide groups was found to be the most effective against *S. aureus*, showing a maximum zone of inhibition of 30 mm (MIC 0.04 µg/mL). **4a** also showed antibacterial activity with a zone of inhibition of 26 mm (MIC 0.4 µg/mL) comparable to the reference drug ciprofloxacin with a zone of inhibition of 26 mm (MIC 0.4 µg/mL) against *S. aureus*. Six more

compounds (**4b-c**, **4f**, and **5b-d**) were found to possess appreciable antibacterial activity with a zone of inhibition greater than 20 mm against *S. aureus*. Interestingly, compounds **4a** and **5a**, both with an unsubstituted phenyl ring at C-3 of pyrazole, displayed a tenfold MIC (0.04 µg/mL) better than the standard drug ciprofloxacin against *B. subtilis*. A comparison within each series suggested that any substituent on the phenyl ring placed at the 3-position of the pyrazole moiety has a negative effect on the antibacterial activity against Gram-positive bacteria, as best results were seen with the naked phenyl ring in each series (compare **4a** with **4a-g**, and **5a** with **5a-g**; Table 1). No definite trend was discernable that could lead to draw a correlation of the activities between series **4** and **5**.

Against Gram-negative bacteria (*P. fluorescens*), only compound **5e** showed a significant activity with a zone of inhibition of 25 mm (MIC 0.4 µg/mL) comparable to the standard drug ciprofloxacin (zone of inhibition 23 mm), albeit with a tenfold better MIC. Against *E. coli*, five compounds (**4e**, **4g 5a**, **5d**, and **5g**) showed good antibacterial activity with a zone of inhibition of 20 mm. However, none of the compounds were found to be as effective as the standard drug ciprofloxacin against *E. coli* (Table 1). Thus, it can be concluded that the synthesized compounds are more effective against the Gram-positive bacteria than the Gram-negative bacteria.

In vitro antifungal activity

All the synthesized compounds were also evaluated for their *in vitro* antifungal activity against the two pathogenic

Table 1 *In vitro* **antibacterial activity and MIC of compounds 4 and 5 using agar well diffusion method**

Compound[a]	Diameter of zone of inhibition in mm (MIC)[b]			
	B. subtilis	*S. aureus*	*P. fluorescens*	*E. coli*
4a	28 ± 0.00 (0.04)	26 ± 0.30 (0.4)	14 ± 0.08 (400)	14 ± 0.46 (400)
4b	20 ± 0.19 (4.0)	24 ± 0.50 (0.4)	15 ± 0.09 (400)	14 ± 0.23 (400)
4c	16 ± 0.19 (40)	24 ± 0.32 (0.4)	-	14 ± 0.23 (400)
4d	16 ± 0.00 (40)	12 ± 0.19 (400)	-	14 ± 0.43 (400)
4e	12 ± 0.40 (400)	16 ± 0.22 (40)	-	20 ± 0.30 (4)
4f	24 ± 0.07 (0.4)	20 ± 0.37 (4.0)	14 ± 0.14 (400)	18 ± 0.33 (40)
4g	14 ± 0.23 (400)	12 ± 0.10 (400)	-	20 ± 0.34 (4)
5a	28 ± 0.09 (0.04)	30 ± 0.15 (0.04)	-	20 ± 0.32 (4)
5b	16 ± 0.32 (40)	25 ± 0.42 (0.4)	16 ± 0.12 (40)	14 ± 0.50 (400)
5c	14 ± 0.18 (400)	22 ± 0.24 (40)	-	18 ± 0.54 (40)
5d	22 ± 0.09 (4.0)	22 ± 0.20 (4.0)	16 ± 0.23 (40)	20 ± 0.12 (4)
5e	14 ± 0.00 (400)	16 ± 0.00 (40)	25 ± 0.13 (0.4)	18 ± 0.23 (40)
5f	12 ± 0.33 (400)	16 ± 0.36 (40)	-	16 ± 0.43 (40)
5g	14 ± 0.32 (400)	12 ± 0.30 (400)	14 ± 0.43 (400)	20 ± 0.21 (4)
Ciprofloxacin	26 ± 0.025 (0.4)	26 ± 0.45 (0.4)	23 ± 0.42 (4.0)	25 ± 0.44 (0.4)

MIC (µg/mL), minimum inhibitory concentration. Hyphens denote no activity. [a]The concentration is 4.0 mg/mL. [b]The values, including the diameter of the well (8 mm), are means of the three replicates.

fungal strains *Candida albicans* (MTCC 227) and *Saccharomyces cerevisiae* (MTCC 170) by agar well diffusion method (Table 2). Fluconazole was used as the reference drug. Most of the tested compounds in each series (4 and 5) showed moderate to good antifungal activity. Compound **4g** was found to be as effective as the standard drug, with a zone of inhibition of 16 mm against *C. albicans*. Against *S. cerevisiae*, **4a** and **5b** (zone of inhibition 28 mm) were found to be the most effective and were better than the standard drug fluconazole (zone of inhibition 24 mm), while the three other compounds (**4d**, **5e**, and **5g**) were found to possess good antifungal activity. Interestingly, some of the newly synthesized compounds (**4a**, **5b**, **5e**, and **5g**) showed multifold reduction in the MIC values against *S. cerevisiae*, making the new derivatives attractive agents for further evaluation.

Experimental

The melting points were determined in open capillaries in an electrical apparatus and were uncorrected. The IR spectra in KBr were recorded with the ABB MB3000 DTGS IR instrument. The ^{1}H NMR spectra were recorded on Bruker instrument (Bruker Scientific Instruments, MA, USA) at 300 MHz, taking DMSO-d_6 as the solvent. The chemical shifts are expressed in δ, ppm. The mass spectra (DART-MS) were recorded on a JEOL AccuTOF JMS-T100LC mass spectrometer having a direct analysis in real time (DART) source in the ES$^+$ mode. The purity of the compounds was checked using ^{1}H

Table 2 *In vitro* **antifungal activity and MIC of compounds 4 and 5 using agar well diffusion method**

Compound[a]	Diameter of zone of inhibition in mm (MIC)[b]	
	Candida albicans	*Saccharomyces cerevisiae*
4a	12 ± 0.43 (400)	28 ± 0.15 (0.04)
4b	12 ± 0.56 (400)	16 ± 0.38 (40)
4c	12 ± 0.54 (400)	16 ± 0.40 (40)
4d	14 ± 0.14 (400)	20 ± 0.45 (4.0)
4e	12 ± 0.45 (400)	18 ± 0.16 (40)
4f	12 ± 0.32 (400)	16 ± 0.27 (40)
4g	16 ± 0.27 (40)	18 ± 0.48 (40)
5a	12 ± 0.32 (400)	16 ± 0.00 (40)
5b	12 ± 0.33 (400)	28 ± 0.28 (0.04)
5c	-	16 ± 0.00 (40)
5d	12 ± 0.23 (400)	18 ± 0.18 (40)
5e	13 ± 0.37 (400)	22 ± 0.44 (4.0)
5f	-	16 ± 0.30 (40)
5g	12 ± 0.43 (400)	20 ± 0.10 (4.0)
Fluconazole	16 ± 0.45 (40)	24 ± 0.50 (40)

MIC (μg/mL), minimum inhibitory concentration. Hyphen denotes no activity.
[a]The concentration is 4.0 mg/mL. [b]The values, including the diameter of the well (8 mm), are means of the three replicates.

NMR and thin layer chromatography on silica gel plates, using a mixture of petroleum ether and ethyl acetate as the eluent. Iodine or UV lamp was used as a visualizing agent. In the following section, these abbreviations are used: 's' for singlet, 'm' for multiplet, and 'ex' for exchangeable proton are used for the NMR assignments; 's' for strong and 'm' for medium are used for the IR assignments.

General procedure for the conversion of 4-formylrazole into 4-arylidene pyrazole derivatives (4 and 5)

To a solution of 4-formylpyrazoles, compound **2** (1 mmol) in ethanol was added to the appropriate pyrazolone **3** (1 mmol) followed by a catalytic amount of triethylamine and refluxed the resulting reaction mixture for 6 to 7 h. After the completion of the reaction, the solution was reduced to 1/4 of its volume and cooled to room temperature. The solid separated out was filtered, washed with water (100 mL) followed by cold ethanol (10 mL), and crystallized from ethanol to afford the target compounds **4** and **5**.

4-{4-[(3-methyl-5-oxo-1-phenyl-1,5-dihydro-4H-pyrazol-4-ylidene)methyl]-3-phenyl-1H-pyrazol-1-yl}benzenesulfonamide (4a)

M.p. 272°C to 275°C, yield 73%; IR (KBr, cm^{-1}): 3,356, 3,267, and 3,256 (m, N-H stretch), 1,674 (s, C=O stretch), 1,589 (s, C=N stretch), 1,497 (s, N-H bend), 1,311 and 1,157 (s, SO$_2$ stretch); ^{1}H NMR (300 MHz, DMSO-d_6): δ 10.23 (s, 1H, C=CH), 8.13 (d, 2H, J = 7.5 Hz, Ar-H), 8.04 (d, 2H, J = 8.4 Hz, Ar-H), 7.95 (d, 2H, J = 8.4 Hz, Ar-H), 7.77 to 7.80 (m, 2H, Ar-H), 7.60 to 7.62 (m, 3H, pyrazole C$_5$-H, Ar-H), 7.52 (s, ex, 2H, SO$_2$NH$_2$), 7.46 (t, 2H, J = 7.5 Hz, Ar-H), 7.21 to 7.23 (m, 1H, Ar-H), 2.23 (s, 3H, CH$_3$); DART MS: m/z 484.30 [M + H]$^+$, C$_{26}$H$_{21}$N$_5$O$_3$SH$^+$ Calcd. 484.13.

4-{4-[(3-methyl-5-oxo-1-phenyl-1,5-dihydro-4H-pyrazol-4-ylidene)methyl]-3-(4-methylphenyl)-1H-pyrazol-1-yl}benzenesulfonamide (4b)

M.p. 158°C to 160°C, yield 74%; IR (KBr, cm^{-1}): 3,742, 3,272, and 3,126 (m, N-H stretch), 1,682 (s, C=O stretch), 1,589 (s, C=N stretch), 1,497 (s, N-H bend), 1,319 and 1,149 (s, SO$_2$ stretch); ^{1}H NMR (300 MHz, DMSO-d_6): δ 10.23 (s, 1H, C=CH), 8.14 (d, 2H, J = 8.7 Hz, Ar-H), 8.04 (d, 2H, J = 8.7 Hz, Ar-H), 7.95 (d, 2H, J = 7.8 Hz, Ar-H), 7.68 (d, 2H, J = 7.8 Hz, Ar-H), 7.53 to 7.54 (m, 3H, pyrazole C$_5$-H, SO$_2$NH$_2$), 7.47 (d, 2H, J = 7.8 Hz, Ar-H), 7.43 (d, 2H, J = 7.5 Hz, Ar-H), 7.21 to 7.24 (m, 1H, Ar-H), 2.43 (s, 3H, CH$_3$), 2.25 (s, 3H, CH$_3$); DART MS: m/z 498.30 [M + H]$^+$, C$_{27}$H$_{23}$N$_5$O$_3$SH$^+$ Calcd. 498.15.

4-{3-(4-methoxyphenyl)-4-[(3-methyl-5-oxo-1-phenyl-1,5-dihydro-4H-pyrazol-4-ylidene)methyl]-1H-pyrazol-1-yl} benzenesulfonamide (4c)

M.p. 156°C to 158°C, yield 76%; IR (KBr, cm^{-1}): 3,372, 3,271, and 3,123 (m, N-H stretch), 1,674 (s, C=O stretch), 1,597 (s, C=N stretch), 1,504 (s, N-H bend), 1,319 and 1,157 (s, SO$_2$ stretch); ^{1}H NMR (300 MHz, DMSO-d_6): δ 10.24 (s, 1H, C=CH), 8.15 (d, 2H, J = 8.1 Hz, Ar-H), 8.04 (d, 2H, J = 7.8 Hz, Ar-H), 7.97 (d, 2H, J = 7.5 Hz, Ar-H), 7.74 (d, 2H, J = 7.8 Hz, Ar-H), 7.55 (s, 1H, pyrazole C$_5$-H), 7.52 (s, ex, 2H, SO$_2$NH$_2$), 7.48 (d, 2H, J = 8.1 Hz, Ar-H), 7.16 to 7.22 (m, 3H, Ar-H), 3.87 (s, 3H, OCH$_3$), 2.28 (s, 3H, CH$_3$); DART MS: m/z 514.29 [M + H]$^+$, C$_{27}$H$_{23}$N$_5$O$_4$SH$^+$ Calcd. 514.15.

4-{4-[(3-methyl-5-oxo-1-phenyl-1,5-dihydro-4H-pyrazol-4-ylidene)methyl]-3-(4-fluorophenyl)-1H-pyrazol-1-yl} benzenesulfonamide (4d)

M.p. 258°C to 260°C, yield 74%; IR (KBr, cm^{-1}): 3,333, 3,225, and 3,132 (m, N-H stretch), 1,674 (s, C=O stretch), 1,597 (s, C=N stretch), 1,504 (s, N-H bend), 1,311 and 1,157 (s, SO$_2$ stretch); ^{1}H NMR (300 MHz, DMSO-d_6): δ 10.25 (s, 1H, C=CH), 8.16 (d, 2H, J = 8.4 Hz, Ar-H), 8.05 (d, 2H, J = 8.7 Hz, Ar-H), 7.96 (d, 2H, J = 8.4 Hz, Ar-H), 7.84 to 7.89 (m, 2H, Ar-H), 7.53 (br s, 3H, pyrazole C$_5$-H, SO$_2$NH$_2$), 7.44 to 7.46 (m, 4H, Ar-H), 7.20 to 7.24 (m, 1H, Ar-H), 2.28 (s, 3H, CH$_3$); DART MS: m/z 502.30 [M + H]$^+$, C$_{26}$H$_{20}$FN$_5$O$_3$SH$^+$ Calcd. 502.13.

4-{3-(4-chlorophenyl)-4-[(3-methyl-5-oxo-1-phenyl-1,5-dihydro-4H-pyrazol-4-ylidene)methyl]-1H-pyrazol-1-yl} benzenesulfonamide (4e)

M.p. 236°C to 238°C, yield 74%; IR (KBr, cm^{-1}): 3,372, 3,271, and 3,123 (m, N-H stretch), 1,674 (s, C=O stretch), 1,589 (s, C=N stretch), 1,497 (s, N-H bend), 1,319 and 1,157 (s, SO$_2$ stretch); ^{1}H NMR (300 MHz, DMSO-d_6): δ 10.23 (s, 1H, C=CH), 8.14 (d, 2H, J = 8.7 Hz, Ar-H), 8.05 (d, 2H, J = 8.7 Hz, Ar-H), 7.95 (d, 2H, J = 8.1 Hz, Ar-H), 7.83 (d, 2H, J = 8.4 Hz, Ar-H), 7.68 (d, 2H, J = 8.4 Hz, Ar-H), 7.53 (s, ex, 2H, SO$_2$NH$_2$), 7.51 (s, 1H, pyrazole C$_5$-H), 7.43 (d, 2H, J = 7.8 Hz Ar-H), 7.21 to 7.24 (m, 1H, Ar-H), 2.27 (s, 3H, CH$_3$); DART MS: m/z 518.26/520.25 [M + H]$^+$/[M + H + 2]$^+$, C$_{26}$H$_{20}$ClN$_5$O$_3$SH$^+$ Calcd. 518.10/520.10.

4-{3-(4-bromophenyl)-4-[(3-methyl-5-oxo-1-phenyl-1,5-dihydro-4H-pyrazol-4-ylidene)methyl]-1H-pyrazol-1-yl} benzenesulfonamide (4f)

M.p. 162°C to 165°C, yield 70%; IR (KBr, cm^{-1}): 3,373, 3,261, and 3,123 (m, N-H stretch), 1,682 (s, C=O stretch), 1,597 (s, C=N stretch), 1,497 (s, N-H bend), 1,311 and 1,157 (s, SO$_2$ stretch); ^{1}H NMR (300 MHz, DMSO-d_6): δ 10.20 (s, 1H, C=CH), 8.11 (d, 2H, J = 8.7 Hz, Ar-H), 8.04 (d, 2H, J = 8.7 Hz, Ar-H), 7.92 to 7.99

(m, 3H, Ar-H), 7.80 (d, 2H, J = 8.1 Hz, Ar-H), 7.67 to 7.74 (m, 3H, Ar-H), 7.61 (s, 1H, pyrazole C$_5$-H), 7.54 (s, ex, 2H, SO$_2$NH$_2$), 7.20 to 7.26 (m, 1H, Ar-H), 2.24 (s, 3H, CH$_3$); DART MS: m/z 562.20/564.19 [M + H]$^+$/[M + H + 2]$^+$, C$_{26}$H$_{20}$BrN$_5$O$_3$SH$^+$ Calcd. 562.05/564.05.

4-{4-[(3-methyl-5-oxo-1-phenyl-1,5-dihydro-4H-pyrazol-4-ylidene)methyl]-3-(4-nitrophenyl)-1H-pyrazol-1-yl} benzenesulfonamide (4g)

M.p. 310°C to 312°C, yield 73%; IR (KBr, cm^{-1}): 3,371, 3,271, and 3,124 (m, N-H stretch), 1,674 (s, C=O stretch), 1,589 (s, C=N stretch), 1,497 (s, N-H bend), 1,335 and 1,157 (s, SO$_2$ stretch); ^{1}H NMR (300 MHz, DMSO-d_6): δ 10.23 (s, 1H, C=CH), 8.44 (d, 2H, J = 8.4 Hz, Ar-H), 8.16 (d, 2H, J = 8.4 Hz, Ar-H), 8.04 to 8.11 (m, 4H, Ar-H), 7.94 (d, 2H, J = 7.8 Hz, Ar-H), 7.56 (s, 1H, pyrazole C$_5$-H), 7.54 (s, ex, 2H, SO$_2$NH$_2$), 7.43 to 7.48 (m, 2H, Ar-H), 7.21 to 7.30 (m, 1H, Ar-H), 2.29 (s, 3H, CH$_3$); DART MS: m/z 529.28 [M + H]$^+$, C$_{26}$H$_{20}$N$_6$O$_5$SH$^+$ Calcd. 529.12.

4-[4-({1-[4-(aminosulfonyl)phenyl]-3-methyl-5-oxo-1,5-dihydro-4H-pyrazol-4-ylidene}methyl)-3-phenyl-1H-pyrazol-1-yl]benzenesulfonamide (5a)

M.p. 248°C to 252°C, yield 73%; IR (KBr, cm^{-1}): 3,340, 3,271, and 3,217 (m, N-H stretch), 1,674 (s, C=O stretch), 1,589 (s, C=N stretch), 1,504 (s, N-H bend), 1,335 and 1165 (s, SO$_2$ stretch); ^{1}H NMR (300 MHz, DMSO-d_6): δ 10.21 (s, 1H, C=CH), 8.14 to 8.19 (m, 4H, Ar-H), 8.05 (d, 2H, J = 8.4 Hz, Ar-H), 7.91 (d, 2H, J = 8.7 Hz, Ar-H), 7.79 to 7.80 (m, 2H, Ar-H), 7.59 to 7.63 (m, 4H, pyrazole C$_5$-H, Ar-H), 7.54 (s, ex, 2H, SO$_2$NH$_2$), 7.36 (s, ex, 2H, SO$_2$NH$_2$), 2.28 (s, 3H, CH$_3$); DART MS: m/z 563.28 [M + H]$^+$, C$_{26}$H$_{22}$N$_6$O$_5$S$_2$H$^+$ Calcd. 563.10.

[4-({1-[4-(aminosulfonyl)phenyl]-3-methyl-5-oxo-1,5-dihydro-4H-pyrazol-4-ylidene}methyl)-3-(4-methylphenyl)-1H-pyrazol-1-yl]benzenesulfonamide (5b)

M.p. 282°C to 285°C, yield 75%; IR (KBr, cm^{-1}): 3,340, 3,248 (m, N-H stretch), 1,682 (s, C=O stretch), 1,589 (s, C=N stretch), 1,497 (s, N-H bend), 1,304 and 1,149 (s, SO$_2$ stretch); ^{1}H NMR (300 MHz, DMSO-d_6): δ 10.19 (s, 1H, C=CH), 8.13 to 8.19 (m, 4H, Ar-H), 8.05 (d, 2H, J = 8.4 Hz, Ar-H), 7.92 (d, 2H, J = 8.4 Hz, Ar-H), 7.68 (d, 2H, J = 7.8 Hz, Ar-H), 7.58 (s, 1H, pyrazole C$_5$-H), 7.52 (s, ex, 2H, SO$_2$NH$_2$), 7.42 (d, 2H, J = 7.5 Hz, Ar-H), 7.34 (s, ex, 2H, SO$_2$NH$_2$), 2.43 (s, 3H, CH$_3$), 2.28 (s, 3H, CH$_3$); DART MS: m/z 577.32 [M + H]$^+$, C$_{27}$H$_{24}$N$_6$O$_5$S$_2$H$^+$ Calcd. 577.12.

4-[4-({1-[4-(aminosulfonyl)phenyl]-3-methyl-5-oxo-1,5-dihydro-4H-pyrazol-4-ylidene}methyl)-3-(4-methoxyphenyl)-1H-pyrazol-1-yl]benzenesulfonamide (5c)

M.p. 320°C to 326°C, yield 74%; IR (KBr, cm^{-1}): 3,317, 3,232, 3,148 and 3,086 (m, N-H stretch), 1,674 (s, C=O stretch), 1,589 (s, C=N stretch), 1,504 (s, N-H bend), 1,335 and 1157 (s, SO_2 stretch); ^{1}H NMR (300 MHz, DMSO-d_6): δ 10.18 (s, 1H, C=CH), 8.12 to 8.19 (m, 4H, Ar-H), 8.04 (d, 2H, J = 8.7 Hz, Ar-H), 7.91 (d, 2H, J = 8.7 Hz, Ar-H), 7.73 (d, 2H, J = 8.7 Hz, Ar-H), 7.57 (s, 1H, pyrazole C_5-H), 7.53 (s, ex, 2H, SO_2NH_2), 7.36 (s, ex, 2H, SO_2NH_2), 7.16 (d, 2H, J = 8.4 Hz, Ar-H), 3.86 (s, 3H, OCH$_3$), 2.28 (s, 3H, CH$_3$); DART MS: m/z 593.30 [M + H]$^+$, $C_{27}H_{24}N_6O_6S_2H^+$ Calcd. 593.12.

4-[4-({1-[4-(aminosulfonyl)phenyl]-3-methyl-5-oxo-1,5-dihydro-4H-pyrazol-4-ylidene}methyl)-3-(4-fluorophenyl)-1H-pyrazol-1-yl]benzenesulfonamide (5d)

M.p. 208°C to 210°C, yield 71%; IR (KBr, cm^{-1}): 3,317, 3,202, 3,148 and 3,070 (m, N-H stretch), 1,674 (s, C=O stretch), 1,589 (s, C=N stretch), 1,504 (s, N-H bend), 1,335 and 1,157 (s, SO_2 stretch); ^{1}H NMR (300 MHz, DMSO-d_6): δ 10.20 (s, 1H, C=CH), 8.14 to 8.19 (m, 4H, Ar-H), 8.05 (d, 2H, J = 8.7 Hz, Ar-H), 7.91 (d, 2H, J = 8.7 Hz, Ar-H), 7.86 (dd, 2H, J = 8.1, 5.4 Hz Ar-H), 7.55 (br s, 3H, pyrazole C_5-H, SO_2NH_2), 7.43 to 7.49 (m, 2H, Ar-H), 7.37 (s, ex, 2H, SO_2NH_2), 2.29 (s, 3H, CH$_3$); DART MS: m/z 581.26 [M + H]$^+$, $C_{26}H_{21}FN_6O_5S_2H^+$ Calcd. 581.10

4-[4-({1-[4-(aminosulfonyl)phenyl]-3-methyl-5-oxo-1,5-dihydro-4H-pyrazol-4-ylidene}methyl)-3-(4-chlorophenyl)-1H-pyrazol-1-yl]benzenesulfonamide (5e)

M.p. 318°C to 320°C, yield 72%; IR (KBr, cm^{-1}): 3,340, 3,256, 3,148 and 3,086 (m, N-H stretch), 1,682 (s, C=O stretch), 1,597 (s, C=N stretch), 1,497 (s, N-H bend), 1,335 and 1,157 (s, SO_2 stretch); ^{1}H NMR (300 MHz, DMSO-d_6): δ 10.20 (s, 1H, C=CH), 8.15 to 8.19 (m, 4H, Ar-H), 8.06 (d, 2H, J = 8.4 Hz, Ar-H), 7.92 (d, 2H, J = 8.7 Hz, Ar-H), 7.84 (d, 2H, J = 8.1 Hz, Ar-H), 7.68 (d, 2H, J = 8.1 Hz, Ar-H), 7.58 (s, 1H, pyrazole C_5-H), 7.54 (s, ex, 2H, SO_2NH_2), 7.36 (s, ex, 2H, SO_2NH_2), 2.31 (s, 3H, CH$_3$); DART MS: m/z 597.25/599.25 [M + H]$^+$/[M + H + 2]$^+$, $C_{26}H_{21}ClN_6O_5S_2H^+$ Calcd. 597.07/599.07.

4-[4-({1-[4-(aminosulfonyl)phenyl]-3-methyl-5-oxo-1,5-dihydro-4H-pyrazol-4-ylidene}methyl)-3-(4-bromophenyl)-1H-pyrazol-1-yl]benzenesulfonamide (5f)

M.p. 330°C to 332°C, yield 69%; IR (KBr, cm^{-1}): 3,742, 3,333 and 3,256 (m, N-H stretch), 1,682 (s, C=O stretch), 1,597 (s, C=N stretch), 1,497 (s, N-H bend), 1,335 and 1,157 (s, SO_2 stretch); ^{1}H NMR (300 MHz, DMSO-d_6): δ 10.19 (s, 1H, C=CH), 8.15 to 8.19 (m, 4H, Ar-H), 8.06 (d, 2H, J = 8.4 Hz, Ar-H), 7.92 (d, 2H, J = 8.4 Hz, Ar-H), 7.82 (d, 2H, J = 7.8 Hz, Ar-H), 7.76 (d, 2H, J = 7.8 Hz, Ar-H), 7.57 (s, 1H, pyrazole C_5-H), 7.54 (s, ex, 2H, SO_2NH_2), 7.35 (s, ex, 2H, SO_2NH_2), 2.31 (s, 3H, CH$_3$); DART MS: m/z 641.19/643.20 [M + H]$^+$/[M + H + 2]$^+$, $C_{26}H_{21}BrN_6O_5S_2H^+$ Calcd. 641.02/643.02.

4-[4-({1-[4-(aminosulfonyl)phenyl]-3-methyl-5-oxo-1,5-dihydro-4H-pyrazol-4-ylidene}methyl)-3-(4-nitrophenyl)-1H-pyrazol-1-yl]benzenesulfonamide (5g)

M.p. 298°C to 300°C, yield 71%; IR (KBr, cm^{-1}): 3,348, 3,248, 3,132 and 3,109 (m, N-H stretch), 1,682 (s, C=O stretch), 1,589 (s, C=N stretch), 1,528 (s, N-H bend), 1,335 and 1,157 (s, SO_2 stretch); ^{1}H NMR (300 MHz, DMSO-d_6): δ 10.21 (s, 1H, C=CH), 8.45 (d, 2H, J = 8.4 Hz, Ar-H), 8.16 to 8.19 (m, 4H, Ar-H), 8.11 (d, 2H, J = 9.0 Hz, Ar-H), 8.07 (d, 2H, J = 8.7 Hz, Ar-H), 7.92 (d, 2H, J = 8.7 Hz, Ar-H), 7.62 (s, 1H, pyrazole C_5-H), 7.55 (s, ex, 2H, SO_2NH_2), 7.36 (s, ex, 2H, SO_2NH_2), 2.33 (s, 3H, CH$_3$); DART MS: m/z 608.27 [M + H]$^+$, $C_{26}H_{21}N_7O_7S_2H^+$ Calcd. 608.09.

Conclusions

In conclusion, we have presented the novel 4-arylidene pyrazole derivatives bearing benzenesulfonamide moiety as potential antimicrobial agents. The reported compounds were conveniently prepared by Knovenagel condensation of 4-formyl pyrazoles with pyrazolones. Some of the tested compounds displayed excellent antibacterial properties against Gram-positive bacteria (*B. subtilis* and *S. aureus*). For instance, compounds **4a** and **5a** were found to be more effective than the reference drug ciprofloxacin. However, against Gram-negative bacteria (*P. fluorescens* and *E. coli*), the level of activity shown by the tested compounds was found to be significantly low as only 2 of the 14 tested compounds displayed activities comparable to the reference drug against *P. fluorescens*, while none of the compounds were found to be highly effective against *E. coli*. All the tested compounds showed moderate antifungal activity against *C. albicans*, while two compounds showed activity better than the reference drug against *S. cerevisiae*. In short, the reported compounds showed remarkable potential as antimicrobial agents and warranted further investigation of their mechanism of actions and binding site. The studies regarding these aspects are being planned with the help of a prospective collaborator.

Abbreviations

DMSO: Dimethylsulfoxide; MIC: Minimum inhibitory concentration; MTCC: Microbial-type culture collection.

Competing interests

The authors declare that they have no competing interests.

Acknowledgements

Defence Research and Development Organization (DRDO), New Delhi, is thankfully acknowledged for the financial support in the form of a research project. One of the authors (PK) is grateful to the Haryana State Council for Science and Technology (HSCST), Panchkula (Haryana), India, for the award of Junior Research Fellowship. The authors are thankful to the Sophisticated Analytical Instrument Facility, Central Drug Research Institute, Lucknow, for the mass spectra analysis.

Author details
[1]Department of Chemistry, Kurukshetra University, Kurukshetra 136119, India.
[2]Department of Microbiology, Kurukshetra University, Kurukshetra 136119, India.

References

1. Bondock S, Fadaly W, Metwally MA (2010) Synthesis and antimicrobial activity of some new thiazole, thiophene and pyrazole derivatives containing benzothiazole moiety. Eur J Med Chem 45:3692–3702
2. Isloor AM, Kalluraya B, Shetty P (2009) Regioselective reaction: synthesis, characterization, and pharmacological studies of some new mannich bases derived from 1,2,4-triazoles. Eur J Med Chem 44:3784–3787
3. Prakash O, Hussain K, Kumar R, Wadhwa D, Sharma C, Aneja KR (2011) Synthesis and antimicrobial evaluation of new 1,4-dihydro-4-pyrazolylpyridines and 4-pyrazolylpyridines. Org Med Chem Lett 1:1–5
4. Aneja DK, Lohan P, Arora S, Sharma C, Aneja KR, Prakash O (2011) Synthesis of new pyrazolyl-2, 4-thiazolidinediones as antibacterial and antifungal agents. Org Med Chem Lett 1:1–15
5. El-Sayed MAA, Abdel-Aziz NI, Abdel-Aziz AAM, El-Azab AS, ElTahir KEH (2012) Synthesis, biological evaluation and molecular modeling study of pyrazole and pyrazoline derivatives as selective COX-2 inhibitors and anti-inflammatory agents. Bioorg Med Chem 20:3306–3316
6. Singh SK, Saibaba V, Rao KS, Reddy PG, Daga PR, Rajjak SA, Misra P, Rao YK (2005) Synthesis and SAR/3D-QSAR studies on the COX-2 inhibitory activity of 1,5-diarylpyrazoles to validate the modified pharmacophore. Eur J Med Chem 40:977–990
7. Lee KY, Kim JM, Kim JN (2003) Regioselective synthesis of 1,3,4,5-tetrasubstituted pyrazoles from Baylis-Hillman adducts. Tetrahedron Lett 44:6737–6740
8. Abdel-Aziz M, Abuo-Rahma El-Din AG, Hassan AA (2009) Synthesis of novel pyrazole derivatives and evaluation of their antidepressant and anticonvulsant activities. Eur J Med Chem 44:3480–3487
9. Hashem AI, Youssef ASA, Kandeel KA, Abou-Elmagd WSI (2007) Conversion of some 2(3H)-furanones bearing a pyrazolyl group into other heterocyclic systems with a study of their antiviral activity. Eur J Med Chem 42:934–939
10. Lv P-C, Li H-Q, Sun J, Zhou Y, Zhu H-L (2010) Synthesis and biological evaluation of pyrazole derivatives containing thiourea skeleton as anticancer agents. Bioorg Med Chem 18:4606–4614
11. Sridhar R, Perumal PT, Etti S, Shanmugan PMN, Prabavathy VR, Mathivanan N (2004) Design, synthesis and anti-microbial activity of 1H-pyrazole carboxylates. Bioorg Med Chem Lett 14:6035–6040
12. Sharma PK, Kumar S, Kumar P, Kaushik P, Kaushik D, Dhingra Y, Aneja KR (2010) Synthesis and biological evaluation of some pyrazolylpyrazolines as anti-inflammatory-antimicrobial agents. Eur J Med Chem 45:2650–2655
13. Rathelot P, Azas N, El-Kashef H, Delmas F, Giorgio CD, Timon-David P, Maldonado J, Vanelle P (2002) 1,3-Diphenylpyrazoles: synthesis and antiparasitic activities of azomethine derivatives. Eur J Med Chem 37:671–679
14. Li X, Liu JL, Yang XH, Lu X, Zhao TT, Gong HB, Hl Z (2012) Synthesis, biological evaluation and molecular docking studies of 3-(1,3-diphenyl-1H-pyrazol-4yl)-N-phenylacrylamide derivatives as inhibitors of HDAC activity. Bioorg Med Chem 20(14):4430–4436
15. Uramaru N, Shigematsu H, Toda A, Eyanagi R, Kitamura S, Ohta S (2010) Design, synthesis and pharmacological activity of non allergenic pyrazolone type antipyretic analgesics. J Med Chem 53:8727–8733
16. Thaker KM, Ghetiya RM, Tala SD, Dodiya BL, Joshi KA, Dubal KL, Joshi HS (2011) Synthesis of oxadiazoles and pyrazolones as a antimycobacterial and antimicrobial agents. Indian J Chem 50B:738–744
17. Chande MS, Barve PA, Suryanarayan V (2007) Synthesis and antimicrobial activity of novel spiro compounds with pyrazolone and pyrazolthione moiety. J Hetero Chem 44:49–53
18. Mariappan G, Saha BP, Satharson L, Haldar A (2010) Synthesis and bioactivity evaluation of pyrazolone derivatives. Indian J Chem 49B:1671–1674
19. Wang XH, Wang XK, Liang YJ, Shi Z, Zhang JY, Chen LM, Fu LW (2010) A cell-based screen for anticancer activity of 13 pyrazolone derivatives. Chin J Cancer 29(12):980–987
20. Chen T, Benmohamed R, Kim J, Smith K, Amanta D, Morimoto RI, Kirsch DR, Ferrante RJ, Silverman RB (2012) ADME-guided design and synthesis of aryloxanyl pyrazolone derivatives to block mutant superoxide dismutase 1 (SOD1) cytotoxicity and protein aggregation: potential application for the treatment of amyotrophic lateral sclerosis. J Med Chem 55(1):515–527
21. Sharma PK, Chandak N, Kumar P, Sharma C, Aneja KR (2011) Synthesis and biological evaluation of some 4-functionalized pyrazoles as antimicrobial agents. Eur J Med Chem 46:1425–1432
22. Sharma PK, Singh K, Kumar S, Kumar P, Dhawan SN, Lal S, Ulbrich H, Dannhardt G (2011) Synthesis and anti-inflammatory evaluation of some pyrazolo[3,4-b]pyridines. Med Chem Res 20:239–244
23. Kumar P, Chandak N, Kaushik P, Sharma C, Kaushik D, Aneja KR, Sharma PK (2012) Synthesis and biological evaluation of some pyrazole derivatives as anti-inflammatory–antibacterial agents. Med Chem Res 21:3396–3405
24. Sharma PK, Kumar S, Kumar P, Kaushik P, Sharma C, Kaushik D, Aneja KR (2012) Synthesis of 1-(4-aminosulfonylphenyl)-3,5-diarylpyrazoline derivatives as potent anti-inflammatory and antimicrobial agent. Med Chem Res 21:2945–2954
25. Kumar S, Namkung W, Verkman AS, Sharma PK (2012) Novel 5-substituted benzyloxy-2-arylbenzofuran-3-carboxylic acid calcium activated chloride channel inhibitors. Bioorg Med Chem 20:4237–4244
26. Chandak N, Bhardwaj JK, Sharma RK, Sharma PK (2012) Inhibitors of apoptosis in testicular germ cells: synthesis and biological evaluation of some novel IBTs bearing sulfonamide moiety. Eur J Med Chem 59:203–208
27. Chandak N, Kumar P, Sharma C, Aneja KR, Sharma PK (2012) Synthesis and biological evaluation of some novel thiazolylhydrazinomethylidene ferrocenes as antimicrobial agents. Lett Drug Des Discov 9(1):63–68
28. Perez C, Pauli M, Bazevque P (1990) An antibiotic assay by the agar well diffusion method. Acta Biol Med Exp 15:113–115
29. Andrews JM (2001) Determination of minimum inhibitory concentrations. J Antimicrob Chemother 48:5–16
30. Knorr L (1884) Einwirkung von acetessigester auf hydrazinchinizinderivate. Chem Ber 17:546–552
31. Knorr L (1886) Synthetische versuche mit dem acetessigester II mittheilung: ueberführung des diacetbernsteinsäureesters und des acetessigesters in pyrrolderivate. Ann Chem 236:290–336

27

Eco-friendly synthesis and antimicrobial activities of some 1-phenyl-3(5-bromothiophen-2-yl)-5-(substituted phenyl)-2-pyrazolines

Ramalingam Sasikala, Kannan Thirumurthy, Perumal Mayavel and Ganesamoorthy Thirunarayanan[*]

Abstract

Background: Green catalyst fly ash: H_2SO_4 was prepared by mixing fly ash and sulphuric acid. Microwave irradiations are applied for solid phase cyclization of 5-bromo-2-thienyl chalcones and phenyl hydrazine hydrate in the presence of fly ash: H_2SO_4 yields, 1-phenyl-3(5-bromothiophen-2-yl)-5-(substituted phenyl)-2-pyrazolines. These pyrazolines were characterized by their physical constants and spectral data. The antimicrobial activities of all synthesized pyrazolines have been studied.

Results: Scanning electron microscopy (SEM) analysis shows the morphology changes between fly ash and the catalyst fly ash: H_2SO_4. The SEM photographs with the scale of 1 and 50 μm show the fly-ash particle is corroded by H_2SO_4 (indicated by arrow mark), and this may be due to dissolution of fly ash by H_2SO_4. The yields of 1-phenyl-3 (5-bromothiophen-2-yl)-5-(substituted phenyl)-2-pyrazolines is more than 75% using this catalyst under microwave heating. All pyrazolines showed moderate activities against antimicrobial strains.

Conclusion: We have developed an efficient catalytic method for synthesis of 1-phenyl-3(5-bromothiophen-2-yl)-5-(substituted phenyl)-2-pyrazolines by solid phase cyclization using a solvent-free environmentally greener catalyst fly ash: H_2SO_4 under microwave irradiation between aryl chalcones and hydrazine hydrate. This reaction protocol offers a simple, economical, environment friendly, non-hazardous, easier work-up procedure, and good yields. All synthesized pyrazoline derivatives showed moderate antimicrobial activities against bacterial and fungal strains.

Keywords: 1-phenyl-3(5-bromothiophen-2-yl)-5-(substituted phenyl)-2-pyrazolines, Fly ash:H_2SO_4, Environmentally benign reaction, IR and NMR spectra, Antimicrobial activities

Background

Pyrazolines are well-known important nitrogen containing five membered heterocyclic bioorganic molecules. The pyrazoline ring protons were bonded with carbon atoms on a spatially different environment. These pyrazolines are used widely in the current decades due to their various biological and pharmacological activities [1]. The α,β-unsaturated ketones can play the role of versatile precursors in the synthesis of the corresponding pyrazolines [2-7]. Numerous methods have been reported for the preparation of pyrazoline compounds. Fischer and Knoevenagel in the nineteenth century studied the reaction of α,β-unsaturated aldehydes and ketones with phenyl hydrazine in acetic acid by refluxing, which became one of the most popular methods for the preparation of 2-pyrazolines [8]. In 1998, Powers et al. [9] have reported the reaction of chalcones with phenyl hydrazine hydrochloride in the presence of sodium hydroxide and absolute ethanol at 70°C, where the longer reaction time is the disadvantage of the reaction. K_2CO_3-mediated microwave irradiation has been shown to be an efficient method for the synthesis of pyrazolines [10]. The regioselective formation of pyrazolines has been synthesized by the reaction of substituted hydrazine with α,β-unsaturated ketones [11,12]. Recently, many organic reactions in aqueous media have been described in the literature [13]. In 2007, Li et al. [14] have synthesized 1,3,5-triaryl-2-pyrazoline with chalcones and phenyl hydrazine hydrochloride in sodium acetate-acetic acid aqueous solution under ultrasound

* Correspondence: drgtnarayanan@gmail.com
Department of Chemistry, Annamalai University, Annamalai Nagar 608 002, India

irradiation. Pyrazolines have been exhibiting various pharmacological activities, such as analgesic [15], anti-inflammatory [16,17], antimicrobial [18,19], anti-amoebic [20,21], antitubercular [22,23], hypoglycemic [24], anti-coagulant [25], antidepressant [26-28], pesticide [29], fungicide [30], antibacterial [31], and anticonvulsant activities [32]. Recent report shows some new pyrazoline-substituted thiazolone-based compounds that exhibit anticancer activity [33]. Apart from biological activities, pyrazolines are also extensively used as synthons in organic synthesis [34-36], as optical brightening agents for textiles, paper, and fabrics, and as a hole-conveying medium in photoconductive materials [37-41]. In this present study, the authors have taken efforts to synthesize a series of 1-phenyl-3(5-bromothiophen-2-yl)-5-(substituted phenyl)-2-pyrazolines from 5-bromo-2-thienyl chalcones and phenyl hydrazine hydrate in presence of fly ash:H_2SO_4. These pyrazolines were characterized by their physical constants and spectral data. The antimicrobial activities of all synthesized pyrazolines have been studied.

Methods

Materials

All chemicals used were purchased from Sigma-Aldrich Corporation (St. Louis, MO, USA) and E-Merck chemical company (Merck Limited, Mumbai, India) Melting points of all pyrazolines have been determined in open glass capillaries on Mettler FP51 melting point apparatus (Mettler-Toledo India Private Limited, Mumbai, India) and are uncorrected. Infrared spectra (KBr, 4,000 to 400 cm^{-1}) have been recorded on AVATAR-300 Fourier transform spectrophotometer (Thermo Nicolet, USA). A BRUKER AMX-500 NMR spectrometer (BRUKER AXS GMBH, Karlsruhe, Germany) operating at 500 MHz has been utilized for recording ^{1}H spectra and 125.75 MHz

for ^{13}C spectra in CDCl$_3$ solvent using TMS as internal standard. Electron impact (70 eV) and chemical ionization mode FAB$^+$ mass spectra have been recorded in VARIAN-SATURN 2200 GC-MS spectrometer (Varian Medical Systems, Palo Alto, CA, USA).

Results and discussion

Fly ash is a waste air pollutant, and it has many chemical species [10,33], such as SiO_2, Fe_2O_3, Al_2O_3, CaO, and MgO, and insoluble residues. The waste fly ash is converted into useful catalyst fly ash: H_2SO_4 by mixing fly ash and sulphuric acid. The sulphuric acid-sulphate ion group and chemical species present in the fly ash have enhanced catalytic activity. During the course of the reactions, these species are responsible for the promoting effects on cyclization between the chalcones and hydrazine hydrate leading to the formation of pyrazolines. In these experiments, the products were isolated, and the catalyst was washed with ethyl acetate, heated to 100°C, and was then reusable for further five run reactions. There was no appreciable change in the percentage of yield of pyrazolines. In this protocol, the reaction gave better yields of the pyrazolines during the condensation without any environmental discharge. The analytical and mass spectral data are presented in Table 1. The infrared (IR) and nuclear magnetic resonance (NMR) spectral data of unknown pyrazolines are presented in Tables 2, and 3.

Infrared spectral study

In the IR spectra of synthesized pyrazolines, the stretching frequency at 1,593 to 1,596 cm^{-1} is assigned to C = N. The frequency at 678 to 688 cm^{-1} is due to the C-S group, and a band at 531 to 569 cm^{-1} is assigned to the C-Br stretching frequency. A collection of medium bands observed in the region 3,028 to 2,854 cm^{-1} is attributed

Table 1 Analytical and mass spectral data of 1-phenyl-3(5-bromothiophen-2-yl)-5-(substituted phenyl)-2-pyrazolines

Entry	Substituent	MF	FW (dalton)	Yield (%)	M.p. (°C)	Mass (m/z)
1	H	$C_{20}H_{17}BrN_2$	365	85	152-153	365[M$^+$], 367[M^{+2}], 287, 285, 221, 209, 142, 79, 77, 68, 65, 41, 28, 14
2	4-Br	$C_{20}H_{16}Br_2N_2$	444	83	148-150	444[M$^+$], 446[M^{+2}], 448[M^{+4}], 365, 363, 229, 222, 201, 155, 142, 77, 68, 41, 28, 14.
3	2-Cl	$C_{20}H_{17}BrClN_2$	399	75	142-144	399[M$^+$], 401[M^{+2}], 403[M^{+4}], 363, 321, 319, 287, 225, 209, 142, 111, 77, 68, 65, 41, 28, 35, 14
4	4-Cl	$C_{20}H_{17}BrClN_2$	399	79	147-149	399[M$^+$], 401[M^{+2}], 403[M^{+4}], 363, 321, 287, 225, 209, 142 77, 65, 41, 28, 14
5	3, 4-(OCH$_3$)$_2$	$C_{22}H_{21}BrN_2O_2$	425	85	140-142	425[M$^+$], 427[M^{+2}], 393, 363, 347, 287, 251, 142, 134, 107, 95, 78, 65, 41, 28, 14
6	4-I	$C_{20}H_{17}BrIN_2$	491	76	146-148	491[M$^+$], 493[M^{+2}], 495[M^{+4}], 412, 363, 347, 287, 269, 229, 203, 142, 126, 77, 42, 28, 14
7	4-(OCH$_3$)	$C_{21}H_{19}BrN_2O$	395	85	128-130	395[M$^+$], 397[M^{+2}], 363, 317, 287, 210, 142, 105, 77, 41, 14
8	4-CH$_3$	$C_{21}H_{19}BrN_2$	379	83	148-149	379[M$^+$], 381[M^{+2}], 365, 287, 235, 210, 142, 91, 77, 41, 14

FW, formula weight; MF, molecular formula; M.p., melting point; m/z, mass-to-change ratio.

Table 2 IR and NMR spectral data of 1-phenyl-3(5-bromothiophen-2-yl)-5-(substituted phenyl)-2-pyrazolines

Entry X	Infrared bands (ν cm^{-1})					^{1}H chemical shifts δ (ppm)					Entry X	^{13}C chemical shifts δ (ppm)				
	C=N	C-S	C-Br	Ar-C and Alip-C	Subst.	Ha (1 H, dd)	Hb (1 H, dd)	Hc (1 H, dd)	Ar-H	Subst.		C$_3$	C$_4$	C$_5$	Ar-C	Subst.
1 H	1,593	679	562	3028-2854	-	3.06 J = 24 Hz	3.77 J = 29 Hz	5.25 J = 19 Hz	6.71-7.34 (12 H, m)	-	1 H	155.60	43.66	64.68	111.77-146.521	-
2 4-Br	1,596	685	5,621	3089-2852	-	3.07 J = 30 Hz	3.82 J = 28 Hz	5.26 J = 24 Hz	6.70-7.51 (11 H, m)	-	2 4-Br	155.56	43.45	64.10	112.13-144.13	-
3 2-Cl	1,595	690	566	3065-2852	-	3.01 J = 23 Hz	3.93 J = 29 Hz	5.66 J = 19 Hz	6.77-7.48 (11 H, m)	-	3 2-Cl	157.50	42.08	61.50	113.28-143.99	-
4 4-Cl	1,594	688	5,31	3046-2852	-	3.10 J = 24 Hz	3.80 J = 29 Hz	5.28 J = 19 Hz	6.75-7.35 (11 H, m)	-	4 4-Cl	155.82	43.70	64.75	113.52-144.40	-
5 3,4-(OCH$_3$)$_2$	1,594	678	569	3073-2873	1,254	3.08 J = 25 Hz	3.76 J = 30 Hz	5.17 J = 19 Hz	6.75-7.36 (11 H, m)	3.83, 3.87	5 3,4-(OCH$_3$)$_2$	155.63	43.81	64.89	111.68-149.74	55.94, 55.98
6 4-I	1,595	680	531	3090-2852	-	3.04 J = 24 Hz	3.78 J = 29 Hz	5.21 J = 20 Hz	6.74-6.69 (11 H, m)	-	6 4-I	156.11	43.52	64.21	93.16-143.45	-
7 4-OCH$_3$	1,596	670	553	3095-2852	1,249	3.07 J = 25 Hz	3.77 J = 31 Hz	5.24 J = 18 Hz	6.75-7.28 (11 H, m)	3.80	7 4-OCH$_3$	155.81	43.75	64.29	113.57-159.13	55.28
8 4-CH$_3$	1,594	680	546	3095-2854	-	3.07 J = 24 Hz	3.77 J = 28 Hz	5.25 J = 19 Hz	6.71-7.34 (11 H, m)	2.31	8 4-CH$_3$	156.10	43.72	64.47	111.68-146.48	21.13

Table 3 The HOMOCOSY and HSQC data δ (parts per million) of 1-phenyl-3(5-bromothiophen-2-yl)-5-(phenyl)-2-pyrazoline (1)

		HOMOCOSY						HSQC		
Proton	Carbon (ppm)	δ H_a at C_4 3.06	δ H_b at C_4 3.77	δ H_c at C_5 5.25	δ Ar-H 6.71-7.34	Proton	Carbon (ppm)	δ C_4 43.66	δ C_5 64.68	δ Ar-H 111.77-46.52
δ H_a at C_4	3.06	-	Bonded	Bonded	-	δ Ha at C4	3.06	Bonded	-	-
δ H_b at C_4	3.77	Bonded	-	Bonded	-	δ Hb at C4	3.77	Bonded	-	-
δ H_c at C_5	5.25	Bonded	Bonded	-	-	δ Hc at C5	5.25	-	Bonded	-
δ Ar-H	6.71-7.34	-	-	-	Bonded	δ Ar-H	6.71-7.34	-	-	Bonded

HOMOCOSY, homonuclear correlation spectroscopy; HSQC, heteronuclear single quantum correlation.

to C-H stretching vibrations of the aliphatic and aromatic groups. These IR bands are supporting evidences for the formation of pyrazolines. The assigned spectral bands of pyrazolines are presented in Table 2.

NMR spectral study

^{1}H NMR spectra

In ^{1}H NMR spectrum of pyrazolines, the doublet of doublet at δ 3.01 to 3.10 with coupling constants $J_1 = 7.5$ Hz and $J_2 = 17$ Hz is assigned to H_a proton of C_4. The doublet of doublet at 3.76 to 3.93 ppm with coupling constants $J_1 = 12.5$ Hz and $J_2 = 17$ Hz is assigned to H_b proton of C_4. Similarly, the doublet of doublet at 5.17 to 5.66 ppm with coupling constants $J_1 = 7.5$ Hz and $J_2 = 12.5$ Hz is assigned to H_c proton of C_5. The aromatic protons appeared in the range of 6.71 to 7.34 ppm. These proton chemical shift (part per million) values were supported for formation of pyrazolines and are presented in Table 2.

^{13}C NMR spectra

In ^{13}C NMR spectrum of pyrazolines, the signals appear in the range 111.77 to 146.52 ppm are due to the aromatic carbons. The signal at downfield region

155.60 ppm are assigned to C = N carbon. Two signals that appeared in the lower frequency region at 43.66 and 64.68 ppm are assigned to the methylene and methyn carbons at C_4 and C_5, respectively. The assigned ^{13}C chemical shift values of all pyrazolines are furnished in Table 2.

HOMOCOSY spectra

In the homonuclear correlation spectroscopy (HOMOCOSY) spectrum of pyrazolines, the possible correlations are furnished in Table 3. The ^{1}H-^{1}H COSY spectrum of parent compound (entry 1) is shown in Figure 1. Both H_a (3.06 ppm) and H_b (3.77 ppm) protons at C_4 show a strong cross peak with the signal at 5.25 ppm. This suggests that the doublet of doublet at 5.25 ppm is due to the H_c proton of C_4. Based on this analysis, the proton chemical shifts (parts per million) of other pyrazolines were assigned and confirmed.

HETCOSY spectra

The HSQC (heteronuclear single quantum correlation) spectrum of synthesized pyrazoline (entry 1) is shown in Figure 2, and their correlations are listed in Table 3. The H_a and H_b protons at C_4 show a cross peak with

Table 4 The antibacterial and antifungal activities of 1-phenyl-3(5-bromothiophen-2-yl)-5-(substitutedphenyl)-2-pyrazolines by disc diffusion method

		Antibacterial activities						Antifungal activities			
Entry	X	Zone of inhibition (mm)					Entry	X	Zone of inhibition (mm)		
		S. aureus	E. coli	K. pneumoniae	S. typhi	Pseudomonas spp.			C. albicans	Mucor spp.	Rhizopus spp.	A. niger
1	H	10	15	20	15	15	1		15	15	15	15
2	4-Br	10	15	20	20	17	2		20	20	20	20
3	2-Cl	15	15	15	5	5	3		15	15	15	15
4	4-Cl	3	10	15	15	15	4		15	15	15	15
5	3,4-$(OCH_3)_2$	17	17	15	17	20	5		17	17	17	17
6	4-I	15	17	20	17	10	6		17	17	17	17
7	4-OCH_3	15	17	20	17	22	7		20	20	20	20
8	4-CH_3	15	10	15	5	5	8		20	15	15	20
Cip	-	17	17	20	22	15	Ket		15	15	15	15

Cip, ciprofloxacin; Ket, ketoconazole.

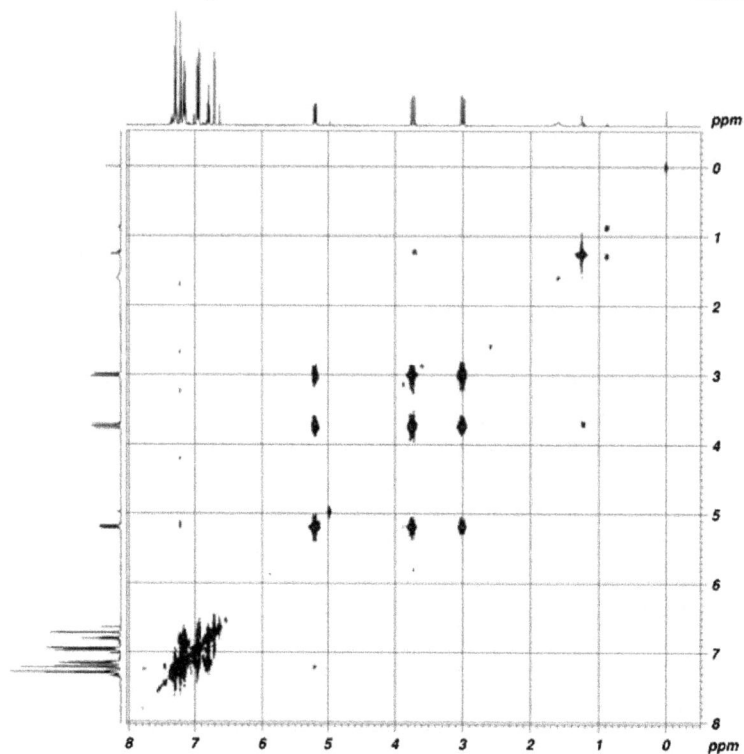

Figure 1 HOMOCOSY spectrum of 1-phenyl-3(5-bromothiophen-2-yl)-5-(phenyl)-2-pyrazoline (1).

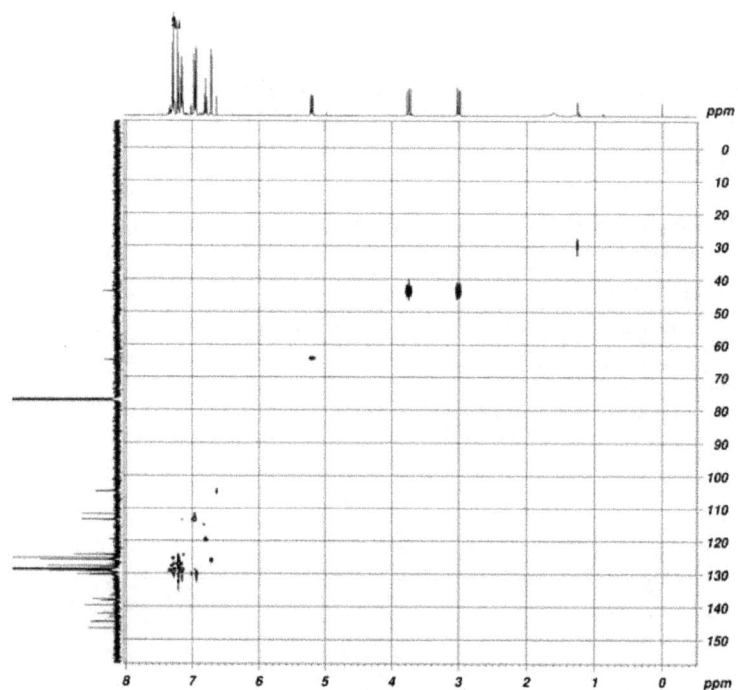

Figure 2 HSQC spectrum of 1-phenyl-3(5-bromothiophen-2-yl)-5-(phenyl)-2-pyrazoline (1).

Staphylococcus aureus

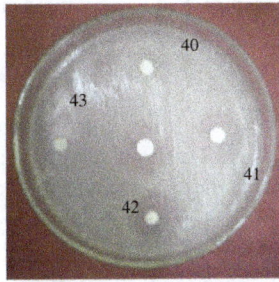 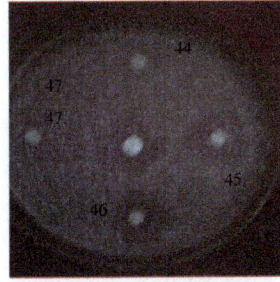

AB1 AB2

Escherichiia Coli

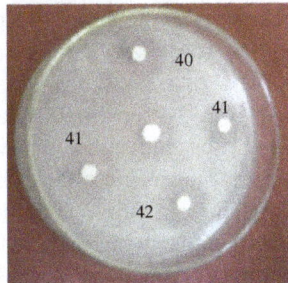 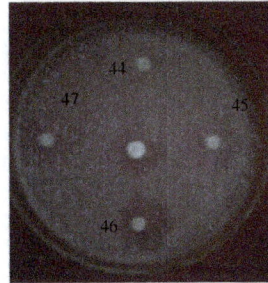

AB3 AB4

Klebsiella pneumonia

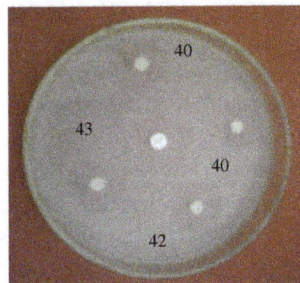 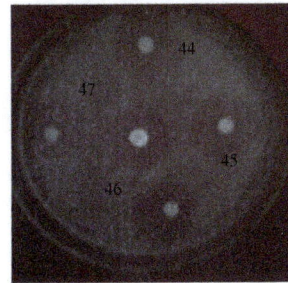

AB5 AB6

Salmonella typhi

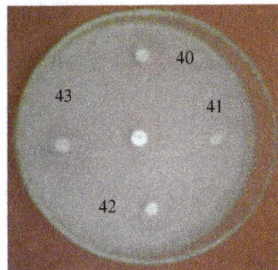 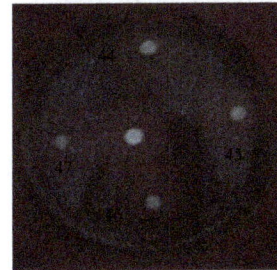

AB7 AB8

Pseudomonas

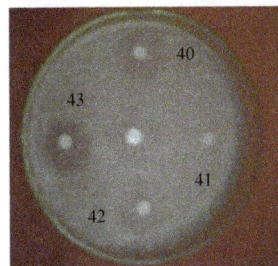 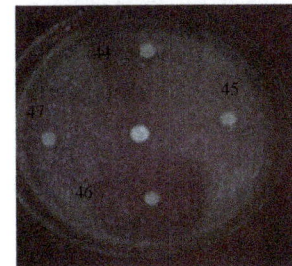

AB9 AB10

Figure 3 (See legend on next page.)

(See figure on previous page.)
Figure 3 Antibacterial activities by zone of inhibition of 1-phenyl-3(5-bromothiophen-2-yl)-5-(substituted phenyl)-2-pyrazoline petri dishes (AB1 to AB10).

the carbon signal at 43.66 ppm, which confirms that this carbon signal is due to C_4 carbon. Similarly, a doublet of doublet at 5.25 ppm is having a strong correlation with the carbon resonance at 64.68 ppm. From this, it is inferred that the carbon signal is due to C_5 carbon. Based on this analysis, the carbon chemical shifts (parts per million) of other pyrazolines were assigned and confirmed.

Antimicrobial activities
Antibacterial activity
Staphylococcus aureus was taken as gram positive strain, and *Escherichia coli*, *Klebsiella pneumoniae*, *Salmonella typhi*, and *Pseudomonas* species were taken as gram negative strains; they have been used for the present study.

Determination of antibacterial activity by disc-diffusion method
Nutrient agar plates were prepared under sterilized conditions and incubated overnight to detect contamination. About 0.2 mL of working stock culture was transferred into separate nutrient broth and spread thoroughly using a glass spreader. Whatman number 1 discs (6 mm in diameter) were impregnated with the test compounds dissolved in DMSO (200 µg/mL) for about half an hour. Commercially available drug disc (ciprofloxacin 10 mg/disc) was used as positive reference standard. Negative control was also prepared by impregnating the disc of same size in dimethyl sulfoxide (DMSO) solvent. The plates were then incubated overnight for 18 to 24 h. Antibacterial activity was evaluated by measuring the zone of inhibition against the test organism.

Determination of minimum inhibitory concentration of test compounds using twofold serial dilution method
Testing was done in the seeded broth (10^{-6} to 10^{-7} cfu/mL). The test compounds were taken at different concentrations ranging from 200, 100, 50, 25, 12.5, 6.25, 3.13, 1.56, 0.78, and to 0.39 µg/mL for finding the minimum inhibitory concentration (MIC) by using seeded broth as diluent. Similarly, the standard solution of ciprofloxacin drug prepared at the concentrations of 200, 100, 50, 25.5, 6.25, 3.13, 1.56, 0.78, and 0.39 µg/mL of sterile distilled water and DMSO were maintained throughout the experiment simultaneously as control.

The study involves a series of 10 assay tubes for the test compounds against each strain. In the first assay tube, 1.6 mL of seeded broth was transferred, and 0.4 mL of the test solution was added, followed

by mixing it thoroughly to obtain a concentration of 200 µg/mL. To the remaining nine assay tubes, 1 mL of seeded broth was transferred, and then, from the first assay tube, per milliliter of the content was pipetted out and added into the second assay tube, followed by mixing thoroughly. This type of dilution was repeated up to the 10th assay tube serially. The same procedure was followed for standard drugs. Duplicates were also maintained; these were done under aseptic conditions.

The racks of assay tubes were placed inside the incubator at $37 \pm 1°C$ for 24 h. After the incubation period, the assay tube concentrations were again streaked into the nutrient agar plate due to turbidity of the drug microorganism mixture. The lowest concentration of the test compounds, which caused apparently a complete inhibition of growth of organisms, was taken as the MIC. The solvent control tube was also observed to find whether there was any inhibitory action. The sterile distilled water and DMSO did not show any inhibition.

The antimicrobial activity of all the synthesized pyrazolines (entries 1 to 8) were examined by disc diffusion and two fold serial dilution methods. Bacterial strains, *viz. S. aureus*, *E. coli*, *K. pneumonia*, *S. typhi*, and *Pseudomonas* species, and fungal strains, *viz. Candida albicans*, *Mucor* species, *Rhizopus* species, *Aspergillus niger*. In the present study, DMSO is used as control, while ciprofloxacin and ketoconazole are used as standards for bacterial and fungal strains, respectively. The zone of inhibition and MIC values of compounds (entries 1 to 8) against both the tested bacterial strains are given in Table 4. The representative photographs of disc diffusion and serial dilution methods are depicted in Figure 3.

The antibacterial activity of all pyrazolines produced a maximum zone of inhibition against all the bacterial strains except compounds 3 and 4 against *S. typhi* and *Pseudomonas* spp., compounds 4 against *S. aureus*, and compounds 7 and 8 against *Pseudomonas* spp. which showed maximum zone of inhibition than the standard (ciprofloxacin).

Antibacterial activity of all synthesized pyrazolines was measured by serial dilution method, and the MICs are presented in Table 5. From Table 5, compounds 1 to 8 showed the growth inhibitory concentration against the tested organism fall in the range of 1.5 to 200 µg/mL. However, compounds 1 to 4 showed the inhibition against all bacterial strains in the range from 25 to 100 µg/mL. The rest of the compounds are more effective against all bacterial strain MICs at 1.5 to 25 µg/mL.

Table 5 The antibacterial and antifungal activities of 1-phenyl-3(5-bromothiophen-2-yl)-5-(substituted phenyl)-2-pyrazolines by serial dilution method

		Antibacterial activities						Antifungal activities			
Entry	X	MIC (µg/mL)					Entry X	MIC (µg/mL)			
		S. aureus	*E. coli*	*K. pneumoniae*	*S. typhi*	*Pseudomonas spp.*		*C. albicans*	*Mucor spp.*	*Rhizopus spp.*	*A. niger*
1	H	25	50	12.5	50	50	1	50	50	50	50
2	4-Br	50	25	3.13	3.13	6.25	2	3.13	3.13	3.13	3.13
3	2-Cl	25	25	25	100	100	3	25	25	25	25
4	4-Cl	200	50	25	25	25	4	25	25	25	3.13
5	3,4-(OCH₃)₂	6.25	6.25	12.5	6.25	3.13	5	6.25	6.25	6.25	6.25
6	4-I	25	6.25	3.13	6.25	50	6	6.25	6.25	6.25	6.25
7	4-OCH₃	12.5	6.25	3.13	6.25	1.5	7	3.13	3.13	3.13	3.13
8	4-CH₃	50	100	50	200	200	8	50	50	50	50
Cip	-	6.25	6.25	3.13	1.5	12.5	Ket	12.5	12.5	12.5	12.5

Cip, ciprofloxacin; Ket, ketoconazole.

Antifungal activity

The following fungal strains *C. albicans*, *Mucor* spp, *Rhizopus* spp, and *A. niger* were used for the present study. Sabouraud dextrose agar (SDA) medium was used for the growth of fungi, and testing was done in Sabouraud dextrose broth (SDB) medium.

The subculture and the viable count were carried out by the same procedure as done in antibacterial studies except for the temperature which should be maintained at $28 \pm 1°C$ for about 72 h. Similarly, for the disc diffusion method, the petri dishes were incubated at $28 \pm 1°C$ for about 72 h. The same concentration of the test compound, solvent (DMSO), and ketoconazole (standard) prepared previously were used for the antifungal studies.

The antifungal activities of synthesized pyrazolines 1 to 4 exhibited a similar inhibition activity as that of the standard (15 mm) against all fungal strains, whereas pyrazoline 2 exhibited against *C. albicans* and *A. niger* (20 mm), and pyrazoline 5 to 8 against all the fungal strains showed maximum zone of inhibition (17 to 20 mm) than the standards (15 mm, ketoconazole). The measured antifungal activities of pyrazolines are presented in Table 4. The representative photographs of disc diffusion methods are depicted in Figure 4.

The antifungal activities of all synthesized pyrazolines were measured by serial dilution method. Among the compounds under study, compounds 1 to 8 were found to be effective against all the fungal strain MICs at 3.13 to 6.25 µg/mL. MIC values of compounds 1 to 4 against all the tested fungal strains are in the range of 25 to 50 µg/mL except for compound 2 against *C. albicans* (12.5 µg/mL) and compound 4 against *A. niger* (3.13 µg/mL). The measured antifungal activities of all compounds are presented in Table 5.

Comparison of potency of compounds 1 to 8 with standard drugs against bacterial and fungal strains from serial dilution method

In order to understand the results of serial dilution method, the potency of synthesized compounds 1 to 8 against tested bacterial and fungal strains are calculated with respect to the reference (standards) using Equation 1:

$$\text{Potency} (\%) = \frac{\text{M IC (mg/mL) of reference compound}}{\text{M IC (mg/mL) of tested compound}} \times 100 \qquad (1)$$

To comprehend it well, the results obtained from the above equation are presented as bar graphs and are shown in Figures 5 and 6.

On comparison with ciprofloxacin compounds 1–4 showed the potency against all the bacterial strains in the range of 25–100%. But, the remaining compounds exhibited lesser potency in the range of 1.5 - 50%.

With reference to ketoconazole, an equal potency is noted for compounds 1 (50%), 3(25%), 5 and 7 (3.13%), 6 and 8 (6.25%) against all the fungal strains. But 12.5% potency is noted for compound 2 against C.albicans and 3.13% is noted for compound 4 against *A. niger*.

Experimental
Preparation and characterization of catalyst

In a 50-mL Borosil beaker (Borosil Glass Works Limited, Mumbai, India), 1 g of fly ash and 0.8 mL (0.5 mol) of sulphuric acid were taken and mixed thoroughly with glass rod. This mixture was heated on a hot air oven at 85°C for 1 h, cooled to room temperature, stored in a Borosil bottle, and tightly capped [42]. This was

Candida albicans

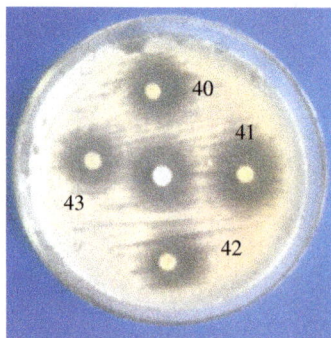

AF1

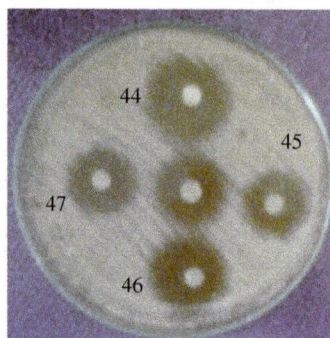

AF2

Mucor.sp

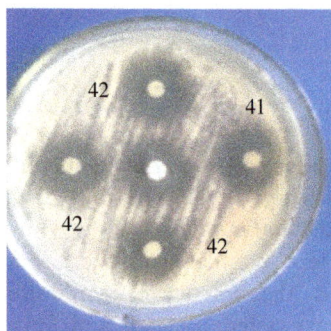

AF3

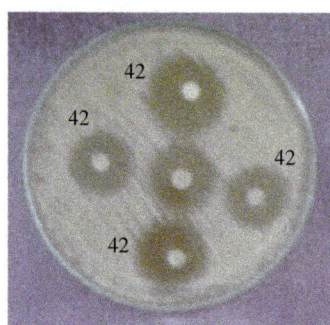

AF4

Rhizopus sp

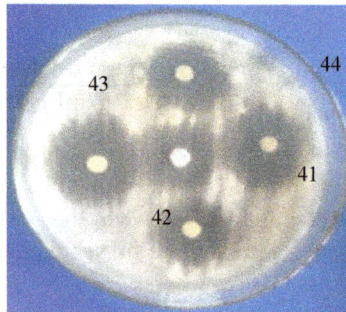

AF5

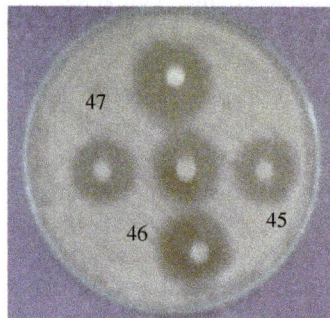

AF6

Aspergillus niger

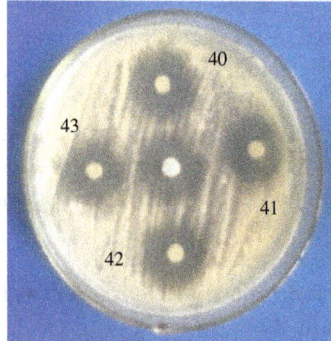

AF7

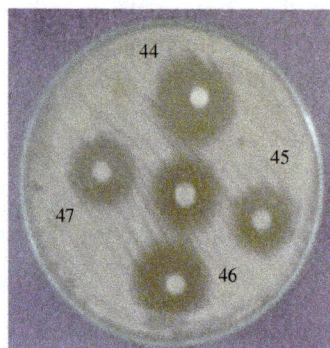

AF8

Figure 4 Antifungal activities of spectrum of 1-phenyl-3(5-bromothiophen-2-yl)-5-(substituted phenyl)-2-pyrazoline pretri dishes (AF1 to AF8).

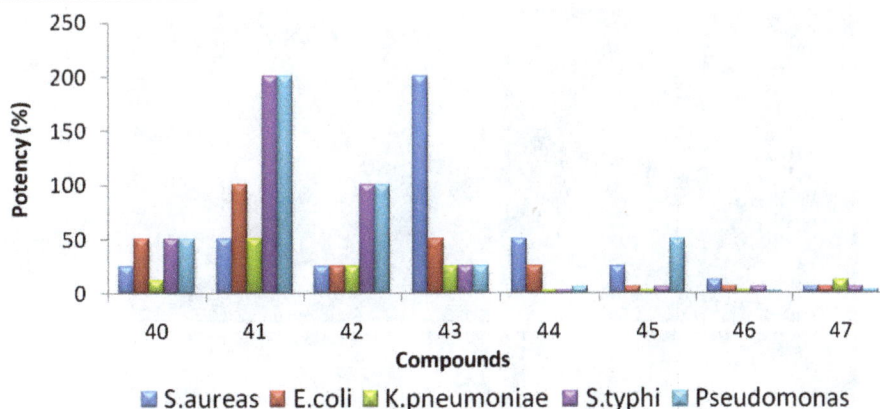

Figure 5 Comparison of potency of pyrazolines with ciprofloxacin (standard) against bacterial strains from serial dilution method.

characterized by infrared spectra and scanning electron microscopy (SEM) analysis.

Infrared spectral data of fly ash: H_2SO_4 is v (per centimeter) with values 3,456(OH); 3,010 (C-H); 1,495, 1,390 (C-S); 1,336, 1,154(S = O) and *op* modes 1,136, 1,090, 976, 890, 850, 820, 667, 658, 620, 580, 498, and 425.

The SEM images of pure fly ash and fly ash:H_2SO_4 at two different magnifications are shown in Figure 7. Figure 1a,b depicted that there is more crystallinity found in pure fly ash. The spherical-shaped particles are clearly seen at both magnifications in Figure 7a,b. Figure 7a reveals the globular structure of pure fly ash (round-shaped particle). This is also seen in Figure 7c,d that some of the particles are slightly corroded by H_2SO_4 (indicated by arrow mark), and this may be due to dissolution of fly ash by H_2SO_4. This will further be confirmed by Figure 7d, the well-shaped particles of pure fly ash. Figure 7b is aggregated to Figure 7d due to the presence of H_2SO_4.

Synthesis of substituted 5-bromo-2-thienyl chalcones

All substituted styryl 5-bromo-2-thienyl ketones were synthesized using the literature procedure [43].

Synthesis of 1-phenyl-3(5-bromothiophen-2-yl)-5-(substituted phenyl)-2-pyrazolines

An appropriate equi-molar quantity of 5-bromo-2-thienyl chalcones, phenylhydrazine hydrochloride (0.2 mmol), and 0.5 g of fly ash:H_2SO_4 was subjected to microwave irradiation for 5 to 6 min in a microwave oven (Scheme 1) (LG Grill, Intellowave, Microwave Oven, LG Electronics, Seoul, South Korea; 160 to 800 W) and then cooled to room temperature. The organic layer was separated with dichloromethane, and the solid product was obtained on evaporation. On recrystallization with benzene-hexane mixture, it gave glittering pale yellow solid. The insoluble catalyst was recycled by washing the solid reagent that remained on the filter by ethyl acetate (8 mL), followed by drying in an oven at 100°C for 1 h, and it was made reusable for further reactions. The analytical and mass spectral data are given in Table 1. Infrared and NMR spectral data of pyrazolines are presented in Table 2. The individual proton and carbon signals were unambiguously assigned by HOMOCOSY and HETCOSY spectral analysis. The ^{1}H-^{1}H COSY and ^{1}H-^{13}C COSY spectral data are presented in Table 3.

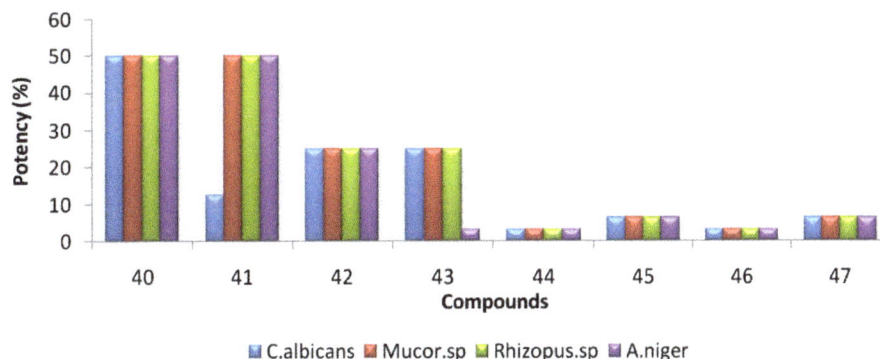

Figure 6 Comparison of potency of pyrazolines with ciprofloxacin (standard) against fungal strains from serial dilution method.

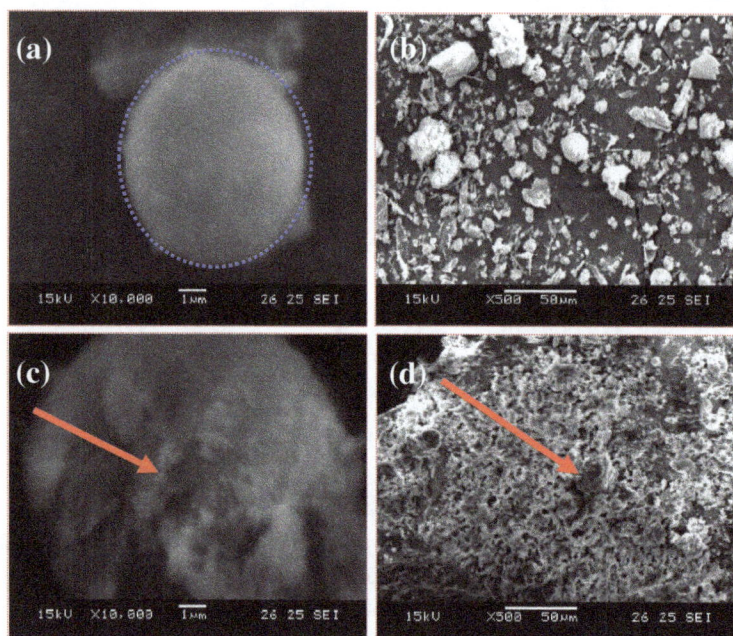

Figure 7 SEM images of pure fly ash and fly ash:H2SO4. (**a**) Pure fly ash (1 μm), (**b**) pure fly ash (50 μm), (**c**) fly ash:H_2SO_4 (1 μm) (red bold arrow, corroded), and (**d**) fly ash:H_2SO_4 (50 μm) (red bold arrow, corroded).

Antibacterial activities

Preparation of test inoculum subculture (preparation of seeded broth)

The strains of *S. aureus*, *E. coli*, *K. pneumoniae*, *Pseudomonas* species, and *S. typhi* were inoculated in conical flasks containing 100 mL of sterile nutrient broth. These conical flasks were incubated at $37 \pm 1°C$ for 24 h. This was referred to as the seeded broth.

Standardization of seeded broth (viable count) dilutions

One mL of 24-h seeded broth of each strain was diluted with 99 mL of sterile normal saline containing 0.05% Tween 80 (drops of Tween 80 in 1,000 mL normal saline). From that, 1 mL is further diluted to 10 mL sterile normal saline. This was continued to 10^{-2}, 10^{-3}, 10^{-4}, 10^{-5}, until 10^{-10} dilution of seeded broth was obtained.

Incubation of nutrient agar petri dishes

The dilutions were studied by inoculating 0.2 mL of each dilution onto the solidified nutrient agar medium by spread plate method, after incubation at $37 \pm 1°C$ for 24 h. The numbers of well-formed colonies on the plates were counted. The seeded broth was then suitably diluted to have been 10^5 to 10^7 microorganisms per milliliter or colony-forming per milliliter. This was designated as the working stock and used for the antibacterial studies.

Preparation of solution of test compounds

The solution of test compounds were prepared by dissolving the same in DMSO in a specific growth bottle and stored in a refrigerator. The solution was removed from the refrigerator 1 h prior to its use and allowed to

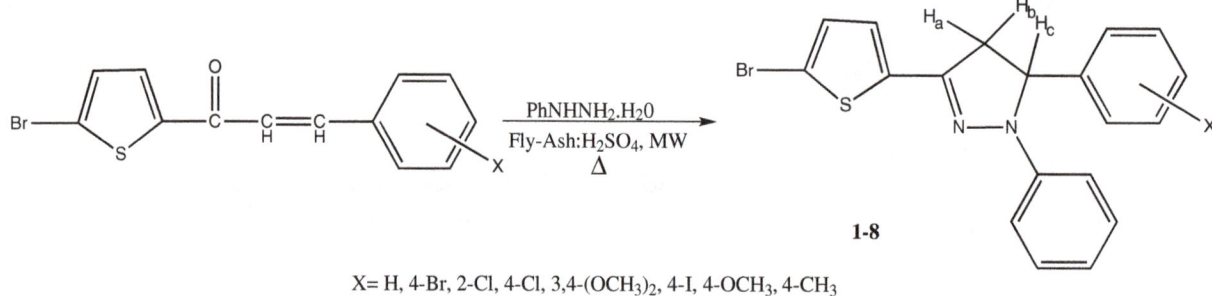

X= H, 4-Br, 2-Cl, 4-Cl, 3,4-$(OCH_3)_2$, 4-I, 4-OCH_3, 4-CH_3

Scheme 1 Synthesis of 1-phenyl-3(5-bromothiophen-2-yl)-5-(substituted phenyl)-2-pyrazolines.

warm up to room temperature. The test compounds were prepared at a concentration of 200 μg/mL. Similarly, the standard drug solution of ciprofloxacin and ketoconazole were used respectively at a concentration of 200 μg/mL for finding the MIC.

Preparation of culture media
The media used for the growth of bacteria were nutrient agar medium and nutrient broth medium. The media were sterilized by autoclaving at a pressure of 15 lbs at 121°C for 20 min.

Nutrient agar medium The nutrient agar medium was prepared by dissolving 28 g of nutrient agar (Hi-media, Mumbai, India) in 1,000 mL of distilled water. The following formula was followed for the preparation of nutrient agar medium: peptone, 1%; NaCl, 0.5%; beef extract, 1%; agar, 2%, and pH, 7.4 ± 0.2.

Nutrient broth medium The nutrient broth medium was prepared by dissolving 13 g of nutrient broth (Hi-media, Mumbai) in 1000 mL of distilled water. The following formula was followed for preparation of nutrient broth medium: peptone 1%; NaCl, 0.5%; beef extract, 1%; agar, 1%; pH, 7.4 ± 0.2.

Antifungal activity
Preparation of culture media SDA medium
The following formula was followed for the preparation of SDA medium: dextrose, 40 g; peptone, 10 g; agar, 15 g; distilled water, 1,000 mL, and pH, 5.4.

SDB broth
The following formula was followed for the preparation of SDB broth: dextrose, 40 g; peptone, 10 g; agar, 15 g; distilled water, 1,000 mL; and pH, 5.4.

Conclusions
We have developed an efficient catalytic method for synthesis of 1-phenyl-3(5-bromothiophen-2-yl)-5-(substituted phenyl)-2-pyrazolines by cyclization of substituted styryl 5-bromo-2-thienyl ketones and phenyl hydrazine hydrochloride using a solvent-free environmentally greener catalyst fly ash: H_2SO_4 under microwave irradiation. This reaction protocol offers a simple, economical, environment friendly, non-hazardous, and easier work-up procedure and good yields. All synthesized pyrazoline derivatives showed moderate antimicrobial activities against the strains used.

Competing interests
The authors declare that they have no competing interests.

Acknowledgments
The authors thank RSIC, IIT, Chennai-600 036 for recording the NMR spectra of all pyrazolines.

References
1. Das BC, Bhowmilk D, Chiranjib B, Mariappan G (2010) Synthesis and biological evaluation of some pyrazoline derivatives. J Pharm Res 3(6):1345–1348
2. Gupta R, Gupta N, Jain A (2010) Improved synthesis of chalcones and pyrazolines under ultrasonic irradiation. Indian J Chem 49B(3):351–355
3. Solankee A, Lad S, Solankee S, Patel G (2009) Chalcones, pyrazolines and aminopyrimidines as antibacterial agents. Indian J Chem 48B(10):1442–1446
4. Revanasiddappa BC, Nagendr Rao R, Subramaniyam EVS, Satyanarayana D (2010) Synthesis and biological evaluation of some novel 1,3,5-trisubstituted pyrazolines. E-J Chem 7(1):295–298
5. Voskiene A, Mickevicius V, Mikulskiene G (2007) Synthesis and characterization of products condensation 4-carboxy-1-(4-styrylcarbonylphenyl)-2-pyrrolidines with hydrazines. ARKIVOC XV:303–314
6. Kataade S, Phalgune U, Biswas S, Wakharkar R, Deshpande N (2008) Microwave studies on synthesis of biologically active chalcones derivatives. Indian J Chem 47B(6):927–931
7. Al-Issa SA, Andis NAL (2005) Solvent free synthesis of chalcones and N-phenyl-2-pyrazolines under microwave irradiation. J Saudi Chem Soc 9(3):687–692
8. Levai A, Jeko J (2007) Synthesis of carboxylic acid derivatives of 2-pyrazolines. ARKIVOC I:134–145
9. Powers DG, Casebier DS, Fokas D, Ryan WR, Troth JR, Coffen DL (1998) Automated parallel synthesis of chalcones based screening libraries. Tetrahedron 54(16):4085–4096
10. Kidwar K, Kukreja S, Thakur R (2006) K_2CO_3-Mediated regioselective synthesis of isoxazoles and pyrazolines. Lett Org Chem 3(2):135–139
11. Katritzky AR, Wang M, Zhang S, Voronkov MV, Steel PJ (2001) Regioselective synthesis of polysubstituted pyrazoles and isoxazoles. J Org Chem 66(20):6787–6791
12. Kuz'menok NM, Koval'chuk TK, Zvonok AM (2005) Synthesis of 5-hydroxy- and 5-amino-1-tosyl-5- phenyl-3-(2-arylvinyl)-4,5-dihydropyrazoles. Syn Lett 3:485–486
13. Li CJ (2008) Organic reactions in aqueous media with a focus on C-C bond formations: a decade update. Chem Rev 105(3):3095–3165
14. Li JT, Zhang XH, Lin ZP (2007) An improved synthesis of 1,3,5-triaryl-2-pyrazolines in acetic acid aqueous solution under ultrasound irradiation. Beli J Org Chem. doi:10.1186/1860-5397-3-13
15. Sahu SK, Banerjee M, Samantray A, Behera C, Azam MA (2008) Synthesis, analgesic, anti-inflammatory and antimicrobial activities of some novel pyrazoline derivatives. Trop J Pharm Res 7(2):961–968
16. Karabasanagouda T, Adhikari AV, Girisha M (2009) Synthesis of some new pyrazolines and isoxazoles carrying 4-methylthiophenyl moiety as potential analgesic and anti-inflammatory agents. Indian J Chem 48B(3):430–437
17. Barsoum FF, Hosni HM, Girgis AS (2006) Novel bis(1-acyl-2-pyrazolines) of potential anti-inflammatory and molluscicidal properties. Bioorg Med Chem 14(11):3929–3937
18. Kumar B, Pathak V, Rani S, Kant R, Tewari IC (2009) Synthesis and antimicrobacterial activity of some bromo-benzothiazolo pyrazolines. Int J Microbiol Res 1(2):20–22
19. Chawla R, Sahoo U, Arora A, Sharma PC, Radhakrishnan V (2010) Microwave assisted synthesis of some novel 1-pyrazoline derivatives as possible antimicrobial agents. Acta Polo Pharm-Drug Res 67(1):55–61
20. Mbarki S, Dguigui K, Hallaoui ME (2011) Construction of 3D-QSAR models to predict antiamoebic activities of pyrazoline and dioxazoles derivatives. J Mater Environ Sci 2(1):61–70
21. Rao NS, Kumar R, Srivastava YK (2009) Microwave induced synthesis and antimicrobial activities of some n1-morpholono ethanoyl-3,5-diaryl-2-pyrazoline derivatives. Rasayan J Chem 2(3):716–719
22. Rahman MA, Siddiqui AA (2010) Pyrazoline derivatives: a worthy insight into the recent advances and potential pharmacological activities. Int J Pharm Sci Drug Res 2(3):165–175
23. Kasabe AJ, Kasabe PJ (2010) Synthesis, antitubercular and analgesic activity evaluation of new 3-pyrazoline derivatives. Int J Pharmacy Pharm Sci 2(2):132–135

24. Sridevi C, Balaji K, Naidu A, Kavimani S, Venkappayya D, Suthakaran R, Parimala S (2009) Synthesis of some phenylpyrazolo benzothiazolo quinoxaline derivatives. Int J Pharm Tech Res 1(3):816–821

25. Levai A, Jeko J (2009) Synthesis of 5-aryl-1-carboxyphenyl-3-(3-coumarinyl)-2-pyrazolines. ARKIVOC VI:63–70

26. Palaska E, Aytemir M, Uzbay IT, Erol D (2001) Synthesis and antidepressant activities of some 3,5-diphenyl-2-pyrazolines. Eur J Med Chem 36(60):539–543

27. Rajendra Prasad Y, Lakshmana Rao A, Prasoona L, Murali K, Ravikumar P (2005) Synthesis and antidepressant activity of some 1,3,5-triphenyl-2-pyrazolines and 3-(2ʹʹ-hydroxynaphthalene-1-ʹʹ-yl)-1,5-diphenyl-2-pyrazolines. Bioorg Med Chem Lett 15(22):5030–5034

28. Zhao PL, Wang F, Zhang MZ, Liu ZM, Huang W, Yang GF (2008) Synthesis, fungicidal and insecticidal activities of β-methoxyacrylate containing N-acetyl pyrazoline derivatives. J Agric Food Chem 56(22):10767–10773

29. Kini S, Gandhi AM (2008) Novel 2-pyrazoline derivatives as potential antibacterial and antifungal agents. Indian J Pharm Sci 70(1):105–108

30. Siddiqui AA, Rahman MA, Shaharyar M, Mishra R (2010) Synthesis and anticonvulsant activity of some substituted 3,5-diphenyl-2-pyrazoline-1-carboxamide derivatives. Chem Sci J 1:1–10

31. Gowramma B, Jubie S, Kalirajan R, Gomathy S, Elango K (2009) Synthesis, anticancer activity of some 1-(Bis N, N-(Chloroethyl)-amino acetyl)-3,5-disubstituted 1,2-pyrazolines. Int J Pharm Tech Res 1(2):347–352

32. Klimova EI, Maartnez Garca M, Klimova Berestneva T, Alvarez Toledano C, Alferdo Toskano R, Ruz Ramres L (1999) The structure of bicyclic ferrocenylmethylene substituted 2-pyrazolines and their reactions with azodicarboxylic acid N-phenylimide. J Org Metal Chem 585(1):106–114

33. Padmavathi V, Sumathi RP, Chandrasekar Babu N, Bhaskar D (1999) 1,3-Dipolar cycloaddition of dipolar reagents to bifunctional olefins in the presence of chloramine-T (CAT). J Chem Res (S):610–611

34. Soni N, Pande K, Kalsi R, Gupta TK, Parmar SS, Barthwal JP (1987) Inhibition of rat brain monoamine oxidase and succinic dehydrogenase by anticonvulsant pyrazolines 56(1):129–132

35. Ferigolo M, Barros HM, Marquardt AR, Tannhauser M (1998) Comparison of behavioral effects of moclobemide and deprenyl during forced swimming. Pharmacol Biochem Behav 60(2):431–437

36. Palaskaa E, Aytemira M, Uzbay IT, Erola D (2001) Synthesis and antidepressant activities of some 3,5-diphenyl-2-pyrazolines. Eur J Med Chem 36:539–543

37. Shader RIMD, Greenblatt DJMD (1999) The reappearance of a monamine oxidase inhibitor (isocarboxazid). J Clin Psychopharm 19(2):106–106

38. Guelfi JD, Strub N, Loft H (2000) Efficacy of intravenous citalopram compared with oral citalopram for severe depression. Safety and efficacy data from a double-blind, double-dummy trial. J Affect Disord 58(3):201–209

39. Gopalakrishnan M, Sureshkumar P, Kanagarajan V, Thanusu J (2005) Aluminium metal powder (atomized) catalyzed Friedel-Crafts acylation in solvent-free conditions: a facile and rapid synthesis of aryl ketones under microwave irradiation. Catal Commun 6(12):753–756

40. Gopalakrishnan M, Sureshkumar P, Kanagarajan V (2007) Easy to execute one pot synthesis of 1,2,4,5-tetrazines catalyzed by activated fly-ash. J Korean Chem Soc 51(6):520–525

41. Thirunarayanan G (2011) Solvent free synthesis, spectral studies and antioxidant activities of some 6-substituted ω-bromo-2-naphthyl ketones and their esters. Indian J Chem 50B(4):593–604

42. Thirunarayanan G, Mayavel P, Thirumurthy K (2012) Fly-ash:H_2SO_4 catalyzed solvent free efficient synthesis of some aryl chalcones under microwave irradiation. Spectrochem Acta 91A:18–22

43. Thirunarayanan G, Mayavael P, Thirumurthy K (2011) National conference on recent trends in green synthesis (RTGS-2011). Alagappa University, Karaikudi, 5–6 August

28

Sunlight-induced rapid and efficient biogenic synthesis of silver nanoparticles using aqueous leaf extract of *Ocimum sanctum* Linn. with enhanced antibacterial activity

Goutam Brahmachari[1*], Sajal Sarkar[1], Ranjan Ghosh[2], Soma Barman[2], Narayan C Mandal[2], Shyamal K Jash[1], Bubun Banerjee[1] and Rajiv Roy[1]

Abstract

Background: Nanotechnology is now regarded as a distinct field of research in modern science and technology with multifaceted areas including biomedical applications. Among the various approaches currently available for the generation of metallic nanoparticles, biogenic synthesis is of increasing demand for the purpose of *green nanotechnology*. Among various natural sources, plant materials are the most readily available template-directing matrix offering cost-effectiveness, eco-friendliness, and easy handling. Moreover, the inherent pharmacological potentials of these medicinal plant extracts offer added biomedical implementations of the synthesized metal nanoparticles.

Results: A robust practical method for eco-friendly synthesis of silver nanoparticles using aqueous leaf extract of *Ocimum sanctum* (Tulsi) as both reducing and capping agent, under the influence of direct sunlight has been developed without applying any other chemical additives. The nanoparticles were characterized with the help of UV-visible spectrophotometer and transmission electron microscopy (TEM). The prepared silver nanoparticles exhibited considerable antibacterial activity. The effects were more pronounced on non-endospore-forming Gram-positive bacteria viz., *Staphylococcus aureus*, *Staphylococcus epidermidis*, and *Listeria monocytogenes* than endospore-forming species *Bacillus subtilis*. The nanoparticles also showed prominent activity on Gram-negative human pathogenic *Salmonella typhimurium*, *Escherichia coli*, *Pseudomonas aeruginosa*, and plant pathogenic *Pantoea ananatis*. A bactericidal mode of action was observed for both Gram-positive and Gram-negative bacteria by the nanoparticles.

Conclusions: We have developed a very simple, efficient, and practical method for the synthesis of silver nanoparticles using aqueous leaf extract of *O. sanctum* under the influence of direct sunlight. The biosynthesis of silver nanoparticles making use of such a traditionally important medicinal plant without applying any other chemical additives, thus offers a cost-effective and environmentally benign route for their large-scale commercial production. The nanoparticles dispersed in the mother solution showed promising antibacterial efficacy.

Keywords: Silver nanoparticles; *Ocimum sanctum*; Sunlight; Antibacterial activity; Mode of action; Nanomedicine

* Correspondence: brahmg2001@yahoo.co.in
[1]Department of Chemistry, Laboratory of Natural Products and Organic Synthesis, Visva-Bharati (a Central University), Santiniketan 731 235, West Bengal, India
Full list of author information is available at the end of the article

Background

Nowadays, nanotechnology is regarded as a distinct field of research in modern science and technology with multidirectional applications [1-7]. Useful application of nanotechnology in medicinal purposes is currently one of the most fascinating areas of research. Metallic nanoparticles (NPs) have also been receiving considerable interest in biomedical applications [1,8]; silver nanoparticles (AgNPs), in particular, are finding applications to the researchers as tools for antibacterial and antifungal [8], anti-inflammatory [9], wound healing [10], radioimaging, retinal neovascularization [11,12], antiviral and antioxidant [13] agents, and also as novel cancer therapeutics, capitalizing on their unique properties to enhance potential therapeutic efficacy [11,12]. In an *in vivo* experiment, silver oxide nanoparticles were found to exhibit notable antitumor efficacies in transplanted Pliss lymphosarcoma tumor models when administered by intravenous injection in the form of aqueous dispersions [14]. Interest in the clinical uses of silver nanoparticles has been facilitated due to their rapid availability as well. The diameters of AgNPs are normally smaller than 100 nm and contain 20 to 15,000 silver atoms per particle [15,16]. Thus, when cells or tissues get exposed to AgNPs, the active surface area of the nanoparticles become significantly large compared to that of the ordinary silver compounds. Such enhanced surface area of metallic nanoparticles is supposed to be responsible for exhibiting remarkably unusual physicochemical properties and biological activities [17]. It is also assumed that promising inhibitory function of AgNPs originates from their interactions with sulfur-containing proteins as well as with phosphorus-containing compounds like DNA inside the microbial membranes [1]. Besides, silver-embedded fabrics are now used in textile industry in manufacturing sporting equipments [18].

Among the various approaches currently available for the generation of metallic nanoparticles, biogenic synthesis that avoids the use of toxic and hazardous chemicals is of increasing demand for the purpose of *green nanotechnology*. It is well-established that biological efficacies of synthesized nanoparticles largely depend on the nature and concentration of capping agent(s) used for stabilizing the nanoparticles. Several matrixes for the biogenic synthesis of such nanoparticles are reported so far, and they include microorganisms such as bacteria [19], fungi [20], enzymes [19], and useful medicinal plant extracts [4,17,21,22]. Among these natural sources, plant materials are the most readily available template-directing matrix offering cost-effectiveness, eco-friendliness, and easy handling much suitable for scaling up processes. Uses of plant materials in generating metallic nanoparticles in both micro- and macroscales are, thus, more advantageous over the microorganism-based methods involving complicated and sensitive cell culture processes. Moreover, the inherent pharmacological potentials of these medicinal plant extracts offer added biomedical implementations of the synthesized metal nanoparticles [23-25].

In compliance with this view, varying extracts of a huge number of medicinal plants such as *Azadirachta indica* [23], *Boswellia ovalifoliolata* [26], *Carica papaya* [27], *Catharanthus roseus* [28], *Cinnamomum camphora* [21], *Citrus aurantium* [29], *Datura metel* [30], *Jatropha curcas, Medicago sativa* [31], *Nelumbo nucifera* (lotus) [32], *Pelargonium graveolens* [33], *Solanum melongena, Tridax procumbens, etc.* have already been used to synthesize and stabilize metallic nanoparticles, very particularly silver (Ag) and gold (Au) nanoparticles [4,19]. However, a little has been carried out on engineering approaches, viz. rapid nanoparticles synthesis using plant extracts and size control of the synthesized nanoparticles [23,29]. Besides, the uses of edible plants are in tremendous demand for the biomedical applications of AgNPs.

In ancient Ayurveda, 'Tulsi' (*Ocimum sanctum* Linn., family: Limiaceae) is known as *the elixir of life* since it promotes longevity and is used in many formulations for the prevention and cure of various ailments [34]. All parts of the plant such as fresh leaves, juice, seeds, and volatile oil are very beneficial to us. The *O. sanctum* plant finds wide applications in the treatment of cough, coryza, hay asthma, bronchial infections, bowel complaints, worm infestations, and kidney stones in traditional systems of medicine [35,36]. *O. sanctum* possesses diverse pharmacological properties that include antioxidant [34], antibiotic, antidiabetic, antiatherogenic, immunomodulatory [34,37], anti-inflammatory [9,37], analgesic, antiulcer [37], and chemo-preventive and antipyretic properties [38]. Tulsi leaf extract reduces blood glucose and cholesterol and promotes immune system function [39], and one of the constituents, β-elemene, has been reported to have potent anticancer property [40]. The major phytochemicals present in *O. sanctum* plant belong to terpenoid, phenolic, tannin, steroid, alkaloid, and saponin class of compounds [41].

That is why *O. sanctum* plant has recently drawn an attention for its possible uses in the biogenic synthesis and stabilization of metal nanoparticles [1,8,42,43]; however, these reported methods suffer from certain shortcomings such as the use of other chemical additives and heating conditions. Hence, development of environmentally more benign, cost-effective, and efficient methodology for the rapid biogenic synthesis of nano-sized metal particles under mild reaction conditions using medicinally significant and edible *O. sanctum* plant as both metal ion reducing and good capping agent is still warranted. We, herein, wish to report for the first time a simple and efficient one-step protocol for the rapid synthesis of AgNPs (7 to 11 nm) by reducing Ag^+ ions in aqueous silver nitrate solution using aqueous fresh leaf extract of *O. sanctum* in the absence of any chemical additive under direct sunlight irradiation with excellent stability. We compared the efficacy of *O. sanctum* with another two medicinal plants, *Citrus limon* Linn. (family: Rutaceae) and *Justicia adhatoda* Linn. (family: Acanthaceae) under the same conditions. Besides, the enhanced antimicrobial activity of the AgNPs plant leaf extract (PLE) against some known pathogenic strains is also evaluated.

Methods

General experimental procedures

Fresh leaves of three medicinal plants Tulsi (*O. sanctum* Linn.), *C. limon* L., and *J. adhatoda* L. were collected in October 2013 at and around Santiniketan, West Bengal, India, and identified by Dr. H. R. Chowdhury (Botany Department, Visva-Bharati University). Voucher specimens are preserved in the Laboratory of Natural Products and Organic Synthesis of this university. The water used as the solvent was previously subjected to deionization, followed by double distillation (first time in alkaline $KMnO_4$). Fresh leaves of the three plants were washed thoroughly with double-distilled water for several times to make it free from dust and were then cut into small pieces. Silver nitrate ($AgNO_3$) (Sigma-Aldrich, Bangalore, India) were used as the source of Ag(I) ion required for the synthesis of Ag nanoparticles. UV-vis absorption spectra were recorded on a Thermo Scientific Spectrascan UV 2700 1 nm double beam spectrophotometer (Thermo Fisher Scientific, Waltham, MA, USA). Sample for transmission electron microscopy (TEM) was prepared by drop-coating the Ag nanoparticles solution onto carbon-coated copper grid. The film on the grid was allowed to dry prior to the TEM measurement in a JEOL TEM-2010 instrument (JEOL Ltd., Akishima-shi, Japan). Solution pH values were measured by Mettler Toledo's pH meter (Mettler-Toledo Inc., Columbus, OH, USA).

Preparation of plant extracts

Fresh and healthy leaves of Tulsi (*O. sanctum*), *C. limon*, and *J. adhatoda* were collected, washed thoroughly with double-distilled water, and were then cut into small pieces. A 10 g of finely cut pieces of leaves of each plant were then transferred into three different 250-mL beakers containing 100 mL distilled water each and boiled for 10 min. After cooling, the aqueous leaf extract obtained from the three different plants were filtered through ordinary filter paper, the filtrates were collected in three separate 100-mL volumetric flasks, and these 10% broth solutions were stored in a refrigerator for further use. On the dilution of the respective mother extract (10%) with requisite amount of distilled water, aqueous extracts of varying concentrations (7%, 5%, and 3%) were used in the present work.

Synthesis of AgNPs and evaluation of reducing potential of the extracts

O. sanctum leaf extracts of varying concentrations (10%, 7%, 5%, and 3%) were then transferred (5 mL each) into four different 100-mL conical flasks containing 45 mL of 10^{-3} M silver nitrate solution so as to make their final volumes to 50 mL each. The resulting solutions were kept under direct sunlight; gradual color change was then noted as an indication of silver nanoparticle formation (Figure 1) confirmed by UV-vis spectrophotometric studies at a regular time interval. Similar procedure was followed also for the other plant extracts.

Analysis of bioreduced silver nanoparticles

UV-vis spectroscopy

To observe the optical property of biosynthesized silver nanoparticles, samples were periodically analyzed with UV-vis spectroscopic studies (Thermo Scientific Spectrascan UV 2700) at room temperature operated at a resolution of 1 nm between 200 and 600 nm ranges.

Transmission electron microscopy

TEM was performed for characterizing the size and shape of biosynthesized silver nanoparticles using JEOL TEM-2010 operated at an accelerating voltage of 300 kV. Prior to analysis, AgNPs were sonicated for 5 min, and a drop of appropriately diluted sample was placed onto carbon-coated copper grid. The liquid fraction was allowed to evaporate at room temperature.

Microorganisms

The bacterial strains used in this study were procured from Microbial Type Culture Collection (MTCC), Institute of microbial technology, Chandigarh, India. The bacterial strains used belonged to both Gram-positive and Gram-negative categories. *Bacillus subtilis* MTCC121 was an endospore former; *Staphylococcus aureus* MTCC96, *Staphylococcus epidermidis* MTCC2639, and *Listeria monocytogenes* MTCC657 were Gram-positive bacteria; *Salmonella typhimurium* MTCC98, *Escherichia coli* MTCC1667, and *Pseudomonas aeruginosa* MTCC741 were human pathogenic Gram-negative bacteria; and *Pantoea ananatis* MTCC2307 was a plant pathogenic Gram-negative bacteria.

Antimicrobial spectrum

Antimicrobial spectra for each concentration (5%, 7%, and 10%) of aqueous leaf extracts of *O. sanctum* as well as silver nano formed by these extracts upon sunlight induction were studied against four Gram-positive and four Gram-negative bacteria described above. Initially, 50 μL of each of the above samples were tested by agar well diffusion for antimicrobial screening [35]. Later, it was confirmed by colony-forming unit CFU counting

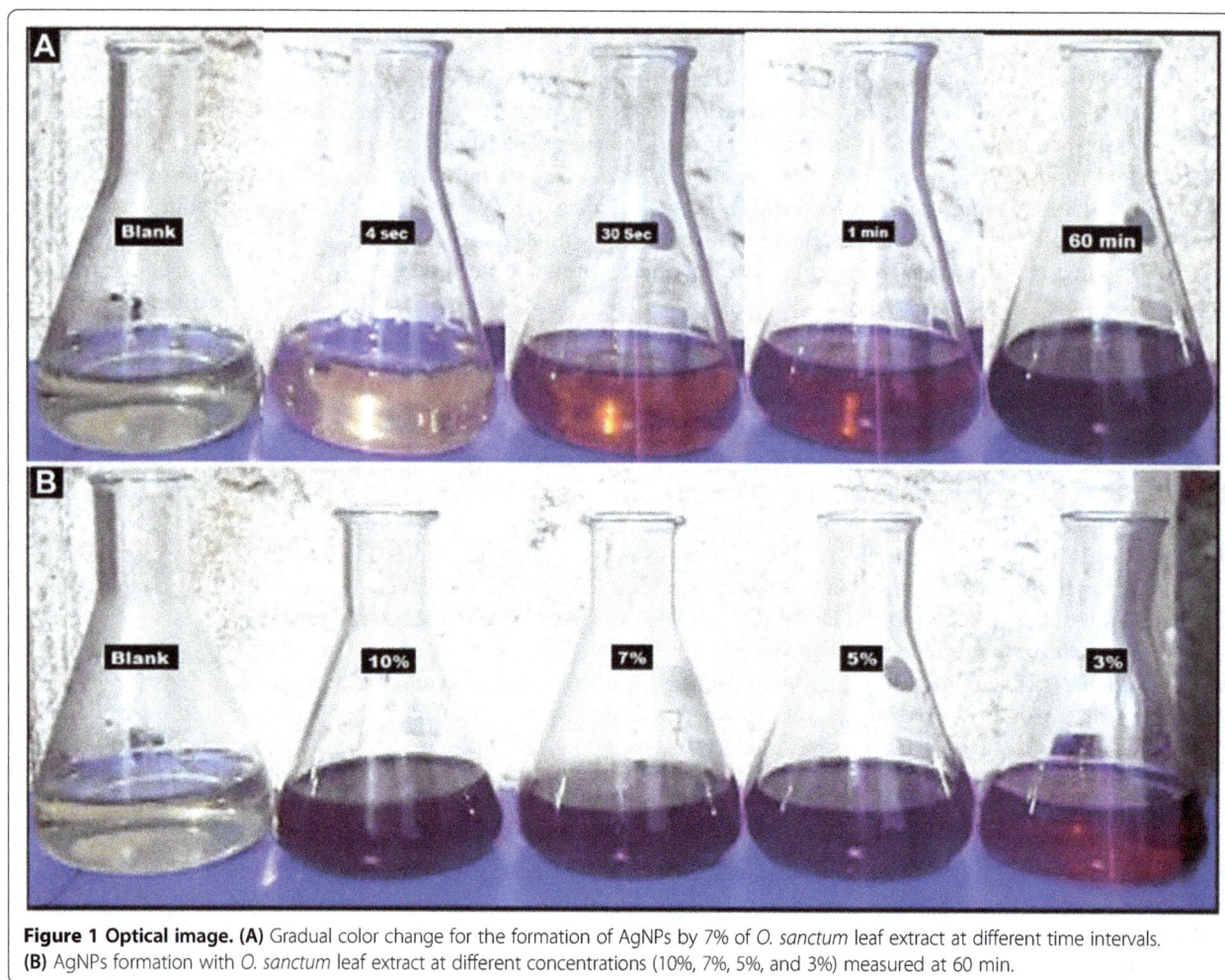

Figure 1 Optical image. (A) Gradual color change for the formation of AgNPs by 7% of *O. sanctum* leaf extract at different time intervals. **(B)** AgNPs formation with *O. sanctum* leaf extract at different concentrations (10%, 7%, 5%, and 3%) measured at 60 min.

method after serial dilution of the bacterial cultures under different treatments.

Antimicrobial mode of action

Antimicrobial mode of action of the silver nano formed by 7% leaf extracts was studied against one Gram-positive *S. aureus* and one Gram-negative *P. aeruginosa*. The study was performed by applying 7% silver nano to the actively growing cultures of the bacteria followed by counting their CFU at regular intervals.

Results and discussion
UV-vis absorbance studies

The addition of fresh leaf extract of *O. sanctum* to silver nitrate solution resulted gradual color change of the solution from transparent to pale yellow, yellow, reddish, and finally to wine-red color due to the production of silver nanoparticles (Figure 1). These color changes arise because of the excitation of surface plasmon vibrations with the silver nanoparticles [44]. Initially, bioproduction of AgNPs was studied with different concentrations (3%, 5%,

7%, and 10%) of aqueous leaf extract of *O. sanctum* with 10^{-3} M AgNO$_3$ solution. UV-visible spectra (Figure 2) indicated the formation AgNPs using these different concentrations of plant leaf extracts on exposure to direct sunlight for a time span of 60 min, and 7% plant leaf extract yielded the best result exhibiting the highest absorption band at 430 nm as a result of surface plasmon resonance (SPR) of silver nanoparticles. Now, we studied the UV-vis absorbance of the reaction mixture with 7% of *O. sanctum* leaf extract with varying time intervals of 1, 3, 8, 15, 30, 60, 90, and 120 min (Figure 3). It was observed that bioreduction of silver ions into nanoparticles started within 3 min and reached at an optimum level within 30 min (optimum absorption at 430 nm), thereby indicating rapid biosynthesis of silver nanoparticles; the absorption band measured at 60 min did not achieve much hike when measured at 90 and 120 min intervals. Broadening of the absorption peak at 430 nm with increase in time indicated the polydispersity of the nanoparticles.

We also verified two other plant leaf extracts such as *C. limon* and *J. adhatoda* (7% aqueous extracts) to compare

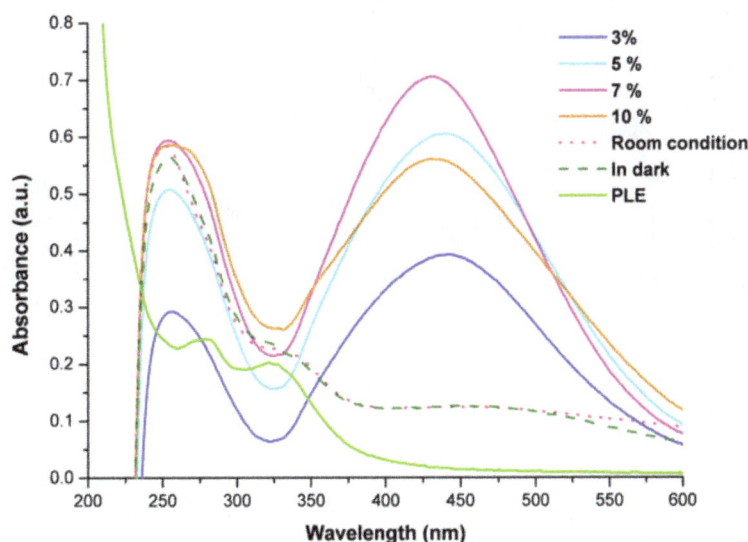

Figure 2 UV-visible spectra for different concentrations of *O. sanctum* Linn. leaf extract (PLE) with 10^{-3} M AgNO₃ measured at 60 min.

the results obtained from *O. sanctum* of the same concentration. The experimental results indicated a clear difference in their efficacy in producing silver NPs; aqueous (7%) leaf extract of only *O. sanctum* produced silver NPs reacting with 10^{-3} M AgNO₃ solution giving rise to the plasmon band at 430 nm (Figure 4).

TEM analysis

While the UV-vis absorption spectral studies provided strong evidence for the formation of silver nanoparticles and their growth kinetics, the shape and size of the resultant nanoparticles are elaborated with the help of TEM analysis. The TEM image at 100-nm scale of the

prepared silver nanoparticles formed by 7% aqueous leaf extract of *O. sanctum* under the influence of direct sunlight is presented in Figure 5. It was observed that Ag nanoparticles were circular in shape with maximum particles in size range within 7 to 11 nm. This particle size range also received support from the appearance of UV-vis absorption band at 430 nm [45].

Bioreduction and stabilization of silver nanoparticles by *O. sanctum* fresh aqueous leaf extract: chemical perspective

From the GC-MS results as reported in literature [46,47], *O. sanctum* fresh aqueous leaf extract is found to contain

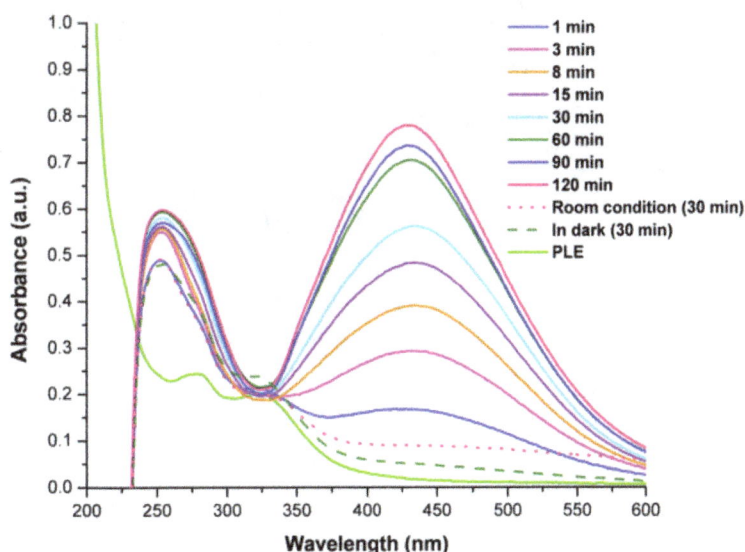

Figure 3 UV-visible spectra for 7% aqueous *O. sanctum* Linn. leaf extract (PLE) with 10^{-3} M AgNO₃ at different time-intervals.

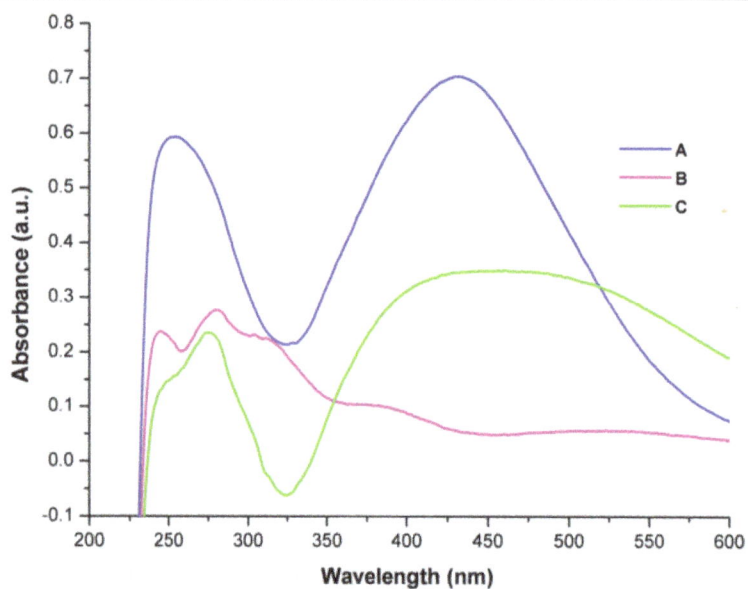

Figure 4 UV-visible spectra of 7% aqueous leaf extract (PLE) of three different plants. (Curve A) *Ocimum sanctum* Linn. (Curve B) *Citrus limon* L. (Curve C) *Justicia adhatoda* L. with 10^{-3} M AgNO$_3$ measured at 60 min.

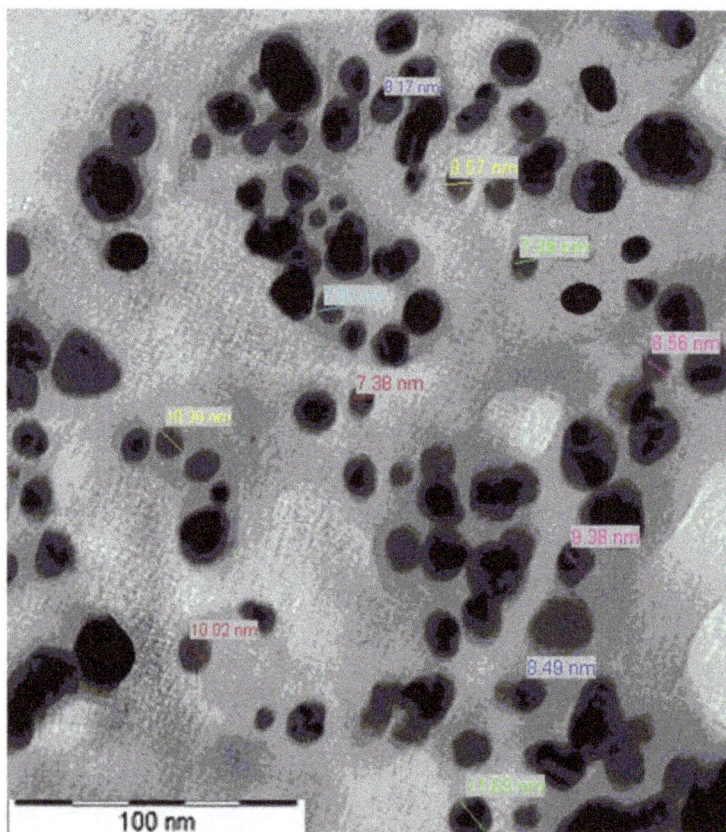

Figure 5 TEM image of biosynthesized silver nanoparticles using *O. sanctum* leaf extract at 100 nm scale.

a variety of organic compounds among which the major components are eugenol, β-caryophyllene, β-elemene, cyclopropylidene, carvacrol, linalool, germacrene, etc. These chemical constituents are supposed to be responsible for photo-induced bioreduction of silver metal ions followed by stabilization of the nanoparticles formed. Since eugenol is the predominant member among the chemical constituents, we do assume a plausible mechanism for the rapid photo-induced bioreduction process (Scheme 1). On sunlight irradiation, the phenolic O-H bond undergoes homolytic cleavage to form hydrogen radical that eventually transfers its electron to a silver ion (Ag^+)-generating silver nanoparticle. The oxygen radical part attains stabilization in the solution through extended conjugation. Hence, H^+ ions are to be formed in the medium and their increasing concentration would affect the pH of the resulting Ag(NPs)-PLE medium. To verify our postulate, we then measured the pH of all types of solutions at 28°C: 1 mM $AgNO_3$ solution (pH 6.54), PLE (pH 5.7), Ag(NPs)-PLE (sunlight, pH 4.8), Ag(NPs)-PLE (room temperature, pH 5.03). To our delight, the simple pH data are quite consistent with our postulation. Due to the presence of phenolic compounds like eugenol, the plant fresh leaf extract recorded moderately acidic pH at 5.7 that became lowered to pH 4.8 on adding silver nitrate solution (1 mM) under sunlight. However, at room temperature, Ag-NP formation is relatively much slower and not so prominent (pH 5.03).

Antimicrobial analyses

Antimicrobial analyses were performed using three different (5%, 7%, and 10%) concentrations of aqueous leaf extracts of O. sanctum as well as the silver nanoparticles formed by them upon sunlight induction from a concentration of 10^{-3} M $AgNO_3$ solution. Only $AgNO_3$ solution at the same concentration was also tested against the bacteria for comparison, and an untreated control of bacterial cultures were also performed. The agar well diffusion experiment was run to perform a qualitative

antimicrobial screening of the samples where clear inhibition zones of varying sizes were observed against all the eight bacteria tested. The other plant extracts at these concentrations did not produce any inhibition zones against these bacteria and are thus not considered for further antimicrobial studies. The preliminary qualitative observations obtained by agar well diffusion were verified quantitatively by CFU count method after treating each bacterial culture with the plant extracts as well as the silver nano formed by them after proper dilution and plating them on their suitable growth media and incubating either at 35°C or 28°C (P. ananatis) for overnight. It has been found that silver nano formed due to sunlight induction produced best result at 7% concentration against the bacteria tested. Its effect was more pronounced on non-endospore-forming Gram-positive S. aureus compared to other bacteria and stopped complete growth of the bacterium. The nanoparticles formed also showed prominent inhibitory activity on other bacteria at this concentration and also the other concentrations but with slightly lower degrees (Table 1). The results in Table 1 clearly depict its strong inhibitory action on the bacteria. This nanoparticle produced remarkable activity on Gram-positive bacterial strains and in particular the non-endospore forming S. aureus, S. epidermidis, and L. monocytogenes. The Gram-negative bacteria were also killed by the silver nano effectively but not at the same pace with Gram-positive members. Only $AgNO_3$ killed the bacteria efficiently from a range of 6×10^8 to 1.5×10^9 CFU to 0.5×10^2 to 1.5×10^3 CFU. Leaf extracts of O. sanctum also could kill the bacteria but with lesser efficiency than the 10^{-3} M silver nitrate solution. The silver nano formed by the leaf extract at its different concentrations showed maximum efficiency, and in particular, the 7% aqueous leaf extract imparted the best antimicrobial action indicating the definite role of tulsi extract as well in enhancing the antibacterial potential. Interestingly, the observed antibacterial potential of AgNPs, formed by 7% aqueous tulsi leaf extract upon

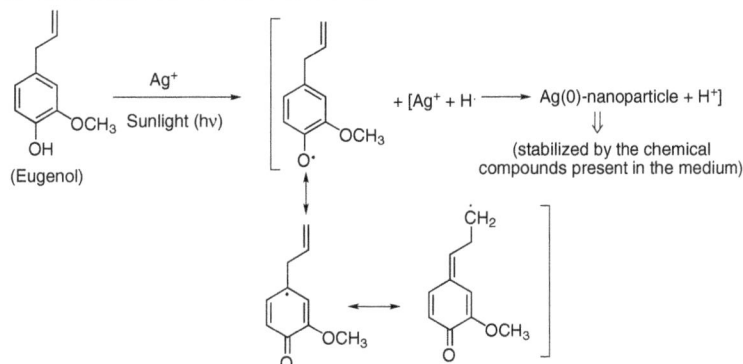

Scheme 1 Plausible photo-induced bioreduction of silver ions to silver nanoparticles by O. sanctum fresh leaf extract.

Table 1 Count of colony forming units of different pathogenic bacteria and the AgNPs

Microorganism	Control (untreated)	10^{-3} M AgNO$_3$ Solution	5% PLE	AgNPs formed by 5% PLE	7% PLE	AgNPs formed by 7% PLE	10% PLE	AgNPs formed by 10% PLE
Staphylococcus aureus	1.2×10^9	0.5×10^2	1.4×10^2	0.01×10^2	1.7×10^2	0	0.7×10^2	0.02×10^2
Bacillus subtilis	6.0×10^8	1.0×10^3	5.2×10^3	0.5×10^2	4.8×10^3	0.3×10^2	3.5×10^3	0.3×10^2
Listeria monocytogenes	7.0×10^8	2.0×10^2	1.2×10^3	0.1×10^2	9.0×10^2	0.09×10^2	5.6×10^2	1.0×10^2
Staphylococcus epidermidis	1.5×10^9	2.0×10^2	5.0×10^2	0.8×10^2	3.7×10^2	0.05×10^2	3.0×10^2	0.08×10^2
Salmonella typhimurium	8.0×10^8	1.5×10^3	6.0×10^3	0.8×10^2	5.5×10^3	0.5×10^2	4.5×10^3	0.7×10^2
Pseudomonas aeruginosa	8.5×10^8	6.0×10^2	7.2×10^3	0.4×10^2	7.0×10^3	0.04×10^2	6.9×10^3	0.4×10^2
Escherichia coli	8.0×10^8	1.3×10^3	2.0×10^3	1.2×10^2	1.5×10^3	0.8×10^2	8×10^2	0.9×10^2
Pantoea ananatis	8.5×10^8	7.0×10^2	4.0×10^3	0.06×10^2	1.7×10^3	0.04×10^2	9×10^2	0.05×10^2

After overnight growth upon treatment with different concentration of aqueous leaf extract of *Ocimum sanctum* and the AgNPs (dispersed in the aqueous leaf extract) formed by them upon sunlight induction. AgNPs, silver nanoparticles dispersed in the aqueous leaf extract; PLE, plant leaf extract.

sunlight exposure, is even higher than almost the same size of AgNPs produced by the conventional methods [48,49]. This is worthy to mention herein that 7% aqueous tulsi leaf extract afforded AgNPs of relatively smaller than those formed by the extracts of other concentrations (3%, 5%, and 10%) tested.

Figure 6 indicates a clear bactericidal mode of action when silver nanoparticles (dispersed in 7% aqueous leaf extract) formed by 7% fresh leaf extract of *O. sanctum* were applied to the actively growing cultures of *S. aureus* and *P. aeruginosa*. A sharp decline in CFU counts from 2×10^6 and 6×10^5 to zero counts with time was observed for *S. aureus* and *P. aeruginosa*, respectively, upon treatment of the silver nanoparticles (dispersed in 7% aqueous

leaf extract). The experimental outcomes unequivocally suggest a potent growth inhibitory activity of the nanoparticles upon both the microorganisms; however, the test material exhibited stronger activity against *P. aeruginosa* than that against *S. aureus*.

Conclusion

In conclusion, we have developed a very simple, efficient, and robust practical method for the synthesis of silver nanoparticles using aqueous leaf extract of *O. sanctum* (Tulsi) as both reducing and capping agent, under the influence of direct sunlight. The biosynthesis of silver nanoparticles making use of such a traditionally important medicinal plant without applying any other chemical

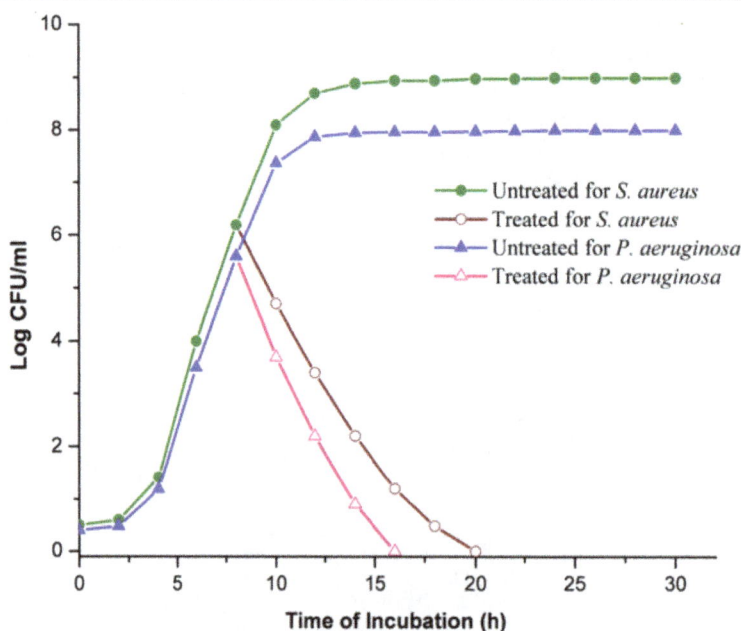

Figure 6 Effect of the treatment of actively growing cells. With AgNPs (dispersed in the aqueous leaf extract) formed by 7% leaf extracts of *O. sanctum* on growth pattern of *Staphylococcus aureus* [(●—●) for untreated and (o—o) for treated] and *Pseudomonas aeruginosa* [(▲—▲) for untreated and (△—△) for treated]. All values are means of three sets of experimental data.

additives, thus offers a cost-effective and environmentally benign route for their large-scale commercial production. The nanoparticles formed are very effective in killing a number of bacteria in a bactericidal mode that include endospore formers, food spoilage pathogens, human as well as plant pathogenic members thus indicating their importance in controlling the growth of such microorganisms.

Competing interests

The authors declare that they have no competing interests.

Acknowledgements

The authors are thankful to the UGC, New Delhi for providing financial assistance under the SAP.

Author details

[1]Department of Chemistry, Laboratory of Natural Products and Organic Synthesis, Visva-Bharati (a Central University), Santiniketan 731 235, West Bengal, India. [2]Department of Botany, Microbiology and Plant Pathology Laboratory, Visva-Bharati (a Central University), Santiniketan 731 235, West Bengal, India.

References

1. Zaheer Z, Rafiuddin R (2013) Bio-conjugated silver nanoparticles: from Ocimum sanctum and role of cetyltrimethyl ammonium bromide. Coll Surf B Biointerfaces 108:90–94
2. Peplow M (2013) Graphene: the quest for supercarbon. Nature 503:327–329
3. Dobrovolskaia MA, McNeil SE (2013) Handbook of immunological properties of engineered nanomaterials. World Scientific Publishing Co Pte Ltd, Singapore
4. Mittal AK, Chisti Y, Banerjee UC (2013) Synthesis of metallic nanoparticles using plant extracts. Biotechnol Adv 31:346–356
5. Prados J, Melguizo C, Perazzoli G, Cabeza L, Carrasco E, Oliver J, Jiménez-Luna C, Leiva MC, Ortiz R, Álvarez PJ, Aranega A (2014) Application of nanotechnology in the treatment and diagnosis of gastrointestinal cancers: review of recent patents. Recent Pat Anticancer Drug Discov 9:21–34
6. Jena BP, Taatjes DJ (2014) Nano cell biology: multimodal imaging in biology and medicine. CRC Press, Taylor & Francis Group, Boca Raton, FL, USA
7. Barends R, Kelly J, Megrant A, Veitia A, Sank D, Jeffrey E, White TC, Mutus J, Fowler AG, Campbell B, Chen Y, Chen Z, Chiaro B, Dunsworth A, Neill C, Malley PO, Roushan P, Vainsencher A, Wenner J, Korotkov AN, Cleland AN, Martinis JM (2014) Superconducting quantum circuits at the surface code threshold for fault tolerance. Nature 508:500–503
8. Rout Y, Behera S, Ojha AK, Nayak PL (2012) Green synthesis of silver nanoparticles using Ocimum sanctum (Tulashi) and study of their antibacterial and antifungal activities. J Microbiol Antimicrob 4:103–109
9. Singh S, Taneja M, Majumamdar DK (2007) Biological activities of Ocimum sanctum L fixed oil—an overview. Ind J Exp Bio 45:403–412
10. Kaler A, Mittal AK, Katariya M, Harde H, Agrawal AK, Jain S, Banerjee UC (2014) An investigation of in vivo wound healing activity of biologically synthesized silver nanoparticles. J Nanopart Res 16:2605, doi:10.1007/s11051-014-2605-x
11. Bhattacharya R, Mukherjee P (2008) Biological properties of naked metal nanoparticles. Adv Drug Deliv Rev 60:1289–1306
12. Kalishwaralal K, Barathmanikanth S, Pandian SR, Deepak V, Gurunathan S (2010) Silver nano—a trove for retinal therapies. J Control Release 145:76–90
13. Hakkim FL, Shankar CG, Girija S (2007) Chemical composition and antioxidant property of holy basil (Ocimum sanctum L.) leaves, stems, and inflorescence and their in vitro callus cultures. J Agric Food Chem 55:9109–9117
14. Rutberg FG, Dubina MV, Kolikov VA, Moiseenko FV, Ignateva EV, Volkov NM, Snetov VN, Stogov AY (2008) Effect of silver oxide nanoparticles on tumor growth in vivo. Dokl Biochem Biophys 421:191–193
15. Lok CN, Ho CM, Chen R, He QY, Yu WY, Sun H, Tam PK, Chiu JF, Che CM (2007) Silver nanoparticles: partial oxidation and antibacterial activities. J Biol Inorg Chem 12:527–534
16. Simi CK, Abraham TE (2007) Hydrophobic grafted and cross linked starch nanoparticles for drug delivery. Bioprocess Biosyst Eng 30:173–180
17. Yen HJ, Hsu SH, Tsai CL (2009) Cytotoxicity and immunological response of gold and silver nanoparticles of different sizes. Small 5:1553–1561
18. Klaus T, Joerger R, Olsson E, Granqvist C-G (1999) Silver-based crystalline nanoparticles, microbially fabricated. Proc Natl Acad Sci USA 96:13611–13614
19. Hebbalalu D, Lalley J, Nadagouda MN, Varma RS (2013) Greener techniques for the synthesis of silver nanoparticles using plant extracts, enzymes, bacteria, biodegradable polymers, and microwaves. ACS Sustainable Chem Eng 1:703–712
20. Srivastava P, Bragança J, Ramanan SR, Kowshik M (2013) Synthesis of silver nanoparticles using haloarchaeal isolate Halococcus salifodinae BK3. Extremophiles 17:821–831
21. Huang J, Li Q, Sun D, Lu Y, Su Y, Yang X, Wang H, Wang Y, Shao W, He N, Hong J, Chen C (2007) Biosynthesis of silver and gold nanoparticles by novel sundried Cinnamomum camphora leaf. Nanotechnology 18:105104–105114
22. Vijayaraghavan K, Nalini SP, Prakash NU, Madhankumar D (2012) One step green synthesis of silver nano/microparticles using extracts of Trachyspermum ammi and Papaver somniferum. Colloids Surf B Biointerfaces 94:14–17
23. Shankar SS, Rai A, Ahmad A, Sastry M (2004) Rapid synthesis of Au, Ag and bimetallic Au core-Ag shell nanoparticles using neem (Azadirachta indica) leaf broth. J Colloid Interf Sci 275:496–502
24. Dar MA, Ingle A, Rai M (2013) Enhanced antimicrobial activity of silver nanoparticles synthesized by Cryphonectria sp evaluated singly and in combination with antibiotics. Nanomed Nanotechnol Biol Med 9:105–110
25. Yu L, Zhang Y, Zhang B, Liu J (2014) Enhanced antibacterial activity of silver nanoparticles/halloysite nanotubes/graphene nanocomposites with sandwich-like structure. Sci Rep 4:4551
26. Ankanna S, Prasad TNVKV, Elumalai EK, Savithramma N (2010) Production of biogenic silver nanoparticles using Boswellia ovalifoliolata stem bark. Dig J Nanomater Bios 5:369–372
27. Jain D, Daima HK, Kachhwaha S, Kothari SL (2009) Synthesis of plant-mediated silver nanoparticles using papaya fruit extract and evaluation of their anti microbial activities. Dig J Nanomater Bios 4:557–563
28. Kannan N, Mukunthan KS, Balaji S (2011) A comparative study of morphology, reactivity and stability of synthesized silver nanoparticles using Bacillus subtilis and Catharanthus roseus (L) G Don. Colloids Surf B Biointerfaces 86:378–383
29. Rajasekharreddy P, Rani PU, Sreedhar B (2010) Qualitative assessment of silver and gold nanoparticle synthesis in various plants: a photobiological approach. J Nanopart Res 12:1711–1721
30. Kesharwani J, Yoon KY, Hwang J, Rai M (2009) Phytofabrication of silver nanoparticles by leaf extract of Datura metel: hypothetical mechanism involved in synthesis. J Bionanosci 3:39–44
31. Gardea-Torresdey JL, Gomez E, Peralta-Videa JR, Parsons JG, Troiani H, Jose-Yacaman M (2003) Alfalfa sprouts: a natural source for the synthesis of silver nanoparticles. Langmuir 19:1357–1361
32. Santhoshkumar T, Rahuman AA, Rajakumar G, Marimuthu S, Bagavan A, Jayaseelan C, Zahir AA, Elango G, Kamaraj C (2011) Synthesis of silver nanoparticles using Nelumbo nucifera leaf extract and its larvicidal activity against malaria and filariasis vectors. Parasitol Res 108:693–702
33. Shankar SS, Ahmad A, Sastry M (2003) Geranium leaf assisted biosynthesis of silver nanoparticles. Biotechnol Prog 19:1627–1631
34. Govind P, Madhuri S (2010) Pharmacological activities of Ocimum sanctum (tulsi): a review. Int J Pharma Sci Rev Res 5:61–66
35. Bauer AW, Kirby WM, Sherris JC, Turck M (1966) Antibiotic susceptibility testing by a standardized single disk method. Am J Clin Pathol 45:493–496
36. Sood S, Narang D, Dinda AK, Maulik SK (2005) Chronic oral administration of Ocimum sanctum Linn augments cardiac endogenous antioxidants and prevents isoproterenol induced myocardial necrosis in rats. J Pharm Pharmacol 57:127–133
37. Pattanayak P, Behera P, Das D, Panda SK (2010) Ocimum sanctum Linn A reservoir plant for therapeutic applications: an overview. Pharmacogn Rev 4:95–105
38. Bhattacharyya P, Bishayee A (2013) Ocimum sanctum Linn (Tulsi): an ethnomedicinal plant for the prevention and treatment of cancer. Anticancer Drugs 24:659–666

39. Mondal S, Varma S, Bamola VD, Naik SN, Mirdha BR, Padhi MM, Mehta N, Mahapatra SC (2011) Double-blinded randomized controlled trial for immunomodulatory effects of Tulsi (*Ocimum sanctum* Linn) leaf extract on healthy volunteers. J Ethnopharmacol 136:452–456

40. Li QQ, Wang G, Zhang M, Cuff CF, Huang L, Reed E (2009) beta-Elemene, a novel plant-derived antineoplastic agent, increases cisplatin chemosensitivity of lung tumor cells by triggering apoptosis. Oncol Rep 22:161–170

41. Baliga MS, Jimmy R, Thilakchand KR, Sunitha V, Bhat NR, Saldanha E, Rao S, Rao P, Arora R, Palatty PL (2013) *Ocimum sanctum* L (Holy Basil or Tulsi) and its phytochemicals in the prevention and treatment of cancer. Nutr Cancer 65:26–35

42. Ramteke C, Chakrabarti T, Sarangi BK, Pandey R-A (2013) Synthesis of silver nanoparticles from the aqueous extract of leaves of *Ocimum sanctum* for enhanced antibacterial activity. J Chem Article ID 278925:7

43. Vijaya PP, Rekha B, Mathew AT, Ali MS, Yogananth N, Anuradha V, Parveen PK (2014) Antigenotoxic effect of green-synthesised silver nanoparticles from *Ocimum sanctum* leaf extract against cyclophosphamide induced genotoxicity in human lymphocytes—in vitro. Appl Nanosci 4:415–420

44. Mulvaney P (1996) Surface plasmon spectroscopy of nanosized metal particles. Langmuir 12:788–800

45. Mallikarjuna K, Narasimha G, Dillip GR, Praveen B, Shreedhar B, Lakshmi CS, Reddy BVS, Raju BDP (2001) Green synthesis of silver nanoparticles using *Ocimmum* leaf extract and their characterization. Dig J Nanomater Bios 6:181–186

46. Devendran G, Balasubramanian U (2011) Qualitative phytochemical screening and GC-MS analysis of *Ocimum sanctum* L leaves. Asian J Plant Sci Res 1:44–48

47. Dohare SL, Shuaib M, Ahmad MI, Naquvi KJ (2012) Chemical composition of volatile oil of *Ocimum sanctum* Linn. Int J Biomed Adv Res 3:129–131

48. Agnihotria S, Mukherjiabc S, Mukherji S (2014) Size-controlled silver nanoparticles synthesized over the range 5–100 nm using the same protocol and their antibacterial efficacy. RSC Adv 4:3974–3983

49. Holla G, Yeluri R, Munshi AK (2012) Evaluation of minimum inhibitory and minimum bactericidal concentration of nano-silver base inorganic anti-microbial agent (Novaron®) against *Streptococcus mutans*. Contemp Clin Dent 3:288–293

Permissions

List of Contributors

Amar Zellagui
Laboratory of Biomolecules and Plant Breeding, Life Science and Nature Department, University of Larbi Ben Mhidi Oum El Bouaghi, Algeria

Noureddine Gherraf
Laboratory of Biomolecules and Plant Breeding, Life Science and Nature Department, University of Larbi Ben Mhidi Oum El Bouaghi, Algeria

Segni Ladjel
Kasdi Merbah University, Ouargla, Algeria

Samir Hameurlaine
Kasdi Merbah University, Ouargla, Algeria

Mohamed Shaaban
Chemistry of Natural Compounds Department, Pharmaceutical Industries Division, National Research Centre, El-Behoos St., Dokki-Cairo 12622, Egypt
Institute of Organic and Biomolecular Chemistry, University of Göttingen, Tammannstrasse 2, D-37077 Göttingen, Germany

Khaled A Shaaban
Institute of Organic and Biomolecular Chemistry, University of Göttingen, Tammannstrasse 2, D-37077 Göttingen, Germany

Mohamed S Abdel-Aziz
Department of Microbial Chemistry, Genetic Engineering and Biotechnology Division, National Research Centre, El-Behoos St., Dokki-Cairo 12622, Egypt

Aruna Jyothi Kora
National Centre for Compositional Characterisation of Materials (NCCCM), Bhabha Atomic Research Centre, ECIL PO, Hyderabad 500 062AP, India

Sashidhar Rao Beedu
Department of Biochemistry, University College of Science, Osmania University, Hyderabad 500 007, AP, India

Arunachalam Jayaraman
National Centre for Compositional Characterisation of Materials (NCCCM), Bhabha Atomic Research Centre, ECIL PO, Hyderabad 500 062AP, India

Joseph W Guiles
Replidyne, Inc., Louisville, CO, USA
CedarburgHauser Pharmaceuticals, Denver, CO, USA

Andras Toro
Replidyne, Inc., Louisville, CO, USA
Mannkind Corporation, Valencia, CA, USA

Urs A Ochsner
Replidyne, Inc., Louisville, CO, USA
Crestone, Inc., Boulder, CO, USA

James M Bullard
Replidyne, Inc., Louisville, CO, USA
Chemistry Department, SCIE. 3.320, The University of Texas-Pan American, 1201 W. University Drive, Edinburg, TX 78541, USA

Mohammad Faheem Khan
Department of Chemistry, HNB Garhwal University, Srinagar (Garhwal), Uttarakhand 246174, India

Nisha Negi
Department of Chemistry, HNB Garhwal University, Srinagar (Garhwal), Uttarakhand 246174, India

Rajnikant Sharma
Department of Chemistry, HNB Garhwal University, Srinagar (Garhwal), Uttarakhand 246174, India

Devendra Singh Negi
Department of Chemistry, HNB Garhwal University, Srinagar (Garhwal), Uttarakhand 246174, India

Howaida I Abd-Alla
Chemistry of Natural Compounds Department, Division of Pharmaceutical Industries, National Research Centre, Dokki, Giza 12622, Egypt

Amal Z Hassan
Chemistry of Natural Compounds Department, Division of Pharmaceutical Industries, National Research Centre, Dokki, Giza 12622, Egypt

Hanan F Aly
Department of Therapeutic Chemistry, National Research Centre, Dokki, Giza 12622, Egypt

Mohamed A Ghani
Red Sea Marine Parks, P.O. Box 363, Hurghada, Red Sea, Egypt

Musiri Maruthai Senthamilselvi
Department of Chemistry, National Institute of Technology, Tiruchirappalli, Tamil Nadu 620 015, India

Devarayan Kesavan
Department of Chemistry, National Institute of Technology, Tiruchirappalli, Tamil Nadu 620 015, India

Nagarajan Sulochana
Department of Chemistry, National Institute of Technology, Tiruchirappalli, Tamil Nadu 620 015, India

Gerlânia de Oliveira Leite
Departamento de Química Biológica, Universidade Regional do Cariri, Crato CE 63105-000, Brazil

Cícera Norma Fernandes
Departamento de Química Biológica, Universidade Regional do Cariri, Crato CE 63105-000, Brazil

Irwin Rose Alencar de Menezes
Departamento de Química Biológica, Universidade Regional do Cariri, Crato CE 63105-000, Brazil

José Galberto Martins da Costa
Departamento de Química Biológica, Universidade Regional do Cariri, Crato CE 63105-000, Brazil

Adriana Rolim Campos
Vice-Reitoria de Pesquisa e Pós-Graduação, Universidade de Fortaleza, Av. Washington Soares, 1321, Fortaleza, Ceará CEP 60811-905, Brazil

Fatemeh Nejatzadeh-Barandozi
Department of Horticulture, Faculty of Agriculture, Khoy Branch, Islamic Azad University, P.O. Box 58168–44799, Khoy, Iran

Amar Zellagui
Laboratory of Biomolecules and Plant Breeding, Life Science and Nature Department, Faculty of Exact Science and Life Science and Nature, University of Larbi Ben Mhidi, Oum El Bouaghi, Algeria

Noueddine Gherraf
Laboratory of Biomolecules and Plant Breeding, Life Science and Nature Department, Faculty of Exact Science and Life Science and Nature, University of Larbi Ben Mhidi, Oum El Bouaghi, Algeria

Salah Rhouati
Laboratory of Natural Products and Organic Synthesis, Department of Chemistry, Faculty of Science, University of Mentouri-Constantine, Constantine, Algeria

Debasish Bandyopadhyay
Department of Chemistry, The University of Texas-Pan American, 1201 West University Drive, Edinburg, TX 78539, USA

Bimal K Banik
Department of Chemistry, The University of Texas-Pan American, 1201 West University Drive, Edinburg, TX 78539, USA

Karna Ji Harkala
Department of Physics and Chemistry, Mahatma Gandhi Institute of Technology, Chaitanya Bharathi, Gandipet, Hyderabad 500075, India

Laxminarayana Eppakayala
Department of Physics and Chemistry, Mahatma Gandhi Institute of Technology, Chaitanya Bharathi, Gandipet, Hyderabad 500075, India

Thirumala Chary Maringanti
Department of Chemistry, College of Engineering, Jawaharlal Nehru Technological University, Hyderabad, Nachupally, Karimnagar 505501, India

Debasish Bandyopadhyay
Department of Chemistry, The University of Texas-Pan American, 1201 West University Drive, Edinburg, TX 78539, USA

Lauren C Smith
Department of Chemistry, The University of Texas-Pan American, 1201 West University Drive, Edinburg, TX 78539, USA

Daniel R Garcia
Department of Chemistry, The University of Texas-Pan American, 1201 West University Drive, Edinburg, TX 78539, USA

Ram N Yadav
Department of Chemistry, The University of Texas-Pan American, 1201 West University Drive, Edinburg, TX 78539, USA

Diana A Zaleta-Pinet
Chemistry, School of Environmental and Life Science, The University of Newcastle, University Drive, Callaghan, NSW 2308, Australia

Ian P Holland
Chemistry, School of Environmental and Life Science, The University of Newcastle, University Drive, Callaghan, NSW 2308, Australia

Mauricio Muñoz-Ochoa
Development Technology Department, Interdisciplinary Centre of Marine Sciences, National Technological Institute, La Paz, Mexico

J Ivan Murillo-Alvarez
Development Technology Department, Interdisciplinary Centre of Marine Sciences, National Technological Institute, La Paz, Mexico

Jennette A Sakoff
Department of Medical Oncology, Calvary Mater Newcastle Hospital, Waratah, NSW 2298, Australia

Ian A van Altena
Chemistry, School of Environmental and Life Science, The University of Newcastle, University Drive, Callaghan, NSW 2308, Australia

Adam McCluskey
Chemistry, School of Environmental and Life Science, The University of Newcastle, University Drive, Callaghan, NSW 2308, Australia

Fariborz Darvishzadeh
Department of Horticulture, Faculty of Agriculture, Garmsar Branch, Islamic Azad University, P.O. Box 58168-44799 Garmsar, Iran

Ali Aminkhani
Department of Chemistry, Khoy Branch, Islamic Azad University, P.O. Box 58168-44799, Khoy, Iran

Ahmed A Al-Amiery
Biotechnology Division, Applied Science Department, University of Technology, Baghdad 10066, Iraq

Yasmien K Al-Majedy
Biotechnology Division, Applied Science Department, University of Technology, Baghdad 10066, Iraq

Heba H Ibrahim
Biotechnology Division, Applied Science Department, University of Technology, Baghdad 10066, Iraq

Ali A Al-Tamimi
Biotechnology Division, Applied Science Department, University of Technology, Baghdad 10066, Iraq

Mahima Pal and Sarvesh Paliwal
Department of Pharmacy, Banasthali University, Banasthali, Tonk, Rajasthan, India

Rajesh Kumar Kesharwani
Division of Applied Science & Indo-Russian Center For Biotechnology [IRCB], Indian Institute of Information Technology, Allahabad 211012, India

Durg Vijay Singh
Department of Bioinformatics, UIET, CSJM University, Kanpur 208024, India

Krishna Misra
Division of Applied Science & Indo-Russian Center For Biotechnology [IRCB], Indian Institute of Information Technology, Allahabad 211012, India

Syed Ibrahim Rizvi
Department of Biochemistry, University of Allahabad, Allahabad 211002, India

Simone Badal
Natural Products Institute, Faculty of Pure and Applied Sciences, University of the West Indies, Mona, West Indies, Jamaica

Winklet Gallimore
Department of Chemistry, Faculty of Pure and Applied Sciences, University of the West Indies, Mona, West Indies, Jamaica

George Huang
Department of Biological Sciences, Clemson University, Clemson SC 29634, USA

Tzuen-Rong Jeremy Tzeng
Department of Biological Sciences, Clemson University, Clemson SC 29634, USA

Rupika Delgoda
Natural Products Institute, Faculty of Pure and Applied Sciences, University of the West Indies, Mona, West Indies, Jamaica

Mohamed MS Nagia
Division of Pharmaceutical Industries, Chemistry of Natural Compounds Department, National Research Centre, El-Behoos st. 33, Dokki, Cairo 12622, Egypt
Institute of Organic and Biomolecular Chemistry, University of Göttingen, Tammannstrasse 2, D-37077 Göttingen, Germany

Mohammad Magdy El-Metwally
Microbial Activity Unit, Microbiology Department, Soil & Water and Environment Research Institute, ARC, Giza, Egypt

Soheir M El-Zalabani
Pharmacognosy Department, Faculty of Pharmacy, Cairo University, Cairo, Egypt

Atef G Hanna
Division of Pharmaceutical Industries, Chemistry of Natural Compounds Department, National Research Centre, El-Behoos st. 33, Dokki, Cairo 12622, Egypt
Institute of Organic and Biomolecular Chemistry, University of Göttingen, Tammannstrasse 2, D-37077 Göttingen, Germany

Abdur Rauf
Institute of Chemical Sciences, University of Peshawar, Peshawar KPK 25120, Pakistan

Ghias Uddin
Institute of Chemical Sciences, University of Peshawar, Peshawar KPK 25120, Pakistan

Jawad Ali
Institute of Chemical Sciences, University of Peshawar, Peshawar KPK 25120, Pakistan

Ramasamy Venkat Ragavan
Centre for Organic and Medicinal Chemistry, VIT University, Vellore 632 014, India

Kalavathi Murugan Kumar
Medical and Biological Computing Laboratory, School of Biosciences and Technology, VIT University, Vellore 632 014, India

Vijayaparthasarathi Vijayakumar
Centre for Organic and Medicinal Chemistry, VIT University, Vellore 632 014, India

Sundaramoorthy Sarveswari
Centre for Organic and Medicinal Chemistry, VIT University, Vellore 632 014, India

Sudha Ramaiah
Medical and Biological Computing Laboratory, School of Biosciences and Technology, VIT University, Vellore 632 014, India

Anand Anbarasu
Centre for Organic and Medicinal Chemistry, VIT University, Vellore 632 014, India
Medical and Biological Computing Laboratory, School of Biosciences and Technology, VIT University, Vellore 632 014, India

Sivashanmugam Karthikeyan
Centre for Organic and Medicinal Chemistry, VIT University, Vellore 632 014, India
Industrial Biotechnology Division, School of Bio Sciences and Technology, VIT University, Vellore 632 014, India

Periyasamy Giridharan
Department of Oncology, HCS & HTS, Piramal Life Sciences Ltd. Guregaon (E), Mumbai 400063, India

Nalilu Suchetha Kumari
Department of Biochemistry, K.S. Hegde Medical Academy, Deralakatte 574 162, India

Priya R Modiya
Department of Pharmaceutical Chemistry, Shri Sarvajanik Pharmacy College, Gujarat Technological University, Arvind Baug, Mehsana 384001, Gujarat, India

Chhaganbhai N Patel
Department of Pharmaceutical Chemistry, Shri Sarvajanik Pharmacy College, Gujarat Technological University, Arvind Baug, Mehsana 384001, Gujarat, India

Kamran J Naquvi
Department of Pharmacognosy and Phytochemistry, Faculty of Pharmacy, Jamia Hamdard, New Delhi 110062, India

Mohammed Ali
Department of Pharmacognosy and Phytochemistry, Faculty of Pharmacy, Jamia Hamdard, New Delhi 110062, India

Javed Ahmad
Department of Pharmacognosy and Phytochemistry, Faculty of Pharmacy, Jamia Hamdard, New Delhi 110062, India

Fathollah Gholami-Borujeni
Social Determinants of Health Research Center and Environmental Health Engineering, School of Health, Urmia University of Medical Science, Urmia, Iran

Poonam Khloya
Department of Chemistry, Kurukshetra University, Kurukshetra 136119, India

Pawan Kumar
Department of Chemistry, Kurukshetra University, Kurukshetra 136119, India

Arpana Mittal
Department of Microbiology, Kurukshetra University, Kurukshetra 136119, India

Neeraj K Aggarwal
Department of Microbiology, Kurukshetra University, Kurukshetra 136119, India

Pawan K Sharma
Department of Chemistry, Kurukshetra University, Kurukshetra 136119, India

Ramalingam Sasikala
Department of Chemistry, Annamalai University, Annamalai Nagar 608 002, India

Kannan Thirumurthy
Department of Chemistry, Annamalai University, Annamalai Nagar 608 002, India

Perumal Mayavel
Department of Chemistry, Annamalai University, Annamalai Nagar 608 002, India

Ganesamoorthy Thirunarayanan
Department of Chemistry, Annamalai University, Annamalai Nagar 608 002, India

Goutam Brahmachari
Department of Chemistry, Laboratory of Natural Products and Organic Synthesis, Visva-Bharati (a Central University), Santiniketan 731 235, West Bengal, India

Sajal Sarkar
Department of Chemistry, Laboratory of Natural Products and Organic Synthesis, Visva-Bharati (a Central University), Santiniketan 731 235, West Bengal, India

Ranjan Ghosh
Department of Botany, Microbiology and Plant Pathology Laboratory, Visva-Bharati (a Central University), Santiniketan 731 235, West Bengal, India

Soma Barman
Department of Botany, Microbiology and Plant Pathology Laboratory, Visva-Bharati (a Central University), Santiniketan 731 235, West Bengal, India

Narayan C Mandal
Department of Botany, Microbiology and Plant Pathology Laboratory, Visva-Bharati (a Central University), Santiniketan 731 235, West Bengal, India

Shyamal K Jash
Department of Chemistry, Laboratory of Natural Products and Organic Synthesis, Visva-Bharati (a Central University), Santiniketan 731 235, West Bengal, India

Bubun Banerjee
Department of Chemistry, Laboratory of Natural Products and Organic Synthesis, Visva-Bharati (a Central University), Santiniketan 731 235, West Bengal, India

Rajiv Roy
Department of Chemistry, Laboratory of Natural Products and Organic Synthesis, Visva-Bharati (a Central University), Santiniketan 731 235, West Bengal, India

www.ingramcontent.com/pod-product-compliance
Lightning Source LLC
Chambersburg PA
CBHW080655200326
41458CB00013B/4859